EDITION 2

CASE STUDIES IN
CRITICAL
CARE NURSING
A Guide for Application and Review

NOTICE

Pharmacology is an ever-changing field. Standard safety precautions must be followed, but as new research and clinical experience broaden our knowledge, changes in treatment and drug therapy may become necessary or appropriate. Readers are advised to check the most current product information provided by the manufacturer of each drug to be administered to verify the recommended dose, the method and duration of administration, and contraindications. It is the responsibility of the appropriately licensed health care provider, relying on experience and knowledge of the patient, to determine dosages and the best treatment for each individual patient. Neither the Publisher nor the editor assumes any liability for any injury and/or damage to persons or property arising from this publication.

The Publisher

EDITION 2

CASE STUDIES IN
CRITICAL
CARE NURSING

A Guide for Application and Review

SHEILA DRAKE MELANDER, RN, DSN, ACNP-C, FCCM

Associate Professor of Nursing and Coordinator of the Acute Care Nurse
  Practitioner Program
University of Southern Indiana
Supplemental Staff
Surgical Intensive Care Unit, Deaconess Hospital
Evansville, Indiana

W.B. SAUNDERS COMPANY

A Harcourt Health Sciences Company

Philadelphia, London, New York, St. Louis, Sydney

W.B. SAUNDERS COMPANY

A Harcourt Health Sciences Company
The Curtis Center
Independence Square West
Philadelphia, Pennsylvania 19106

Vice-President, Nursing Editorial Director: Sally Schrefer
Executive Editor: Barbara Nelson Cullen
Associate Developmental Editor: Eric Ham
Project Manager: John Rogers
Project Specialist: Kathleen L. Teal
Designer: Kathi Gosche

Library of Congress Cataloging-in-Publication Data

Case studies in critical care nursing : a guide for application and review / [edited by]
Sheila Drake Melander.—2nd ed.

p. ; cm.

Rev. ed. of: Review of critical care nursing. c1996.
Includes bibliographical references and index.

ISBN 0–7216–8996–5

1. Intensive care nursing—Case studies. I. Title: Critical care nursing. II. Melander,
   Sheila Drake. III. Review of critical care nursing.
   [DNLM: 1. Critical Illness—nursing—Case Report. 2. Critical Care—Case Report. WY
   154 C3367 2001]

RT120.I5 C37 2001   610.73'61—dc21

00–034499

CASE STUDIES IN CRITICAL CARE NURSING:
A GUIDE FOR APPLICATION AND REVIEW
Second Edition   ISBN 0–7216–8996–5

Printed in the United States of America

00 01 02 03 04 GW/FF 9 8 7 6 5 4 3 2 1

CONTRIBUTORS

CINDA ALEXANDER, MSN, CCRN,
CNRN, CNOR, CRNFA
Tri-State Neurological
Evansville, Indiana
*Subarachnoid Hemorrhage with Aneurysm;
Head Trauma and Subdural Hematoma;
Epidural Hematoma*

SHARON ANGLE, RN, MSN
Administrative Director of Quality
Management/Compliance Officer
Shore Memorial Hospital
Nassawadox, Virginia
Acute Respiratory Distress Syndrome

CONNIE COOPER, RN, MSN
Instructor
University of Southern Indiana
Evansville, Indiana
Assistant Professor
DePaul University
Chicago, Illinois
Acquired Immunodeficiency Syndrome

ANNE G. DENNER, MS Biology, BSN
Former Instructor in Biology
University of Southern Indiana
Evansville, Indiana
Adrenal Crisis; Diabetic Ketoacidosis

PHYLLIS ANN EGBERT, MSN,
RNC, ACNP, CNN
Clinical Coordinator/Nurse Practitioner
Renal Care Group/Vanderbilt
Dialysis Clinic
Nashville, Tennessee
*Chronic Renal Failure and Renal
Transplantation*

LINDA K. EVINGER, RN,
MSN, C-OGNP
Instructor
School of Nursing and Health
Professions
University of Southern Indiana
Evansville, Indiana
Esophageal Varices

CYNTHIA S. GOODWIN, RN, MSN
Instructor
School of Nursing and Health Professions
University of Southern Indiana
Evansville, Indiana
Gastrointestinal Bleeding

JUDITH A. HALSTEAD, RN, DNS
Associate Professor and Director of
Instructional Services and Resources
School of Nursing and Health
Professions
University of Southern Indiana
Evansville, Indiana
Pulmonary Contusion

DEBRA L. HARMON, RN, MSN, CCRN
Nursing Instructor
Department of Nursing
University of Southern Indiana
Evansville, Indiana
*Cardiac Shock in Anterior Wall Myocar-
dial Infarction; Multiple Organ
Dysfunction Syndrome*

BRIAN W. HIGGERSON, RN,
MSN, FNP, CCRN
Adjunct Faculty
School of Nursing and Health
Professions
University of Southern Indiana
Evansville, Indiana
Abdominal Aortic Aneurysm

KAREN L. JONES, RNC, BSN, MSN
Director of Clinical Operations
Ohio Valley Heart Care
Evansville, Indiana
Coronary Artery Bypass Graft

JOAN E. KING, RN, PhD, ACNP
Program Director for the Acute Care
Nurse Practitioner Program
Associate Professor of Nursing
Vanderbilt University School of Nursing
Nashville, Tennessee
Congestive Heart Failure;
Blunt Abdominal Trauma

PAM B. KOOB, RN, PhD, CFNP
Nurse Practitioner, Private Practice
Hopkinsville, Kentucky
Carotid Endarterectomy

ALICE LOWE, RN, BSN
Deaconess Hospital
Evansville, Indiana
Percutaneous Transluminal Coronary
Angioplasty and Thrombolytic Therapy
in Myocardial Infarction

SHEILA DRAKE MELANDER, RN, DSN,
ACNP-C, FCCM
Associate Professor of Nursing
and Coordinator of the Critical Care
BSN Nursing Course
University of Southern Indiana
Supplemental Staff
Evansville Indiana
Acute Respiratory Distress Syndrome;
Pulmonary Contusion; Chronic
Obstructive Pulmonary Disease
with Pneumonia; Percutaneous
Transluminal Coronary Angioplasty
and Thrombolytic Therapy in Myocardial
Infarction; Coronary Artery Bypass
Graft; Non–Q-Wave Myocardial
Infarction; Acute Renal Failure

AMY REESE RAMIREZ, RN, BSN,
MSW, MSN, FNP
Family Nurse Practitioner
University of Southern Indiana
Evansville, Indiana
Non–Q-Wave Myocardial Infarction;
Acute Renal Failure

LYNN RODGERS, RNC, MSN, CCRN,
CNRN, ACNP
Staff Nurse in CUICU
Deaconess Hospital
Evansville, Indiana
Peritonitis; Sepsis/Septic Shock

COLLEEN R. WALSH, RN, MSN, ONC,
ACNP-C
Instructor
University of Southern Indiana
Evansville, Indiana
Adjunct Assistant Professor
University of South Alabama
College of Nursing
Mobile, Alabama
Syndrome of Inappropriate Secretion of
Antidiuretic Hormone

MARY ANN WEHMER, RN,
MSN, CNOR
Nursing Instructor
School of Nursing and Health
Professions
University of Southern Indiana
Evansville, Indiana
Pulmonary Embolism

ANN H. WHITE, CNA, RN,
MBA, PhD
Associate Professor of Nursing
University of Southern Indiana
Evansville, Indiana
Acute Pancreatitis; Burns

ACKNOWLEDGMENT

I'd like to take this opportunity to thank specific people in my life who have supported me throughout the publishing process of this text. I'd like to begin by thanking the talented contributors of the case studies. Without each contributor, whose expertise is clearly reflected through each of their case studies, this project would not have been possible. I would also like to thank Dr. Nadine Coudret, Dean of the School of Nursing and Health Professions, and Charles Anstett, Coordinator of Computer and Internet Services, for their assistance, support, and encouragement throughout this project.

Finally, to my husband Chuck and my two children Ryan and Matthew, I want to take this moment to tell you how much I appreciate your continuous patience, love, and support. God has truly blessed me by bringing each of you into my life.

Sheila Drake Melander

FOREWORD

Recently, a faculty member at a local nursing school was working with students in our ICU. We got into a discussion about an assignment that she had given the Junior level students. Those students handed in papers that were clearly "cut and paste" from information available on the Internet. We both remarked that technology is increasingly making information easily accessible, but the "cut and paste" method may not provide the best learning tool for students. What is needed in our environment today are educators and educational tools that go beyond the traditional knowledge-based instructional approach and promote the active process of learning. It is a challenge for educators at all levels to find methods of learning in this technologic time that are valid, exciting, and practical. In short, it is time for an educational revolution. There is no better place for this revolution than in our methods of educating nurses.

It has been said that knowledge is knowing a fact, but wisdom is knowing what to do with it. We are often very good at knowing facts. Much of our testing and evaluation focuses on knowing facts. Measurement of the PR interval and the action and indications of heparin are important facts to know in caring for critically ill patients. However, so much of what it is that nursing does goes beyond the facts and beyond acquiring knowledge. This case study book offers the reader the opportunity to gain wisdom, to know what to do with those facts and reach a level beyond knowledge. The case studies allow the reader to do more than problem solve, they also encourage critical thinking, a vital skill for the future. Critical thinking can identify ways not only to solve problems but to prevent problems. It helps the learner maximize their potential and efficiency in order to make an optimal contribution to their patients and their profession.

How better to develop the necessary skill of critical thinking than to provide an active, experiential learning through case studies? The cases presented are actual practice-based scenarios. They allow the reader to analyze "reality-based" data about a patient situation and then challenge the reader with questions about the nursing care for that patient. Answers for the scenario-based questions are provided for comparison but also to challenge the reader to explore options, analyze controversies, and consider going beyond the initial response providing a link to other learning resources.

The world around us is changing in quantum leaps. Nursing needs highly developed critical thinking skills that will help us adapt to new situations, make competent decisions, and foster life-long learning. This text is a tool to help us obtain those skills so needed in acquiring wisdom in nursing for now and for the future.

Mary G. McKinley, RN, MSN, CCRN
Past President, AACN
Clinical Nurse Specialist for Critical Care
Ohio Valley Medical Center
Wheeling, West Virginia

PREFACE

Case Studies in Critical Care Nursing was compiled with the intent of capturing actual patient data from a critical care setting. The data were then placed in a scenario that recaptured patient events as they actually occurred. Patient scenarios were sought that represented common diagnoses seen in six body systems—respiratory, cardiovascular, renal, neurologic, gastrointestinal, and endocrine—and in multisystems. The 28 chapters are grouped according to body systems for quick reference. These cases were compiled with one goal in mind: to create a tool for use with critical care students that provides a true perspective of patient needs in the critical care setting. Students can study actual patient situations and apply critical thinking skills in discussions of current treatment modalities, effectiveness of treatments and medications prescribed, alternative care options, the necessity for diagnostic tests ordered, and the impact of hemodynamic values on patient care and the "real-life" necessity for hemodynamic monitoring.

The case study application text represents a different approach to education of critical care nurses. In each scenario, students follow the patient from entrance into the health care setting through his or her discharge from the acute care setting. Students are challenged to use critical thinking skills to accurately answer the case study questions that accompany each case and provide solutions to the patient's problem. Students can then study answers to those same questions written by the author of the chapter. Students should then be well versed in current diagnostic procedures, laboratory data requirements, pharmacologic needs, and treatment modalities for that particular disease entity.

This text is appropriate for the baccalaureate or graduate student and for use in the hospital setting in critical care training. It may also serve as a review tool for nurses preparing for the CCRN examination. The answers to the case study questions provide a detailed account of each disease studied. Educators can choose the questions appropriate for the student's level or can adapt their expectations of the depth of the student's answers.

Health care needs are quickly changing, and we must prepare nurses to change and adapt with the health care system. Students who are challenged to think critically while still in the classroom setting can translate those skills into the clinical care setting to better meet the changing needs of the critically ill patient. It is hoped that this text will increase students' knowledge of the needs of the critically ill patient and enhance education in the clinical setting.

Sheila Drake Melander

CONTENTS

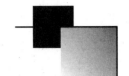

CHAPTER 1

ACUTE RESPIRATORY DISTRESS SYNDROME

Sharon Angle, RN, MSN • Sheila Drake Melander, RN, DSN, ACNP-C, FCCM

CASE PRESENTATION

Postoperative Day 3

Mr. Embry, a 62-year-old, 68-kg (150-lb) white man, had undergone an anterior colon resection for rectal polyps and had an uneventful postoperative course until the evening of the third postoperative day. He was monitored with telemetry and had no unusual complaints. At 10 PM on the third postoperative day, he began to complain of not feeling "right." Assessment of the patient revealed hypotension and shortness of breath. Within minutes, he became confused and agitated. The shortness of breath worsened (he began gasping for air), and he experienced severe hypoxia. He was intubated and transferred to the intensive care unit (ICU). Initial assessment indicated the following:

BP	60/40 mm Hg	pH	7.3
HR	160 bpm	P_{CO_2}	46 mm Hg
Respirations	12-35 breaths/min	P_{O_2}	104 mm Hg
Temperature	38.8° C (101.8° F)	HCO_3^-	22 mmol/L

On arrival in the ICU, mechanical ventilation in the synchronized intermittent mandatory ventilation (SIMV) mode was begun.

Fio_2	90%
SIMV rate	6
Tidal volume	800 ml

Mr. Embry was given a 500-ml bolus of normal saline. He received dopamine (Intropin) 3 to 5 µg/kg/min for renal perfusion and was given vancomycin (Vancocin IV) 1 g intravenously every 12 hours for prophylaxis against staphylococcal infection. A pulmonary artery catheter (Swan-Ganz) was inserted, and the patient's pulmonary capillary wedge pressure was 12 mm Hg.

His fraction of inspired oxygen (Fio_2) increased from 90% to 100%, tidal volume (V_T) was 800 ml, and SIMV was 6 with total respiration of 16 breaths/min. At this time, a positive end-expiratory pressure (PEEP) of 5 cm H_2O was added, and he continued to receive pressure support of 7 cm H_2O. He was given several boluses of normal saline and continued to receive the dopamine infusion. The ventilator settings just outlined were continued. The following arterial blood gas (ABG) values were obtained 2 hours after the ventilator settings were changed:

pH	7.42	Po_2	75.2 mm Hg
Pco_2	46 mm Hg	HCO_3^-	28.9 mmol/L

Postoperative Day 5

PEEP was increased to 10 cm H_2O, and V_T was increased to 1000 ml.

BP	130/60 mm Hg	pH	7.43
HR	120 bpm	Pco_2	46.2 mm Hg
Respirations	10 breaths/min	Po_2	86.8 mm Hg
Temperature	38.3° C (101° F)	HCO_3^-	30.5 mmol/L

After these changes, Mr. Embry's oxygen levels gradually stabilized and he was weaned from ventilatory support. His urinary output also increased significantly after administration of the fluid boluses. Ten days after intubation, Mr. Embry was extubated and received oxygen by nasal cannula.

ACUTE RESPIRATORY DISTRESS SYNDROME

Questions

1. What is ARDS?
2. Discuss the pathophysiologic changes associated with ARDS.
3. What are the pathophysiologic phases of ARDS?
4. How is ARDS diagnosed?
5. What are some medical complications seen with ARDS?
6. What laboratory findings are diagnostic for ARDS?
7. What radiologic changes are seen with ARDS?
8. What changes are seen in pulmonary function studies with ARDS?
9. Tissue hypoxia is a major finding in ARDS. Describe signs and symptoms found on assessment that would be seen with ARDS in the following systems: central nervous, cardiovascular, pulmonary, renal, gastrointestinal/hepatic, and musculoskeletal.
10. What is the goal of treatment for ARDS?
11. What are the principal treatments for ARDS? List and describe the types of ventilatory support available.
12. Describe nonventilatory means of pulmonary support.
13. What are some of the pharmacologic interventions used in ARDS?

14. What role does hemodynamic monitoring play in the management of ARDS?
15. Describe appropriate nursing diagnoses seen with ARDS.
16. What is the nurse's overall goal in caring for the patient with ARDS?

ACUTE RESPIRATORY DISTRESS SYNDROME

Questions and Answers

1. What is ARDS?

ARDS refers to acute respiratory distress syndrome, a set of manifestations presenting in the most extreme form of an acute lung injury that is associated with a wide range of causes or associated conditions (Hudson & Steinberg, 1999). ARDS was first described 30 years ago during the Vietnam War (Bucher & Melander, 1999); however, the first widely used or standardized definition was not published until 1994 by an America-European Consensus Conference (Wyncoll & Evans, 1999). This definition describes ARDS as "a syndrome of inflammation and increased permeability associated with a constellation of clinical, radiologic, and physiologic abnormalities that could not be explained by left atrial hypertension" (Wyncoll & Evans, 1999).

2. What are the pathophysiologic changes associated with ARDS?

Pathophysiologic changes with ARDS are precipitated by some type of injury to the lungs, either direct or indirect, and may come from various sources. When the body is injured, a systemic inflammatory response syndrome (SIRS) is triggered. This takes the normal local inflammatory response that occurs with an injury and moves it from a local to a systemic response (Bucher & Melander, 1999). There are many triggers for the SIRS response. The most common triggers found with ARDS are infection and trauma (Wyncoll & Evans, 1999). Other events may trigger SIRS. These events include the following: hypoxemia, major surgery, burns, and conditions with tissue necrosis (Bucher & Melander, 1999). When SIRS is triggered, the inflammatory process affects the alveolar epithelium (Zimmerman et al, 1999). Damage of the epithelium of the alveolar capillary membrane causes an increase in permeability. This increase in permeability results in an accumulation of protein-rich fluid in the alveoli, causing edema (Bucher & Melander, 1999).

The increase in alveolar fluid deactivates surfactant in the lungs. Without the surfactant, there is a decrease in alveolar tension, which causes the alveoli to collapse (Bucher & Melander, 1999). The alveolar collapse creates a breakdown in the barrier and gas exchange functions in the lungs (Hudson & Steinberg, 1999). The damage to the lung creates a further triggering of SIRS. As the process progresses, there is a fibroproliferation with deposits of collagen in the lungs, leading to lung remodeling (Hudson & Steinberg, 1999). These deposits cause a further disruption of gas exchange, which leads to decreased elasticity of the lungs (Bucher & Melander, 1999).

As the alveoli collapse, there is a further disruption of gas exchange and a ventilation-perfusion imbalance occurs because of an insufficient number of alveoli open to participate in gas exchange (Bucher & Melander, 1999). As the process continues and additional alveoli become dysfunctional, the patient no longer responds to oxygen therapy. This hypoxemia leads to activation of the inflammatory process by the lungs (Bucher & Melander, 1999).

3. What are the pathophysiologic phases of ARDS?

Bucher and Melander (1999) describe three phases of ARDS. The first phase is associated with alveolar edema. Buildup of fibrin and leukocyte debris causes damage to the interstitium. Phase two is marked by persistent capillary and endothelial damage. There is a proliferation of type II cells and the beginning of squamous cell transformation. The third phase is more chronic in nature and is characterized by fibroproliferation with a thickening of the interstitium and an increase in type II cells and fibrosis.

4. How is ARDS diagnosed?

Understanding risk factors and identifying a history of a precipitating event that would trigger SIRS and the development of ARDS are key in identifying the onset of ARDS. Knowledge of a precipitating event, the presence of diffuse pulmonary infiltrates, and refractory hypoxemia are characteristics that would lead to a diagnosis of ARDS (Wyncoll & Evans, 1999).

5. What are some medical complications seen with ARDS?

Mortality from ARDS is greater than 50%, although improvements have been seen in recent years, probably because of better management protocols and ventilatory management (Wyncoll & Evans, 1999). Nosocomial infections, especially pneumonia, and development of stress ulcers are a threat. Prevention of these infections is an important goal in the treatment of patients with ARDS (Wyncoll & Evans, 1999). Respiratory alkalosis and acidosis are problems at varying times during the course of ARDS. In addition, barotrauma, hypotension, volutrauma, sepsis, and multisystem organ failure have all been cited as complications associated with ARDS (Baudouin, 1998; Bucher & Melander, 1999).

6. What laboratory findings are diagnostic for ARDS?

Blood gas measurements are both diagnostic and treatment management tools in ARDS. They are used in the pulmonary treatment for ARDS through management of acid-base balance and arterial oxygenation in conjunction with assessment parameters and trends over time (Bucher & Melander, 1999). ABG measurements are used to calculate a ratio of Fio_2 to the arterial partial pressure of oxygen (Pao_2) (Pao_2/Fio_2 ratio). With ARDS, this ratio drops to less than 200 mm Hg regardless of the amount of PEEP used (Bucher & Melander, 1999).

7. **What radiologic changes are seen with ARDS?**

The hallmark of ARDS is the protein-rich fluid, which accumulates in the alveoli and interstitial spaces as a result of increased permeability. The alveoli become so filled with debris that they can no longer function and are no longer responsive to oxygen therapy. This is evident on the chest x-ray films as the characteristic finding of bilateral diffuse infiltrates or total whiteout (Bucher & Melander, 1999).

8. **What changes are seen in pulmonary function studies with ARDS?**

As a result of the many infiltrates, ARDS presents with changes in pulmonary function studies. The functional residual capacity decreases secondary to the microatelectasis and edema associated with the lung injury and the minute ventilation increases (Bucher & Melander, 1999). The patient will begin to develop a right-to-left shunt and then the alveolar to arterial gradient will begin to increase. Within 2 weeks of extubation, restorative impairments and abnormalities in diffusing capacity begin to subside and continued improvement is noted at 3 and 6 months with maximum improvement at 1 year (Hudson & Steinberg, 1999).

9. **Tissue hypoxia is a major finding in ARDS. Describe signs and symptoms found on assessment that would be seen with ARDS in the following systems: central nervous, cardiovascular, pulmonary, renal, gastrointestinal/hepatic, and musculoskeletal.**

Central Nervous System
Changes in oxygen leading to hypoxemia result in changes in the acid-base balance, which affect the level of consciousness, causing restlessness, fearfulness, agitation, confusion, and a sense of impending doom. As the disease process progresses, the patient becomes increasingly lethargic and less responsive as decompensation continues (Bucher & Melander, 1999).

Pulmonary
Early in the disease process, there is an increase in respiration and dyspnea with crackles resulting from the fluid shifts occurring in the alveolar spaces. There is a cough with foamy, thick sputum production because of the protein, with hemoptysis from the inflammatory process. Initially, the patient is alkalotic as a result of tachypnea. With increasing hypoxemia, responsiveness is decreased and the patient may develop cyanosis, pallor, and diaphoresis. As the disease progresses, crackles and wheezes are very evident on physical examination. With further progression, the breath sounds become absent. Absence of breath sounds is an ominous sign because it signals the collapse of the alveoli. As the process continues, the patient may become acidotic (Bucher & Melander, 1999).

Cardiovascular
As hypoxia increases, there is evidence of tachycardia and arrhythmias. These are seen as a result of the increased cardiac output. The patient's cardiac output will be

increased in an effort to compensate for the decreased oxygen saturation (Bucher & Melander, 1999).

Renal

As the body attempts to compensate for changes in cardiac output and decreased perfusion, the next system to be affected is the renal system. Because of the decreased cardiac output, blood flow through the kidneys will decrease, resulting in a reduction in urine output.

Gastrointestinal

As other systems in the body begin to become affected, blood will be diverted from nonvital organs to assist in the compensatory mechanisms. The gastrointestinal (GI) tract is one system in which this will occur. As a result of decreased blood flow, the bowel can become ischemic and the patient could experience GI bleeding. An ischemic bowel is also an area where translocation of bacteria can occur. This would be an added risk factor for the development of infection, sepsis, or septic shock.

10. What is the goal of treatment for ARDS?

Because the damaged alveoli cannot be treated directly, the treatments are primarily supportive in nature (Bucher & Melander, 1999). The primary goal is to optimize oxygen delivery to the tissues and identify and treat the condition precipitating the development of ARDS (Bucher & Melander, 1999). Treatment efforts for ARDS are to facilitate the restoration of the alveolar capillary membrane integrity (Bucher & Melander, 1999).

Identification of the underlying illness that precipitated ARDS and any complications resulting from that illness or injury becomes important in controlling ARDS (Baudouin, 1998). Other goals should be prevention of nosocomial infection, especially nosocomial pneumonia, and stress ulcers and maintenance of good nutritional status and fluid balance (Wyncoll & Evans, 1999).

11. What are the principal treatments for ARDS? List and describe the types of ventilatory support available.

The principal treatments for the patient with ARDS are ventilatory support and therapy for the underlying precipitating event. The major supportive therapy for ARDS is positive-pressure ventilation. Use of positive-pressure ventilation helps decrease workload and atelectasis (Bucher & Melander, 1999). Collapsing alveoli and the increase in membrane permeability cause an impairment in gas exchange. This leads to decreased elasticity of lung tissue. As a result higher pressures are needed to distend the lung (Bucher & Melander, 1999).

High pressures and volume may lead to additional lung injury. To prevent additional lung injury, other methods of ventilation, including high-frequency jet ventilation, pressure-controlled inverse ratio ventilation, and pressure-controlled ventilation without the inverse ratio, have been tried.

High-frequency jet ventilation has been used in the last 10 years to maintain gas exchange and decrease lung injury (Velmahos et al, 1999). High-frequency jet ventilation has been used effectively in the pediatric population, but results in adult patients have been conflicting (Velmahos et al, 1999). High-frequency jet ventilation allows the use of smaller volumes by creating constant airway pressure throughout the respiratory cycle (Bucher & Melander, 1999).

Inverse ratio ventilation has become popular as a mode of ventilatory support to help provide improvement in gas exchange. According to Yanos, Watling, and Verhey (1998), there has been no definitive proof that inverse ratio ventilation has improved gas exchange. Pressure-controlled inverse ratio ventilation reverses the normal pattern of breathing seen with ventilatory support and causes expiration to be greater than inspiration.

Pressure-controlled ventilation without inverse ratio is used to deliver a preset pressure instead of volume. There is no reversal of the inspiratory/expiratory ratio. Pressure-controlled ventilation without inverse ratio is used to support the patient's own breathing by delivering a preset volume with each patient-initiated breath (Bucher & Melander, 1999).

12. Describe nonventilatory means of pulmonary support.

Extracorporeal membrane oxygenation (ECMO) is a form of pulmonary support without the use of a ventilator. ECMO has been more widely used in the neonatal arena. Masiakos, Islam, Doody, Schnitzer, and Ryan (1999) describe the use of ECMO in nonneonatal acute respiratory failure. It is used most commonly when all other conventional therapies have failed and the patient has a recoverable pulmonary insufficiency (Masiakos et al, 1999). ECMO provides support when the supplemental oxygen, PEEP, and pressure ventilation limits reach the point where continued use will cause irreversible damage and fibrosis of the lung (Masiakos et al, 1999).

13. What are some of the pharmacologic interventions used in ARDS?

The pharmacologic agents used depend on the underlying processes being treated. Dopamine and dobutamine may be used to support cardiovascular dynamics by increasing cardiac output and hence blood pressure. Often because sepsis is a significant precipitating event and because of the risk of nosocomial infections, antibiotic therapy is a key pharmacologic intervention. Neuromuscular blocking agents and sedatives are also widely used to aid with ventilatory support. Glucocorticoids may be used because of their ability to inhibit the inflammatory response at all levels (Meduri, 1999).

14. What role does hemodynamic monitoring play in the management of ARDS?

Mechanical ventilation, which is a main component of therapy for the patient with ARDS, may have a great effect on cardiac output. The use of hemodynamic monitoring can help determine the effects of mechanical ventilation and PEEP on cardiac output as well assist in the management of fluid volume. Hemodynamic monitoring can also help the health care professional differentiate between ARDS and congestive heart failure (Bucher & Melander, 1999). Hemodynamic monitoring can also be used to evaluate whether the current therapy modalities are effective.

15. Describe appropriate nursing diagnoses seen with ARDS.

Nursing diagnoses vary according to which body systems are affected and which complications occur with ARDS. The most common nursing diagnoses associated with ARDS include the following (Bucher & Melander, 1999):

- Impaired tissue perfusion
- Alteration in cardiac output
- Ineffective breathing patterns
- Ineffective airway clearance
- Impaired gas exchange
- Alteration in nutrition
- Anxiety
- Alteration in communication
- High risk for infection
- High risk for impaired skin integrity

16. What is the nurse's overall goal in caring for the patient with ARDS?

The nurse has many roles in the care of the patient with ARDS. One of the first roles is to assist in the use of ventilation modalities to improve gas exchange and to monitor the patient's response to these. A second very important role is for the nurse to continually be watching for potential complications through the nursing assessment and to intervene to prevent the many complications associated with ARDS. A third role is to be supportive and provide palliative care for the patient while other treatment modalities are being used.

Acute Respiratory Distress Syndrome

References

Baudouin, S. (1998). Improved survival in ARDS: chance, technology or experience? *Thorax,* *53*(4), 237-238.

Bucher, L., & Melander, S. (Eds.). (1999). *Critical care nursing.* Philadelphia: Saunders.

Hudson, L. D., & Steinberg, K. P. (1999). Epidemiology of acute lung injury and ARDS. *Chest, 116*(1, Suppl.), 74S-82S.

Masiakos, P., Islam, S., Doody, D., Schnitzer, J., & Ryan, D. (1999). Extracorporeal membrane oxygenation for nonneonatal acute respiratory failure. *Archives of Surgery, 134,* 375-380.

Meduri, G. U. (1999). Levels of evidence for the pharmacologic effectiveness of prolonged methylprednisolone treatment in unresolving acute respiratory distress syndrome. *Chest, 116*(1, Suppl.), 116S-118S.

Velmahos, G. C., Chan, L. S., Tatevossian, R., Cornwell, E. E., III, Dougherty, W. R., Escudero, J., & Demetriades, D. (1999). High frequency percussive ventilation improves oxygenation in patients with ARDS. *Chest, 116*(2), 440-446.

Wyncoll, D., & Evans, T. (1999). Acute respiratory distress syndrome. *The Lancet, 354*(9177), 497-501.

Yanos, J., Watling, S., & Verhey, J. (1998). The physiologic effects of inverse ratio ventilation. *Chest, 114*(3), 834-838.

Zimmerman, G. A., Albertine, K. H., Carveth, H. J., Gill, E. A., Grissom, C. K., Hoidal, J. R., Imaizumi T., Maloney, C. G., McIntyre, T. M., Michael, J. R., Orme, J. F., Prescott, S. M., & Topham, M. S. (1999). Endothelial activation in ARDS. *Chest, 116*(1), 18S-24S.

CHAPTER 2

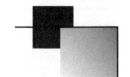

PULMONARY EMBOLISM

Mary Ann Wehmer, RN, MSN, CNOR

CASE PRESENTATION

Janet Leigh, a 62-year-old woman, was admitted to the hospital for an exploratory laparotomy for abdominal pain. The admission history and physical examination revealed a healthy white woman who smokes a pack of cigarettes a day. Mrs. Leigh had no history of medical problems or abnormalities except for obesity and the absence from work with bed rest for the last week because of pain. She is married and has three children. She denied taking any medications except for hormone replacement therapy (HRP) and a multiple vitamin. Her preoperative diagnostic data were the following:

BP	160/84 mm Hg	RBCs	$5.0 \times 10^6/mm^3$
HR	77 bpm	WBCs	$5000/mm^3$
Respirations	16 breaths/min	Platelets	$148,000/mm^3$
Temperature	37.1°C (98.9°F)	PT	14 sec
Hgb	15 g/dl	PTT	40 sec
Hct	42%	Urine analysis	Normal

Day of Surgery

Mrs. Leigh's surgical procedure involved lysis of numerous adhesions and removal of the left ovary for an ovarian tumor. The tumor was sent for pathologic examination to rule out a malignancy. Results of the permanent pathologic report are pending. Mrs. Leigh tolerated the general anesthesia and 2-hour surgical procedure without incident.

She was transferred to a medical-surgical floor from the postanesthesia care unit. Her vital signs remained stable. An intravenous (IV) infusion of 5% dextrose in 0.45% normal saline was infusing at 125 ml/hr, and she was to be given nothing by mouth (NPO). Her pain was managed with patient-controlled administration of morphine via a 2-mg bolus dose every 12 minutes for a maximum dose of 10 mg every hour. If postoperative nausea and vomiting occurred, she could receive ondansetron hydrochloride (Zofran) 4 mg IV every 3 to 4 hours.

Mrs. Leigh was informed about the need to get out of bed for pulmonary hygiene and the prevention of postoperative complications such as pneumonia and atelectasis, paralytic ileus, and deep vein thrombosis (DVT). Mrs. Leigh experienced a lot of pain, which resulted in nausea and vomiting when she was assisted in a transfer from the side-of-the-bed sitting position to sitting in a chair at the bedside. She was treated for the nausea and vomiting and returned to bed. Later that day, she refused to get up because of her previous experience with pain and nausea. Deep (diaphragmatic) breathing 10 times every 2 hours and leg exercises were encouraged while she was awake.

Postoperative Day 1

Mrs. Leigh's vital signs remained stable with the exception of the presence of a low-grade fever. Bowel sounds were hypoactive in all four quadrants, and because of nausea; NPO status was continued, but she could have ice chips. Laboratory values remained normal with the exception of a slight decrease in the hemoglobin (12 g/dl) and hematocrit (45%). Mrs. Leigh continued to complain of incisional pain with nausea. So far she had had two episodes of vomiting. Mrs. Leigh used her patient-controlled analgesia frequently and requested Zofran for the nausea and vomiting. When encouraged to get out of bed, she responded, "I hurt too much and then throw up." An abdominal binder was ordered to assist in supporting her abdominal muscles when she changed positions, coughed, or vomited. An incentive spirometer was ordered.

Postoperative Day 2

After the initial morning assessment, the registered nurse (RN) assisted Mrs. Leigh to the bedside commode and then helped her return to bed. When the RN checked on her later that morning, she found Mrs. Leigh to be very restless and apprehensive. She was complaining of shortness of breath (SOB), chest pain that worsened on inspiration, and right calf pain. Upon assessment, her nurse found crackles in the left lower lobe, labored respirations, diaphoresis, and an erythematous, warm, and tender right calf with a dusky colored lower leg and foot. Mrs. Leigh's vital signs were the following:

BP	170/90 mm Hg	Respirations	36 breaths/min
HR	124 bpm	Temperature	37.8° C (100.1°F)

Mrs. Leigh was placed in a semi-Fowler position, and oxygen was started at 4 L/min through a nasal cannula. The physician was notified, and the stat orders of arterial blood gas (ABG) measurements, an electrocardiogram (ECG), ultrasound of the right leg, a chest x-ray film, and a Doppler study of the right leg were completed. Following are the results of these tests:

pH	7.52	Chest x-ray study	Bibasilar
$Paco_2$	27 mm Hg	ECG	Sinus tachycardia
Pao_2	78 mm Hg	Doppler study	Right DVT
Sao_2	95%		

A heparin bolus of 5000 U was administered, followed by a continuous infusion of 1400 U/hr. A ventilation-perfusion ($\dot{V}/\dot{Q}$) scan revealed perfusion defects of the left lower lobe with normal ventilation. A pulmonary embolism (PE) with DVT in the right leg was suspected. Mrs. Leigh was transferred to the intensive care unit and a pulmonary angiogram was performed that verified the diagnosis.

That evening, Mrs. Leigh's respiratory distress worsened, requiring intubation and mechanical ventilation. The following hemodynamic values were then obtained:

pH	7.58	Sao$_2$	80%
Paco$_2$	24 mm Hg	PT	17.1 sec
Pao$_2$	60 mm Hg	aPTT	49.2 sec

PULMONARY EMBOLISM

Questions

1. Discuss in detail venous thrombosis as the origin of a PE, its prevention, and treatment. Briefly discuss other potential sources of PE.
2. Compare the action and monitoring of unfractionated heparin and low-molecular-weight heparin (LMWH). Identify advantages of LMWH.
3. Identify the elements of Virchow's triad and the pathophysiology of its development into PE.
4. List other predisposing factors or conditions for DVT. Identify which risk factors or conditions for DVT applied to Mrs. Leigh.
5. Describe the pathophysiology of the pulmonary and hemodynamic alterations that occur as a result of PE.
6. What are clinical manifestations of PE and which signs and symptoms did Mrs. Leigh exhibit?
7. What differential and diagnostic tests are used to determine PE? What did Mrs. Leigh's studies show?
8. Describe medical and nursing assessment and interventions to be used in the prevention of PE?
9. Develop a list of nursing diagnoses appropriate for Mrs. Leigh in the acute phase of the PE event.
10. List the nursing responsibilities for Mrs. Leigh and other patients with acute PE events.
11. What guidelines are available for Mrs. Leigh's anticoagulation therapy in the treatment of PE?
12. Describe three other fibrinolytic therapy modalities that may be used in the management of PE.

PULMONARY EMBOLISM

Questions and Answers

1. Discuss in detail venous thrombosis as the origin of a PE, its prevention, and treatment. Briefly discuss other potential sources of PE.

Venous Thrombosis

Ninety percent of PEs originate from a venous thromboembolism (VTE) in the deep veins of the lower extremity. Most VTEs evolve from the popliteal, femoral, and iliac veins, but other sites include the pelvic veins, right ventricle, and upper extremities (Alspach, 1998). Two million Americans develop DVT annually (Hirsch & Hoak, 1996). Clinical manifestations of DVT are a positive Homans' sign (may be unreliable if the patient had a positive Homans' sign before the DVT), calf asymmetry with swelling and pain in the affected extremity, and a dusky coloring of the site (McCance & Huether, 1998).

Noninvasive lower extremity studies for assessment of DVTs exist, but they are not very sensitive to DVTs. Noninvasive tests that detect venous thrombosis include ultrasound and Doppler studies, impedance plethysmography, and the I-fibrinogen leg scan. Doppler ultrasonography indicates blood flow by measuring sound waves as they are reflected off red blood cells (RBCs). Impedance plethysmography measures electrical resistance changes when a blood pressure cuff is rapidly deflated. In the I-fibrinogen leg scan, fibrinogen is tracked with a radioisotope so that when the fibrinogen attaches to the thrombus, it becomes visible.

A more sensitive test for DVTs is the venogram, but this is an invasive test. Dye is injected into the vein so that the shape of the vessel is displayed via radiography (WellnessWeb, 1998).

DVTs dislodge in about 7 to 10 days after an injury, when the clot begins to dissolve, with sudden movement (especially with the first ambulation after several days of immobility), deep leg muscle massage, and with vascular pressure changes that occur with straining, sneezing, coughing, and so on (Rodgers, 1999). Once DVT is diagnosed, unfractionated heparin is administered for hospitalized patients and a LMWH can be administered to outpatients. The unfractionated heparin dosage is adjusted until the activated partial thromboplastin time (aPTT) is prolonged two times the control while the dose for LMWH is calculated by the patient's body weight (Graber, 1999).

The potential for recurrence of DVT depends on the status of the individual's risk factors. If risk factors are reversed or decreased, recurrence within the first year is less than if risk factors remain the same. Most patients have normal noninvasive lower extremity studies after 3 months, and 90% have normal studies by 1 year, indicating resolution of the clot but not necessarily a fully competent normal vein. If a patient develops postthrombotic syndrome, the rate of recurrence becomes even higher (Lipchik & Presberg, 1996).

Fat Emboli

The initial presentation of a fat embolus is more difficult to recognize because vasoactive substances are released from fatty emboli that produce bronchospasm and asthmalike symptoms. Petechiae on the neck, anterior chest, axilla, and conjunctivae are often seen with PE originating from fat emboli (Rodgers, 1999). Significant patient historical data usually are associated with multiple skeletal fractures and traumatic injury to the long bones and pelvis in the last 48 hours. The pathophysiology is believed to be associated with toxic free fatty acid liberated from fat globules that were released from the bone marrow into the venous circulation (Lipchik & Presberg, 1996).

Air Emboli

Air emboli are a major concern in operative procedures that require a patient to be in the sitting position. Procedures such as a cervical laminectomy or suboccipital craniotomy have an increased risk for air emboli that can enter the venous system when venous tracts are transected during exposure of the wound and surgical repair or removal. Extra perioperative measures for early detection and treatment of air emboli include Doppler monitoring, arterial line monitoring, and central venous catheter (CVC) and/or pulmonary artery catheter (PAC) placement. If an air embolus is suspected, attempts are made to keep the embolus from passing through the right ventricle into the pulmonary circulation. A large syringe may be used to aspirate blood and the air embolus from the CVC or PAC. Positive pressure is added to the ventilation, and the patient is placed in a "right-side-up" lateral position.

Catheter Emboli

A CVC or PAC is a risk factor for the development of DVT, although clinically significant VTEs occur less often from subclavian and axillary vein thrombosis (Lipchik & Presberg, 1996). Secondary injury to the vascular wall occurs from mechanical or chemical trauma that activates the coagulation cascade and inflammatory process to set up for thrombi formation (Erdman, Rodvold, & Friedenberg, 1997). To decrease the chance of DVT development, the maintenance protocol for central lines includes a heparin flush every 8 hours.

Right Atrial or Ventricular Emboli

Atrial fibrillation or flutter causes ineffective pumping of blood through the right atrium. The disrupted muscular activity leads to the stasis of blood flow. Blood contains serum and RBCs, white blood cells (WBCs), and platelets that circulate through the vessels, but when blood flow is stagnated, platelets come in contact with the vessel wall lining and begin to agglutinate and thus start the formation of a thrombus.

Amniotic Fluid Emboli

Although rare, amniotic fluid emboli can occur with amniocentesis, abruptio placenta, or abortion when the amniotic fluid passes into the venous circulation. PE from amniotic fluid occurs with a rapid onset of hyperemia, hypotension, and disseminated intravascular coagulopathy. According to Lipchik and Presberg (1996), the pathophysiology of amniotic fluid in the venous system is believed to be related to one or all of the following:

- Amniotic fluid in the venous system stimulates the aggregation of platelets and factor X activation.
- Particles of fetal ruins may migrate into the venous circulation to stimulate another mechanism.
- Amniotic fluid can enter into the venous system and migrates into the smaller pulmonary lumina where obstruction occurs.

Tumor Emboli

In 1865, Trousseau associated the development of VTE with the presence of an occult malignancy. Lipchik and Presberg (1996) stated that when an otherwise healthy patient develops a DVT, it is reasonable to direct examinations for possible malignancy of the gastrointestinal tract, lung, breast, or reproductive organs (Lipchik & Presberg, 1996). Likewise the assessment of DVT should also include signs of an occult malignancy. The relationship between cancer and VTE is that certain types of carcinoma affect the production of thrombin and thus the development of a thrombus.

Septic Emboli

Bacterial or viral infections can infect a clot that breaks off and causes obstruction in the pulmonary artery circulation. Patients with PE from this origin are likely to have SOB, fever, hemoptysis, and a productive cough. Septic emboli occur more often with infected indwelling implants and catheters and after obstetrical/gynecologic surgical procedures (Lipchik & Presberg, 1996).

2. **Compare the action and monitoring of unfractionated heparin and low-molecular-weight heparin (LMWH). Identify advantages of LMWH.**

LMWH has been found to be safer and as effective as unfractionated heparin in preventing PE (Nilsson et al, 1997). Unfractionated heparin inactivates thrombin and factor Xa, which are clotting enzymes. Heparin-induced thrombocytopenia that occurs after 5 days of heparin therapy is seen more often with unfractionated heparin, which has a narrow therapeutic range, than with LMWH, which inactivates only factor Xa (Hirsh et al, 1998).

Monitoring of unfractionated heparin anticoagulation therapy consists of the timely drawing of blood for aPTT assessment at 6 hours after bolus and initiation of the continuous IV infusion. Blood should be drawn at approximately the same time every morning for monitoring of aPTT levels during heparin therapy administration. The aPTT should be maintained at a therapeutic range equivalent to 0.3 to 0.7 U/ml of the antifactor Xa heparin level. The antifactor Xa assay has been suggested to be more useful than the aPTT in monitoring heparin therapy because it is more specific to the effects of heparin and is not influenced by coagulation factors (Hyers et al, 1998). Because heparin assays are more costly than aPTT assessments, the assay is recommended only when the aPTT response is less than the lower limit of therapeutic range despite heparin dosages of 40,000 U/24 hr (Hirsh & Hoak, 1996). The recommended therapeutic aPTT for PE is 1.5 to 2.5 times the control value (Erdman, Rodvold, & Fridenberg, 1997).

LMWH requires no monitoring of the clotting status, and dosages are adjusted to the patient's weight as recommended by the product manufacturer. Monitoring of the clotting status is not required because (1) the plasma recovery and clearance of LMWH are independent of the plasma concentration and dose, (2) LMWH binds less to the plasma protein, and (3) the half-life of LMWH is two to four times that of unfractionated heparin. The greater safety of LMWH is believed to be related to its lesser dose variability and longer half-life than unfractionated heparin (Nunnelee, 1997).

3. **Identify the elements of Virchow's triad and the pathophysiology of its development into PE.**

Elements of Virchow's Triad

Virchow's triad refers to Virchow's 1856 theory that three predisposing factors are involved in venous thrombus formation. The three factors include the following three situations.

- *Venous wall intimal injury:* A natural defense mechanism to injury in the intima of the venous wall stimulates the formation of a clot to stop the flow of blood from the vasculature. Injury to the venous wall exposes collagen, which initiates (1) the activation and aggregation of platelets at the injured site and (2) the release of tissue factor III, which leads to formation of a fibrin plug (Launius & Graham, 1998).

Venous wall intimal injury can result from direct insults to the vessel such as mechanical impairment in surgery (especially obstetrical and orthopedic procedures), spontaneous rupture, or DVT; infections involving viruses or bacteria; hypoxia; or elevated levels of cholesterol and plaque formation.

- *Decreased blood flow or stasis:* Stagnation of blood flow disrupts the normal laminar or central flow through the vessel. As the blood flows along the intima wall, the flow of blood and naturally occurring anticoagulants is slowed. The decreased blood flow or stasis allows blood cells to contact the endothelial lining, preventing the dilution of clotting factors (Launius & Graham, 1998). Together the decreased flow of anticoagulants and collection of clotting factors cause the patient to be prone to clot formation. In addition, clot formation leads to prostacyclin depletion, which impairs the activation of coagulation factors and reduces production of platelet coagulation inhibitors.

Venous blood return to the heart is disrupted when the action of voluntary and involuntary muscles and venous valves is halted as in the following conditions: prolonged immobility; atrial fibrillation, decreased cardiac output, or congestive heart failure; obesity; pregnancy; sickle cell disease; systemic lupus erythematosus; polycythemia; and sepsis. PEs occur four times more often in the lower lobes of the lungs, where the blood flow is sluggish (Rodgers, 1999). Venous stasis has appeared to be the most important factor of Virchow's triad that predisposes patients for PE (Thelan, Urden, Laugh, & Stacy, 1998).

- *Hypercoagulability of blood:* Hypercoagulability decreases the resistance to clot formation in the vascular bed. The lowered threshold for thrombus formation is related to a release of cytokines that indirectly enhance thrombin's clotting activity (Rodgers, 1999). Patients may have a primary or secondary predisposition for hypercoagulability that does not cause a DVT until an added stressor stimulates the hypercoagulable state.

A genetic defect in the protein C and/or heparin-antithrombin III anticoagulant pathways usually causes primary or idiopathic hypercoagulability. Secondary or acquired hypercoagulable states are caused by physiologic and disease processes that increase the risk for clot formation (Launius and Graham, 1998). Acquired hypercoagulable states can occur with polycythemia, pregnancy, oral contraceptive and estrogen use, systemic lupus erythematosus, and malignancy.

Pathophysiology in the Development of PE

As a result of thrombus formation, phlebitis (inflammation of the vein) occurs. When phlebitis occurs in superficial veins, disruption of blood flow is not a serious problem. Blood from the swollen and inflamed vein is redirected through other superficial veins. When phlebitis occurs in the deep veins, blood flow is disrupted because rerouting mechanisms do not occur and blood flow is sluggish or pooled at the inflamed site. Blood flow is further disrupted as (1) the thrombus attaches to venous valves and (2) the thrombus travels into smaller circumferences (Rodgers, 1999).

DVT and PE are clearly associated and exhibit the same beginning disease process. Lipchik and Presberg (1996) stated that a high-probability $\dot{V}/\dot{Q}$ mismatch occurred in 40% of patients with DVT without PE symptoms, indicating that DVT and PE display the same initial disease process (Lipchik & Presberg, 1996). On autopsy, 75% of DVTs were associated with signs of PE. Lung scans confirmed that 70% of patients with a symptomatic PE have had an asymptomatic DVT (Rodgers, 1999).

One of the most common causes of a clinical PE is a dislodged DVT breaking free from the venous wall. The embolus travels through the right side of the heart into the main pulmonary artery and into the pulmonary circulation or until the clot blocks a segment of smaller diameter arteries. PEs occur in both lungs 65% of the time, in the right lung 25% of the time, and in the left lung 10% of the time (Rodgers, 1999).

4. List other predisposing factors or conditions for DVT. Identify which risk factors or conditions for DVT applied to Mrs. Leigh.

Other Predisposing Conditions for DVT

- According to Lipchik and Presberg (1996), patients who are younger than 40 years of age with no other risk factors and who have had a surgical procedure that lasts less than 30 minutes are at low risk with 0.5% chance for developing VTE. Patients who are older than 40 years of age and have had a surgical procedure that lasts more than 30 minutes are at moderate risk with a 2% to 10% chance for VTE development. High-risk groups with a 20% chance for developing VTE include those who are older than 65 years of age, have been immobilized for a prolonged period, have had a prior SVT or myocardial infarction, are obese, have congestive heart failure (CHF), and are undergoing surgery for hip fractures, hip and knee joint replacements, pelvic or lower extremity trauma, and malignancy (Lipchik & Presberg, 1996).
- The top four risk factors for development of PE in hospitalized patients were identified as DVT, more than 7 days of immobilization, obesity, and postoperative status. The frequency of PE is 40% with surgical procedures on the back and extremities, 20% with head and neck procedures, 15.8% with abdominal procedures, and 9.4% with thoracic procedures (Rodgers, 1999).
- Additional risk factors identified for development of PE are smoking, long trips (2 hours or more), and prolonged inactivity.

Mrs. Leigh's risk factors and conditions are as follows:

- 62 years old
- Pack-a-day smoker
- Bed rest for 1 week preoperatively
- Obesity
- HRP
- High normal values preoperatively for blood pressure, hemoglobin (Hgb), hematocrit (Hct), RBCs, prothrombin time (PT), and aPTT
- Pelvic surgical procedure lasting 2 hours
- Possible malignancy
- Postoperative pain and nausea/vomiting resulting in resistance to ambulate
- Slight decrease of Hct postoperatively to 45% related to postoperative dehydration (NPO status and vomiting)

5. **Describe the pathophysiology of the pulmonary and hemodynamic alterations that occur as a result of PE.**

Pathophysiology of the Pulmonary and Hemodynamic Alterations

PE can impair the $\dot{V}/\dot{Q}$ efforts of the pulmonary system by affecting the dead space, bronchi, and alveoli. Compensatory vascular shunting leads to pulmonary artery hypertension and right-sided ventricular failure. When these compensatory efforts are imposed on an already compromised cardiac system or in a massive occlusion, decreased cardiac output, right-sided ventricular failure, and pulmonary infarction can occur.

Increased Dead Space and $\dot{V}/\dot{Q}$ Mismatch

Alveolar-capillary gas exchange does not occur distal to the point at which the embolus lodges (Hartshorn, Sole, & Lamborn, 1997). When nonperfused alveoli are being ventilated, ventilatory efforts are wasted, and the area not being perfused is dead space. This situation creates a $\dot{V}/\dot{Q}$ mismatch when the following primary and secondary events occur:

- Diminished oxygen is available to local tissue (hypoxia).
- The blood being circulated to all body cells is low in oxygen (hypoxemia).
- Carbon dioxide cannot enter the affected alveoli (alveolar hypocarbia).
- The level of systemic carbon dioxide increases (hypercapnia).
- Varying degrees of hyperventilation increase the partial pressure of oxygen in arterial blood (Pao_2) but do not affect the alveolar-arterial (A-a) gradient elevation.

Bronchial Constriction

The bronchial constriction occurs from alveolar hypocarbia that causes ventilation to be shunted to perfused areas of the lung. Platelet aggregation at the site of the occlusion causes a release of thromboxane A_2 and serotonin that further constricts airways and the pulmonary artery (Rodgers, 1999).

Atelectasis

Atelectasis occurs after bronchoconstriction when the production of surfactant decreases proportionately with the length of time that alveoli are not perfused. Galvin and Choi (1999) stated that alveolar surface tension decreases within 2 to 3 hours after a PE obstruction and the production of surfactant is severely slowed within 12 to 15 hours (Galvin & Choi, 1999). Twenty-four hours after the obstruction of perfusion, surfactant production and alveolar type II cell nutrition are depleted, leading to atelectasis.

Pulmonary Arterial Hypertension

Patients who have had a massive PE (obstruction of more than 50% of the pulmonary vascular bed) are likely to demonstrate pulmonary hypertension (Thelan et al, 1998). Pulmonary arterial hypertension could be described as an ineffective but adaptive response of shunting blood from nonfunctional to functional alveoli. As a result, hyperventilation occurs in an effort to perfuse and ventilate the lungs (Hartshorn et al, 1997). These two compensatory mechanisms circulate the entire cardiac output to the unaffected areas of the lungs, which leads to increased pulmonary artery pressure and resistance (Thelan et al, 1998).

Right-Sided Ventricular Failure

When pulmonary hypertension develops, the pulmonary artery diastolic-occlusive pressure gradient widens and the workload of the right ventricle increases until right-sided ventricular failure occurs. The normal right ventricle can compensate at levels of a systolic pressure of 65 mm Hg or a mean pulmonary artery pressure up to 40 mm Hg. Lipchik and Presberg (1996) stated that after these limits are reached, right-sided ventricular failure results.

Depending on the degree of right-sided heart failure, systemic symptoms may occur such as neck vein distension, peripheral edema, ascites, and hepatomegaly. With decompensation of the right ventricle, a fixed-split P_2 heart sound may result from delayed closure of the pulmonic valve. A diastolic murmur from pulmonary insufficiency indicates further right-sided ventricular decompensation (Thelan et al, 1998). Decreased cardiac output leads to decreased perfusion of the coronary arteries, brain, and kidneys (Rodgers, 1999).

Decreased Cardiac Output

Backward and forward effects result from right-sided ventricular failure. The right atrial pressure increases as blood backs up into the right atrium and the amount of blood entering the left ventricle decreases resulting in decreased cardiac output (Rodgers, 1999). The two compensatory mechanisms that respond to the decreased cardiac output include (1) an increased Pao_2 resulting from the increased ventilatory efforts and (2) stimulation of the sympathetic nervous system, chemoreceptors, and baroreceptors. A normal pulmonary artery occlusive pressure in an acute PE event indicates normal left ventricular pressure.

Pulmonary Infarction

Pulmonary infarction (PI) occurs with 10% to 15% of PEs because of the extensive collateral circulation to the lungs. Patients at risk for PI include those with preexisting cardiopulmonary disease that compromises circulation. Signs of infarction, such as hemoptysis, occur 24 to 48 hours after the PE event, which is not necessarily 24 hours from the clinical presentation of the PE. Consequences of PI include changes in the pulmonary artery pressure and circulation that cause more PE events. Hemorrhage, effusion, and eventually fibrosis and scarring will be the results (Rodgers, 1999). Pulmonary resection may be required for large areas of necrosis or abscess.

6. What are clinical manifestations of PE and which signs and symptoms did Mrs. Leigh exhibit?

Clinical Manifestations of PE

Clinical manifestations of a PE depend on the size of the affected vessel, the extent of obstruction, the type of embolus, and preexisting comorbidity. According to Brashers and Davey (1998), clinical manifestations of the initial insult depend on whether the following are present:

- A single or multiple pulmonary emboli occurred that may be chronic or recurrent.
- An embolus occurred without infarction and thus there was no permanent damage and it was not severe.

- A massive occlusion occurred and a major artery for pulmonary circulation was occluded.
- An embolus occurred with infarction and thus some portion of lung tissue died (Brashers & Davey, 1998).

Clinical signs and symptoms of PE such as dyspnea, pleuritic chest pain, hemoptysis, acute right-sided heart failure, and cardiovascular collapse can be difficult to distinguish from other respiratory and cardiovascular causes. The Pulmonary Embolism Prospective Investigation of Pulmonary Embolism Diagnosis (PIOPED) study identified signs and symptoms of patients with angiographically proven PE who had no preexisting pulmonary or heart disease (Lipchik & Presberg, 1996). The most common symptoms were dyspnea (identified 73% of the time), pleuritic chest pain that increased during inspiration (identified 66% of the time), and cough (identified 37% of the time). All of these symptoms can occur in a number of other medical diagnoses. The most common physical sign was tachypnea, which was identified 70% of the time. Rales occurred in 51% of patients, but tachycardia, fever, and phlebitis occurred in fewer than 50% of the patients (Rodgers, 1999).

Other clinical manifestations of PE may include the following:

- Wheezing related to bronchoconstriction
- Cyanosis and decreased breath sounds related to pleuritic chest pain and ventilation defects
- Hypotension related to ineffective sympathetic stimulation
- Accentuated pulmonic heart sounds and systolic murmurs related to ventricular compromise and increased pulmonary artery pressure
- Diaphoresis and tachycardia related to release of catecholamines
- Jugular venous distension and edema related to right-sided ventricular failure
- Phlebitis and fever related to inflammation

Mrs. Leigh's signs and symptoms were the following:

- Unexplained restlessness and apprehension after postoperative ambulation
- SOB and labored respirations
- Chest pain that worsened on inspiration
- Right calf pain with erythema, warmth, and tenderness and a dusky colored leg and foot
- Crackles in the left lower lobe
- Diaphoresis

7. What differential and diagnostic tests are used to recognize PE? What did Mrs. Leigh's studies show?

Differential Diagnostic Tests

After assessment of the history and physical examination, tests should be conducted to establish a baseline status to make a differential diagnosis from other disease processes such as cardiovascular diseases (ischemic cardiac chest pain, pericarditis, or dissecting aortic aneurysm), pulmonary diseases (pneumonia, pleural effusion, or pleuritis), and gastrointestinal disorders (gastric or duodenal ulcer, gastritis, or esophageal rupture) (Dietzen, 1997). Baseline tests should include (1) complete blood count to check for inflammation (WBCs and sedimentation rate) and the hydration status (Hgb and Hct); (2) SMA; (3) PT and aPTT; (4) chest x-ray study; (5) ECG; (6) ABG measurements to check for decreased or increased Pao_2, increased A-a gradient, and elevated pH indicative of respiratory alkalosis; and (7) pulmonary function studies to determine reduced forced expiratory volume in 1 second and peak expiratory flow rates (Alspach, 1998).

Konstadt (1999) described the use of transesophageal echocardiography (TEE) to differentiate an intraoperative PE from an acute cardiovascular collapse. A central PE that occurs in the main, right, or left pulmonary artery is associated with cardiovascular collapse and can be visualized with TEE. Additional noninvasive studies for future use in the diagnosis of PE include fiberoptic and intravascular pulmonary ultrasound, computed tomography (CT) using contrast media, digital subtraction angiography, magnetic resonance imaging (MRI), and radiolabeled platelets (Erdman et al, 1997).

Diagnostic Studies

Lung scintigraphy ($\dot{V}/\dot{Q}$ scan) is performed (1) to differentiate PE from bronchogenic or lymphangitic carcinomas and congenital vascular abnormalities and (2) to determine the probability that a $\dot{V}/\dot{Q}$ mismatch exists (Dietzen, 1997; Galvin & Choi, 1999). In the PIOPED study, lung scans were found to be sensitive and reliable in differentiating a normal $\dot{V}/\dot{Q}$ from a $\dot{V}/\dot{Q}$ mismatch. An even distribution of radiotracers for ventilation and perfusion throughout both lung fields without defects indicates normal perfusion and rules out PE (Ward & Faitelson, 1996). When ventilation tracers are normal in multiple segmental defects of abnormal perfusion, a $\dot{V}/\dot{Q}$ mismatch or a high probability for PE exists. An exception to the high reliability in the scan occurs in a patient who has had a previous embolus with abnormal perfusion studies before scanning. When the scan does not fit into the high-probability or normal $\dot{V}/\dot{Q}$ groups, the scan is considered nondiagnostic and an investigation for a DVT should follow (Galvin & Choi, 1999).

Pulmonary angiography is the gold standard test for PE because it can detect emboli as small as 0.5 mm (Erdman et al, 1997). The pulmonary vasculature is viewed under fluoroscopy after an iodine contrast medium has been injected via a peripheral catheter threaded through the right side of the heart. Reliable signs of a PE include an abrupt termination of a pulmonary artery vessel or an intraluminal-filling defect.

Mrs. Leigh's Studies

Elevated vital signs were related to tissue hypoxia and compensatory efforts.

BP	170/90 mm Hg	Respirations	36 breaths/min
HR	124 bpm	Temperature	37.8° C (100.1° F)

Initial ABG measurements revealed respiratory alkalosis and the attempted response to blow off CO_2.

pH	7.52	Pao_2	78 mm Hg
$Paco_2$	27 mm Hg	Sao_2	95%

Later ABG measurements revealed alkalosis with a further drop in the Pao_2. The aPTT was within the therapeutic range for anticoagulation.

pH	7.58	Sao_2	80%
$Paco_2$	24 mm Hg	PT	17.1 sec
Pao_2	60 mm Hg	aPTT	49.2 sec

8. Describe medical and nursing assessment and interventions to be used in the prevention of PE?

Early Assessment

In the United States, PEs are responsible for 100,000 deaths annually and are the third leading cause of death (Brashers & Davey, 1998). Evaluation of risk factors is an important step in early diagnosis and treatment of PE because more than 90% of patients with PE have clinical predisposing factors (Galvin & Choi, 1999). VTEs from the legs and pelvis are responsible for the development of more than 90% of PEs (Brashers & Davey, 1998). Significant historical information should include predisposing factors for VTEs such as hypercoagulable states and antiphospholipid syndrome. Patients who are young and have a history of thrombotic events, unresolved thrombotic resolution, or a familial history of thrombotic events may be at risk (Lipchik & Presberg, 1996). Inherited deficiencies in antithrombin III, protein S, and protein C also increase a patient's susceptibility to venous clot formation.

Prophylaxis for VTE

Knowledge of current guidelines for prophylaxis can be used for identifying at-risk patients. Guyatt, Cook, Sackett, Eckman, and Pauker (1998) state the recommendations or guidelines for prophylactic treatment of VTE that were established from the 1998 American College of Chest Physicians Consensus Conference on Antithrombotic Therapy. These recommendations were system-atically graded according to the methodologic strength of supporting research and the trade-off of benefits versus risks for treatment. Methodologic strength was graded on a scale of A, large randomized trials or meta-analysis with consistent results; B, randomized trials with inconsistent results; and C, observational studies. Two categories compare the trade-off of estimated treatment effects: 1, most patients, regardless of values, would make the same choice because the trade-off for benefits against risks is clear, and 2, patients, with different values, would have different preferences because the trade-off of benefit versus risk is not as clear (Guyatt et al, 1998).

Clagett et al (1998) stated the following recommendations for prophylactic treatment decisions considering specific circumstances and clinical risk factors (CRFs) for VTE in average patients with typical estimated benefits and risks.

Medical or Surgical Condition	Recommendation for Prophylaxis of VTE	Grade of Recommendation
General surgery	Aspirin not recommended	
Low risk (younger than 40 years, no CRFs, minor procedure)	Early ambulation	C1
Moderate risk (older than 40 years, no CRFs, major procedure)	Either low-dose unfractionated heparin (LDUH), LMWH, intermittent pneumatic compression (IPC), or elastic stockings (ES)	A1
Higher risk (older than 40 years, CRFs, major procedure)	LDUH or higher-dose regimen of LMWH	A1
Higher risk and prone to wound infections or hematomas	IPC	A1
Very high risk (multiple CRFs)	LDUH or LMWH combined with IPC	B1
Selected very high risk	Perioperative warfarin (with warfarin therapy the international normalized ratio [INR] should be 2-3)	A2
Orthopedic procedures	Limit use of inferior vena cava (IVC) filter placement to high-risk patients when other prophylaxis is not feasible	C2
Elective total hip replacement (THR)	*Start either:* (1) LMWH 12-24 hr postoperatively (2) Warfarin therapy preoperatively or immediately after operation or (3) Adjusted-dose heparin preoperatively and ES or IPC	A1

Adapted from Clagett et al, 1998.

Medical or Surgical Condition	Recommendation for Prophylaxis of VTE	Grade of Recommendation
Elective total knee replacement (TKR)	LMWH Warfarin or IPC	A1
Duration of prophylaxis for elective THR and TKR is uncertain	7-10 days duration with LMWH or warfarin	A1
	Emerging data suggest benefits from 29-35 days duration of LMWH Routine duplex ultrasound screening not recommended for asymptomatic patients postoperatively	A2
Hip fracture surgical procedures	Either preopera-tive LMWH or preoperative or immediate postoperative warfarin therapy	A2
Elective neurosurgical procedures		
Intracranial procedures	IPC with or without ES; LMWH and LDUH may be acceptable alternatives	A1
	If high risk, a combination of pharmacologic and physical treatments may be more effective that either one alone	B1
Acute spinal cord injury	LMWH	B1
	IPC and ES may have benefit if used with LMWH or if anticoagulant agents are contraindicated	C1

Medical or Surgical Condition	Recommendation for Prophylaxis of VTE	Grade of Recommendation
	Rehabilitation phase: continuing LMWH or converting to full-dose oral anticoagulation may provide protection	C2
Trauma patients with CRF	Start LMWH as soon as safe and not contraindicated	A1
	If administration of LMWH is delayed, use IPC	C1
	If high risk or suboptimal prophylaxis, screen with duplex ultrasonography; if DVT is demonstrated and anticoagulation is contraindicated, insert IVC filter	C2
Medical conditions Myocardial infarction	LDUH Full anticoagulation	A1
	IPC and ES if heparin is contraindicated	C1
Ischemic stroke and lower extremity paralysis	LDUH and LMWH	A1
	IPC plus ES are probably effective	B1
General medical patients with CRFs and especially those with pulmonary infections and/or CHF	LDUH or LMWH	A1
Patients with long-term indwelling CVCs	Warfarin 1 mg/day or LMWH daily	A1
Patients with spinal puncture or epidural catheters for regional analgesia or anesthesia	Use LMWH with caution	C1

Preventative Nursing Interventions

1. Preoperatively
   - Demonstrate and have patient return demonstrate turn, cough, deep breathing, and leg exercises.
2. Postoperatively
   - Encourage and monitor these exercises and the use of the incentive spirometer 10 times every 2 hours while awake.
   - Assist in early ambulation.
   - Provide pain management.
     –Pharmacologic interventions
         Have patient identify effectiveness of pain coverage on a pain scale of 1 to 10.
         Follow-up if pain coverage is not adequate, especially in the first 24 to 48 hours.
         Encourage patients to use pain relief agents before pain peaks.
         Explain the need of restful sleep for the production of growth hormones and healing.
         Medicate before increasing activities.
         Provide for a "win-win" situation.
     –Nonpharmacologic interventions for pain relief
         Position and reposition frequently (every 1 to 2 hours).
         Provide incisional supports such as abdominal binder, folded bath blanket or towels, and so on.
         Use healing touch and or music therapy.
   - Avoid impedance of blood flow in the lower extremities.
       No pillows below the knee.
       No crossing the legs.
       Promote venous return.
       Use elastic pneumatic compression stockings.

9. **Develop a list of nursing diagnoses appropriate for Mrs. Leigh in the acute phase of the PE event.**

   - Ineffective gas exchange
   - Anxiety
   - Ineffective breathing pattern
   - Alteration in tissue perfusion
   - Alteration in comfort: pain
   - Risk for decreased cardiac output
   - Risk for fluid volume excess
   - Knowledge deficit

10. **List the nursing responsibilities for Mrs. Leigh and other patients with acute PE events.**

    Acute Phase
    - Administer oxygen and elevated head of bed.
    - Keep patient in bed and avoid unnecessary movement.
    - Attempt to relieve anxiety and remain with patient and reassure/explain.
    - Administer a narcotic analgesic and monitor the patient's status.
    - Complete vital signs, differential tests (ABGs, ECG, and chest x-ray), and diagnostic tests as soon as possible.

- Monitor for subsequent PE events and be prepared to assist the patient in compensatory efforts.
- Have intubation and ventilatory equipment readily available.
- Monitor for pulmonary hypertension and right-sided ventricular failure (jugular vein distension, peripheral edema, arrhythmias, and tachypnea).
- Monitor cardiac output (tachycardia, hypotension, decreased cardiac output, and shock).
- Monitor PT (INR) and aPTT levels and assume that samples are drawn on time for accurate results. Assess for signs of bleeding.

After the Acute Phase
- Teaching after PE
- Need for lifestyle changes
- Signs and symptoms of DVT and the need for appropriate intervention
- Oral anticoagulation teaching regarding the medication, signs of hemorrhage, and control testing

11. What guidelines are available for Mrs. Leigh's anticoagulation therapy in the treatment of PE?

Anticoagulant Therapy
Heparin has been proven effective in the treatment of PE and should begin as soon as a PE is suspected and unless heparin is contraindicated. The 1998 American Heart Medical/Scientific Statement on the Management of DVT and PE states that a bolus of heparin 5000 U should be followed by a subcutaneous injection of 17,500 U twice daily, or an IV infusion of 1400 U/hr, or a weight-adjusted dosage regimen. Weight-adjusted heparin dosing includes a bolus of 80 U/kg, followed by an IV infusion of 18 U/kg/hr (Hirsh & Hoak, 1996).

Warfarin (Coumadin), an oral anticoagulant, should be started within 24 hours of the initiation of heparin therapy. The PT is used to monitor the depression of factors II, VII, and X (three of the four vitamin K–dependent procoagulant clotting factors). The effects of warfarin take effect according to the half-life of the three factors. The initial PT reflects the depression of factor VII while the depression of factors II and X occur later (Hirsh et al, 1998). For this reason, heparin therapy is continued for about 5 days after the initiation of warfarin or when the warfarin dosage has kept the INR in the therapeutic range for 2 consecutive days.

Traditionally, the PT has been stated as a ratio of the patient's time to the control time. Because response of thromboplastins varies depending on the source of the laboratory reagent used, confusion in determination of an appropriate therapeutic range has occurred and the recommended dosage of warfarin has been inadequate to maintain a therapeutic level. As a result of the differences in reagents and confusion in the therapeutic level for the PT, the INR is now recognized as a standardized means to report therapeutic levels and to monitor warfarin therapy. A therapeutic INR range of 2 to 3 is recommended for most uses of warfarin. Because the efficacy of the drug is reduced when the INR is less than 2, a target rate in the middle of the therapeutic range should be maintained. For example if the range is 2 to 3, a 2.5 target should be maintained and if the range is 2.5 to 3.5, a target of 3.5 should be maintained (Hirsh et al, 1998).

Anticoagulant Therapy Guidelines
According to Hyers et al (1998), grade A1 recommendations or guidelines for treatment of VTE or PE from the 1998 American College of Chest

Physicians Consensus Conference on Antithrombotic Therapy include the following:

- IV heparin or an adjusted-dose subcutaneous heparin can be used to prolong the aPTT to a range corresponding to 0.3-0.6 IU/ml by an aminolytic anti-XA assay or a plasma heparin level of 0.2-0.4 IU/ml protamine sulfate.
- LMWH can be used in place of unfractionated heparin with PE when the patient is in a stable condition.
- If the PE is not massive, heparin or LMWH should be continued for at least 5 days, with oral anticoagulant therapy overlapping the heparin therapy for at least 4 to 5 days.
- If the PE was massive, a longer duration for heparin therapy may be used.

Heparin therapy can be discontinued when the INR (used to monitor the warfarin therapy) is at a level of 2 for 2 consecutive days.

- The duration of oral anticoagulants should prolong the PT to a target INR of 2.5 or a range of 2 to 3 and be continued for 3 months. If oral anticoagulants cannot be used, LMWH with or without unfraction-ated adjusted-dose heparin should be used so that the aPTT is pro-longed to therapeutic plasma heparin level.

Other graded recommendations consist of the following:

- The duration for anticoagulant therapy should be 3 to 6 months in patients with time-limited or reversible risk factors and for at least 6 months in patients with a first-time idiopathic DVT event (grade A2 recommendation).
- Patients with continued risk factors for VTE or recurrent venous throm-bosis (RVT) events should receive therapy indefinitely (grade C2 recommendation).
- Placement of an IVC shunt is recommended for patients who have com-plications with or contraindications for anticoagulant therapy, recur-rent VTE with adequate anticoagulation therapy, concurrent surgical pulmonary embolectomy or endarterectomy, and chronic recurrent PE with pulmonary hypertension (no grade for recommendation) (Hyers et al, 1998).

12. Describe three other fibrinolytic therapy modalities that may be used in the management of PE.

Thrombolytic Therapy
Thrombolytic therapy is used to dissolve PE in patients who are hemodynamically unstable and intolerant of the obstruction. Thrombolytic agents include activase (tissue plasminogen activator), streptokinase, or urokinase, but other agents are currently being developed and researched. Although thrombolytic agents lyse the obstruction in the acute event, mortality does not seem to be different from nonthrombolytic treatment. Weaknesses of thrombolytic therapy include cost, increased risk of hemorrhage, limited use when surgery may be indicated, and the time-event relationship (Lipchik & Presberg, 1996).

Inferior Vena Cava Interruption and Filters

Ligation and clips can be used for IVC interruption, but the Greenfield filter is often preferred. The complication rate for IVC filters that is placed transvenously under fluoroscopy is low, but venous stasis can occur. IVC interruption and IVC filters prevent recurrences of major PE but not minor recurrent events or emboli that may generate from sites other than the lower extremities (Lipchik & Presberg, 1996).

Pulmonary Embolectomy

According to Hyers et al (1998), pulmonary embolectomy should be reserved for emergency treatment of PE by an experienced cardiac surgical team. Shock and cardiac arrest account for the high operative mortality rates that range from 10% to 75% with cardiopulmonary bypass standby and 50% to 94% in patients with cardiac arrest.

Candidates may have the following parameters: (1) massive PE (affects more than 50% of the pulmonary circulation), (2) shock and hemodynamically unstable condition despite resuscitative and anticoagulant therapy, and (3) a contraindication for or failed thrombolytic therapy. Postoperative complications include severe neurologic defects, acute respiratory distress syndrome, acute renal failure, and mediastinitis (Hyers et al, 1998).

PULMONARY EMBOLISM

References

Alspach, J. G. (Ed.). (1998). *American Association of Critical-Care Nurses: Core curriculum for critical care nursing* (5th ed.). Philadelphia: Saunders.

Brashers, V. L., & Davey, S. S. (1998). Alterations in pulmonary function. In K. L. McCance & S. E. Huether (Eds.), *Pathophysiology: The biologic basis for disease in adults and children* (pp. 1158-1200). St Louis: Mosby.

Clagett, G. P., Anderson, F. A., Geerts, W., Heit, J. A., Knudson, M., Lieberman, J. R., Meerli, G. J., & Wheeler, H. B. (1998). Prevention of venous thromboembolism. *Chest, 114*(5, Suppl.), 531S-561S.

Dietzen, D. L. (1997). Pulmonary embolus. In R. E. Rakel (Ed.), *Saunders manual of medical practice* (pp. 142-144). Philadelphia: Saunders.

Erdman, S. M., Rodvold, K. A., & Friedenberg, W. R. (1997). Thromboembolic Disorders. In J. T. DiPiro, R. L. Talbert, G. C. Yee, G. R. Matzke, B. G. Wells, & L. M. Posey (Eds.), *Pharmacotherapy: A pathophysiologic approach* (3rd ed., pp. 399-433). Stamford, CT: Appleton & Lange.

Galvin, J. G., & Choi, B. S. (1999). Clinical presentation pulmonary embolus [WWW document]. URL http://www.vh.org/Providers/Tesxtbooks/ElectricPE/Text/ClinPresent.html.

Graber, M. A. (1999). Pulmonary medicine: Pulmonary embolism and deep vein thrombosis [WWW document]. URL http://www.vh.org/Providers/ClinRef/FPHandbook/Chapter03/01-3.html.

Guyatt, G. H., Cook, D. J., Sackett, D. L., Eckman, M., & Pauker, S. (1998). Grades for recommendation for antithrombotic agents. *Chest, 114*(5, Suppl.), 441S-469S.

Hartshorn, J. C., Sole, M. L., & Lamborn, M. L. (1997). *Introduction to critical care nursing* (2nd ed.). Philadelphia: Saunders.

Hirsh, J., Dalen, J. E., Anderson, D. R., Poller, L., Bussey, H., Ansell, J., Deykin, D., & Brandt, J. T. (1998). Oral anticoagulants: Mechanism of action, clinical effectiveness, and optimal therapeutic range. *Chest, 114*(5, Suppl.), 445S-469S.

Hirsh, J., & Hoak, J. (1996). Management of deep vein thrombosis and pulmonary embolism [WWW document]. URL http://www.americanheart.org/Scientific/statements/1996/069601.html.

Hirsh, J., Warkentin, T. E., Raschke, R., Granger, C. Ohman, E. M., & Dalen, J. E. (1998). Heparin and low-molecular-weight heparin. *Chest, 114*(5, Suppl.), 489S-510S.

Hyers, T. M., Agnelli, G., Hull, R. D., Weg, J. G., Morris, T. A., Samama, M., & Tapson, V. (1998). Antithrombotic therapy for venous thromboembolic disease. *Chest, 114*(5, Suppl.), 561S-578S.

Konstadt, S. (1999). Diagnostic dilemma [WWW document]. URL http://www.jcardioanesthesia.com/abs13_1/v13n1p105.html (visited March 17, 1999).

Launius, B.K., & Graham, B. D. (1998). Understanding and preventing deep vein thrombosis and pulmonary embolism. *AACN Clinical Issues, 9*(1), 91-99.

Lipchik, R. J., & Presberg, K. W. (1996). Venous thromboembolism and other pulmonary vascular diseases. In J. Noble, H. L. Green, W. Levinson, G. A. Modest, & M. J. Young (Eds.), *Textbook of primary care medicine* (2nd ed., pp. 1603-1627). St Louis: Mosby.

McMance, K. L., & Huether, S. E. (1998). *Pathophysiology: The biologic basis for disease in adults and children.* St Louis: Mosby.

Nilsson, P. E., Bergqvist, D., Benoni, G., Bjorgell, O., Fredin, H., Hedlund, U., Nicolas, S., & Nylander, G. (1997). The post-discharge prophylactic management of the orthopedic patient with low-molecular-weight heparin: Enoxaparin. *Orthopedics, 20*(Suppl.), 22-25.

Nunnelee, J. D. (1997). Low-molecular-weight heparin. *Journal of Vascular Nursing, 15*(3), 94-96.

Rodgers, M. L. (1999). Common respiratory problems: pulmonary embolism, pneumothorax, and thoracic pulmonary surgery. In L. Bucher & S. Melander (Eds.), *Critical care nursing* (pp. 465-507). Philadelphia: WB Saunders.

Thelan, L., Urden, L., Laugh, M., & Stacy, K. (1998). *Critical care nursing: Diagnosis and management.* (3rd ed., rev.). St Louis: Mosby.

Ward, V. L., & Faitelson, B. B. (October, 1996). Pulmonary embolus [WWW document]. URL http://brighamrad.harvard.edu/Cases/bwh/hcache/182/full.html (visited March 17, 1999).

WellnessWeb. URL http://www.wellweb.com (visited 1998).

CHAPTER 3

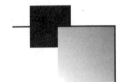

PULMONARY CONTUSION

Judith A. Halstead, RN, DNS • Sheila Drake Melander, RN, DSN, ACNP-C, FCCM

CASE PRESENTATION

Mr. Hays, a 23-year-old man, was involved in a late-night motor vehicle accident when he apparently fell asleep at the wheel. His car left the road, striking a tree head-on at approximately 35 miles per hour. He was not wearing a seat belt. Mr. Hays was arousable at the scene and slightly disoriented, but he was able to follow commands. He complained of chest and back pain. Oxygen at 2 L via nasal cannula and two peripheral intravenous lines were started before the patient was transported to the nearest hospital. On arrival at the emergency department, Mr. Hays was alert and cooperative but anxious. He was able to communicate without difficulty and complained of right-sided chest pain, which he described as "rib pain," and some slight difficulty breathing. Marked ecchymosis in the right chest area with medial to lateral progression was noted. The following are his diagnostic data on admission:

BP	176/94 mm Hg	pH	7.43
HR	138 bpm	P_{O_2}	100 mm Hg
Respirations	32 breaths/min and slightly labored	P_{CO_2}	37 mm Hg
		K^+	3.1 mmol/L
Temperature	37.2° C (99° F)		

Arterial blood gas measurements with the patient receiving 2 L of oxygen by nasal cannula were the following:

HgB	120 g/dl
Hct	36.3 vol/dl
WBCs	10,500/mm³

The chest x-ray film revealed four fractured ribs on the right side and two fractured ribs on the left side and was otherwise unremarkable. Findings from computed tomographic (CT) scans of the head, chest, and abdomen were normal, and findings from the electrocardiogram were normal except for a sinus tachycardia. Physical examination revealed symmetric chest expansion, a midline trachea, bruising of the right chest and flank, and some facial bruising. Auscultation of the lungs revealed fine crackles in the right lung and clear breath sounds in the left lung field. Mr. Hays was transferred to the telemetry unit for monitoring.

The physician ordered the following:

5% dextrose in 45% normal saline at 75 ml/hr
Clear liquids
Accurate intake and output
Cefazolin 1 g intravenously every 8 hours
Patient-controlled analgesia for pain: morphine sulfate 1 mg/1 ml, 1 mg every 10 minutes with lockout, not to exceed 20 mg in 4 hours
Repeat chest x-ray study in 12 hours

The repeat chest radiograph revealed patchy, irregular areas of density in the right lung indicative of a right pulmonary contusion. Mr. Hays received education regarding the extent of his injuries and the potential dangers they may present. He was taught to use the incentive spirometer and instructed to use it hourly. Mr. Hays progressed satisfactorily and was discharged from the hospital on the second day.

PULMONARY CONTUSION

Questions

1. Describe the mechanism of injury resulting in a pulmonary contusion.
2. Discuss the pathophysiology of a pulmonary contusion.
3. How is respiratory functioning affected by blunt chest trauma and the development of a pulmonary contusion?
4. What assessment findings may be indicative of a pulmonary contusion?
5. What methods are required for the diagnosis and monitoring of a pulmonary contusion?
6. What is the nurse's responsibility in the diagnosis of a pulmonary contusion?
7. What are the most common complications of a pulmonary contusion?
8. Describe the treatment for a patient who has a flail chest.
9. Identify the appropriate nursing interventions for a patient with a pulmonary contusion.
10. What discharge instructions would be appropriate for Mr. Hays?
11. What nursing diagnoses might be appropriate for the care of a patient with a pulmonary contusion?

PULMONARY CONTUSION

Questions and Answers

1. Describe the mechanism of injury resulting in a pulmonary contusion.

Pulmonary contusions typically are a result of a blunt trauma and can be potentially life-threatening. Pulmonary contusions are present in 30% to 70% of patients who experience blunt chest trauma (Karlet, 1997). The blunt forces causing pulmonary contusions are most commonly the result of motor vehicle accidents and falls (Karlet, 1997). Patients injured through assault, explosives, or other traumatic events may also develop pulmonary contusions (Alspach, 1998). Chest trauma rarely occurs in isolation, and the patient should be assessed for associated injuries. Men younger than 40 account for most trauma patients (Karlet, 1997).

2. Discuss the pathophysiology of a pulmonary contusion.

The rapid chest compression and decompression that occur in blunt chest trauma causes a disruption in the pulmonary vasculature, tissue, and alveoli (Ruth-Sahd, 1997). This disruption allows blood to enter the alveoli and interstitium, resulting in alveolar hemorrhage and interstitial edema (Farrar, 1998; Karlet, 1997). The symptoms of pulmonary contusion typically are insidious but progressive in nature. Evolution of symptoms may occur over hours or even days after an injury is sustained (Farrar, 1998). The nurse should suspect a pulmonary contusion in any patient who has experienced a blunt trauma, even in the absence of symptoms, and assess the patient accordingly. Interstitial edema can gradually develop within the first 6 hours of injury, ultimately resulting in perfusion without ventilation, which leads to intrapulmonary shunting, hypoxemia, and respiratory distress (Farrar, 1998).

3. How is respiratory functioning affected by blunt chest trauma and the development of a pulmonary contusion?

Blunt chest trauma usually bruises the lung tissue; however, pulmonary tears or lacerations may be seen, especially if rib fractures are present, which is likely in approximately 50% of patients with blunt chest trauma. Approximately 5% to 13% of patients experiencing major chest trauma develop a flail chest (Karlet, 1997). In a pulmonary contusion, the initial chest injury results in alveolar hemorrhage and interstitial edema (Farrar, 1998; Karlet, 1997). Disruption of the alveolar-capillary unit leads to increased pulmonary vascular resistance and decreased pulmonary blood flow, resulting in the development of a ventilation-perfusion imbalance with hypoxia and hypercapnia (Ruth-Sahd, 1997). Decreased lung compliance can also develop, and ventilatory support may be required (Farrar, 1998; Karlet, 1997). Atelectasis can develop in the area of injury as a result of fluid retention and development of infection (Ruth-Sahd, 1997). Although pulmonary contusion typically is a secondary diagnosis, close monitoring, assessment of the patient, and identification of subtle changes in the patient's condition are extremely important. Other significant injuries associated with blunt chest trauma, which may be present along with a pulmonary contusion, include pneumothorax; hemothorax; cardiac contusion; trachea, bronchi, or diaphragm trauma; and great vessel trauma (Alspach, 1998; Lawkowski-Jones, 1999).

4. What assessment findings may be indicative of a pulmonary contusion?

Physical findings may include ecchymosis at the site of impact, chest abrasions, guarding of the site, hemoptysis, dullness to percussion, and moist crackles (Alspach, 1998; Farrar, 1998; Karlet, 1997). Other findings may include dyspnea, reduced chest expansion and breath sounds, tachypnea, tachycardia, and a partial pressure of oxygen in arterial blood (Pao$_2$) of less than 60 mm Hg on room air (Alspach, 1998). When a pulmonary contusion occurs with a flail chest, paradoxical chest movement (Harrahill, 1998), subcutaneous emphysema, and increased pain are also normal occurrences (Alspach, 1998).

5. What methods are required for the diagnosis and monitoring of a pulmonary contusion?

The hallmark sign of pulmonary contusion is arterial and venous hypoxemia after chest trauma (Ruth-Sahd, 1997). Several pulmonary parameters, in addition to the partial pressure of oxygen in arterial and venous blood (Pao$_2$ and Pvo$_2$), can be used to measure tissue oxygenation and monitor the patient's ventilation and perfusion. The hemoglobin saturation of venous blood (Svo$_2$) will identify subtle changes in tissue oxygenation and perfusion at the cellular level before any changes are seen clinically. Arterial and venous oxygen content (Cao$_2$ and Cvo$_2$) are necessary to calculate some measures of cardiac output and estimate intrapulmonary shunting (Ahrens, 1996; Ruth-Sahd, 1997). The alveolar-arterial oxygen difference (P(A-a)o$_2$) identifies pulmonary diffusion capacity and is a reliable indicator of pulmonary contusion. A low Pao$_2$, wide P(A-a)o$_2$, and radiologic changes confirm the presence of pulmonary contusion (Ruth-Sahd, 1997).

Initial chest x-ray findings may be normal and not indicative of the degree of lung injury (Farrar, 1998; Karlet, 1997; Ruth-Sahd, 1997). Radiologic changes vary depending on the seriousness of the injury, but typically, they can range from patchy, irregular, localized areas of consolidation to complete consolidation of one or both lungs reflecting intraalveolar hemorrhage. In severe contusions, the lung will appear larger because of edema and will push the diaphragm down. Several chest x-ray studies over hours to days are usually necessary as the contusion fully develops (Ruth-Sahd, 1997). It may take 2 or 3 weeks for resolution of the contusion (Karlet, 1997).

CT scan is one of the most accurate methods for assessing pulmonary damage in trauma. The CT scan can identify small tears and lacerations by allowing transverse sections of the lung to be studied (Ruth-Sahd, 1997).

6. What is the nurse's responsibility in the diagnosis of pulmonary contusion?

The diagnosis of pulmonary contusion depends on physical examination findings, tissue oxygenation measures, and chest x-ray and CT results (Ruth-Sahd, 1997). Assessment of patients who have experienced blunt trauma requires expert clinical skills to diagnose the potential and actual problems that may develop (Klein, 1996). The diagnosis is often delayed until signs of complications occur as a result of associated injuries and because of a lack of radiographic changes and external evidence of injury (Klein, 1996; Ruth-Sahd, 1997). Through physical assessment, history taking, and monitoring of laboratory and diagnostic data, the nurse can (1) identify acute respiratory problems, (2) anticipate potential future changes in the patient's condition, (3) understand the underlying pathophysiology of the signs and symptoms, and (4) develop an appropriate plan of care for the client (Brooks-Brunn, 1999).

7. What are the most common complications of pulmonary contusion?

Pneumonia, which can develop insidiously, is the most common complication caused by decreased clearance of bacteria from the lung (Ruth-Sahd, 1997). Prevention is best achieved by monitoring for infection through daily chest radiographs, white blood cell counts, vital sign measurements, and sputum culture. Aggressive pulmonary physiotherapy is also important (Karlet, 1997).

Other potential complications include acute respiratory distress syndrome (Farrar, 1998; Ruth-Sahd, 1997), pulmonary edema, atelectasis, and pulmonary emboli (Ruth-Sahd, 1997).

8. Describe the treatment for a patient who has a flail chest.

The major goals of treatment for the patient who has a flail chest include promoting and maintaining optimal tissue oxygenation, implementing aggressive pulmonary physiotherapy, and ensuring adequate pain control (Harrahill, 1998). Specific treatment and nursing interventions for a patient who has a flail chest include the following:

1. Anticipating the need for endotracheal intubation and mechanical ventilation (Farrar, 1998; Harrahill, 1998; Klein, 1996) and chest tube insertion (Klein, 1996)
2. Administering IV fluids (crystalloids) at a rate that maintains a urine output of 30 ml/hr, and normal hemodynamic values, being careful not to overhydrate client (Harrahill, 1998; Karlet, 1997; Klein, 1996; Ruth-Sahd, 1997)
3. Managing pain through the use of patient-controlled analgesia, an epidural catheter, or intercostal nerve block (Harrahill, 1998)
4. Implementing aggressive pulmonary physiotherapy through the use of incentive spirometry, turning and postural drainage, suctioning, early ambulation, and "HUFF" coughing (Harrahill, 1998)

9. Identify the appropriate nursing interventions for a patient with a pulmonary contusion.

Ruth-Sahd (1997) identified the following nursing interventions as essential to the care of a patient with a pulmonary contusion:

1. Maintaining the patient's arterial blood gases through supportive oxygen therapy, and maintaining mechanical ventilation with positive end-expiratory pressure setting (patients who have contusion of more than 28% of their lung tissue are likely to require ventilatory support)
2. Observing the airway for obstruction, clots, or bloody mucus
3. Using saline irrigation with frequent suctioning of the endotracheal tube
4. Turning the patient frequently to promote adequate ventilation
5. Positioning the patient who has unilateral chest trauma with the injured side up to improve ventilation-perfusion
6. Placing the patient in the semi-Fowler's position to decrease pressure on the diaphragm and increase inspiratory capacity

7. Achieving adequate pain control, because pain can promote hypoventilation and atelectasis
8. Monitoring the patient closely for complications, especially pneumonia

10. What discharge instructions would be appropriate for Mr. Hays?

Discharge instructions for the patient with a pulmonary contusion must include information regarding potential changes in respiratory status. The patient should be instructed to report immediately to the physician any change in respiratory status such as tightness in the chest, increased sputum production, difficulty breathing deeply, or elevated temperature. Continued use of incentive spirometry, adequate fluid intake, and maintenance of mobility are other important self-care activities that the patient should implement at home to prevent the development of complications. It is crucial that patients understand that any change in respiratory status, as identified previously, may be indicative of developing respiratory complications.

11. What nursing diagnoses might be appropriate for the care of a patient with a pulmonary contusion?

Nursing diagnoses appropriate for the care of the patient with pulmonary contusion include the following:

- Ineffective airway clearance related to decreased pulmonary compliance
- Impaired gas exchange related to interstitial hemorrhage
- Ineffective breathing pattern related to decreased pulmonary compliance
- Anxiety related to unusual muscular effort required for breathing
- Activity intolerance related to hypoxemia

PULMONARY CONTUSION

References

Ahrens, T. (1996). Respiratory monitoring. In J. Clochesy, C. Bleu, S. Cardin, A. Whittaker, & E. Rudy (Eds.), *Critical care nursing* (2nd ed., pp. 245-261). Philadelphia: Saunders.

Alspach, J. G. (1998). *American Association of Critical-Care Nurses core curriculum for critical care nursing* (5th ed.). Philadelphia: Saunders.

Brooks-Brunn, J. (1999). Respiratory assessment. In L. Bucher & S. Melander (Eds.), *Critical care nursing* (pp. 369-388). Philadelphia: Saunders.

Farrar, J. (1998). Trauma. In M. Kinney, S. Dunbar, J. Brooks-Brunn, N. Molter, & J. Vitello-Cicciu (Eds.), *American Association of Critical-Care Nurses: Clinical reference for critical care nursing* (4th ed., pp. 1111-1112). St Louis: Mosby.

Harrahill, M. (1998). Flail chest: A nursing challenge. *Journal of Emergency Nursing, 24*(3), 288-289.

Karlet, M. (1997). AANA Journal course: Update for nurse anesthetists: Thoracic trauma. *Journal of the American Association of Nurse Anesthetists, 65*(1), 73-80.

Klein, D. (1996). Patients with trauma. In J. Clochesy, C. Breu, S. Cardin, A. Whittaker, & E. Rudy (Eds.), *Critical care nursing* (2nd ed., pp. 1341-1352). Philadelphia: Saunders.

Lawkowski-Jones, L. (1999). Trauma. In L. Bucher & S. Melander (Eds.), *Critical care nursing* (pp. 1094-1095). Philadelphia: Saunders.

Ruth-Sahd, L. (1997). Pulmonary contusions: Management and implications for trauma nurses. *Journal of Trauma Nursing, 4*(4), 90-98.

CHAPTER 4

CHRONIC OBSTRUCTIVE PULMONARY DISEASE WITH PNEUMONIA

Sheila Drake Melander, RN, DSN, ACNP-C, FCCM

CASE PRESENTATION

Mr. Stevens, a 62-year-old retired coal miner, has been experiencing a productive cough off and on for approximately 3 years. He decided to come to the emergency department because he has had difficulty in his breathing pattern on exertion. He stated that he has had several bouts of chest colds during the past few years, but this time he said that he "can't seem to shake this round." His wife stated that he is allergic to penicillin.

During his history, Mr. Stevens stated that he has smoked two packs of cigarettes a day for 25 years. Crackles were noted in the lower bases of his lungs, with an occasional expiratory wheeze. He also said that he had been running a low-grade fever for approximately 2 to 3 days and had experienced chills and general weakness. A chest x-ray film disclosed some consolidation in the right lower lobe. Bronchography revealed nonuniform tapering of the airway. The following are additional diagnostic data:

BP	158/98 mm Hg	P_{CO_2}	54 mm Hg
HR	107 bpm	HCO_3^-	30 mmol/L
Respirations	32 breaths/min	WBCs	20,000 mm^3
Temperature	38.9° C (102° F)	Hct	56%
pH	7.25	Gram stain	Negative
P_{O_2}	52 mm Hg (with room air)		

As a result of Mr. Stevens' arterial blood gas (ABG) levels, he was given 28% oxygen with a Venturi mask. His ABG levels 30 minutes after placement of the mask were as follows:

pH	7.42	P_{CO_2}	48 mm Hg
P_{O_2}	58 mm Hg	HCO_3^-	30 mmol/L

On the basis of these data, Mr. Stevens' diagnosis was chronic obstructive pulmonary disease (COPD) with an acute exacerbation of chronic bronchitis. Sputum cultures revealed a gram-positive organism, *Streptococcus pneumoniae*. Mr. Stevens received erythromycin after a secondary diagnosis of pneumonia was made. He also received theophylline at this time.

Mr. Stevens' condition improved in response to the antibiotic and bronchodilator therapy. He was discharged 3 days later.

CHRONIC OBSTRUCTIVE PULMONARY DISEASE WITH PNEUMONIA

Questions

1. Discuss the pathophysiology involved in the diagnosis of COPD.
2. Mr. Stevens' diagnosis was chronic bronchitis. This is one of the medical diagnoses associated with COPD. Discuss chronic bronchitis and the other two medical diagnoses that belong to the COPD group.
3. Were Mr. Stevens' presenting symptoms among the classic signs and symptoms exhibited by patients with COPD? Compare and contrast symptoms associated with bronchitis and emphysema.
4. Why is Mr. Stevens' temperature of concern?
5. Why was a Venturi mask chosen as the route of administration for oxygen therapy?
6. Is the organism found in Mr. Stevens' sputum cultures a common finding in patients with COPD?
7. Why was Mr. Stevens given erythromycin?
8. What are the contributing factors for the development of pneumonia in Mr. Stevens' case? List other contributing factors along with signs and symptoms associated with pneumonia not present in Mr. Stevens' case.
9. What diagnostic tests are significant in the determination of a diagnosis of pneumonia?
10. Discuss the medical management for a patient who has pneumonia.
11. What is the goal of therapy with theophylline, and what special considerations exist with this treatment for Mr. Stevens?
12. What is the clinical significance of the pH reading, and what is the appropriate range of partial pressure of oxygen (Po_2) values in the patient with COPD?
13. Why were steroids not ordered for Mr. Stevens?
14. Were Mr. Stevens' laboratory results consistent with those expected for a patient with COPD and pneumonia?
15. What other pulmonary function tests would have assisted in the diagnosis of Mr. Stevens' COPD?
16. Had Mr. Stevens' condition deteriorated and not responded to the bronchodilator and antibiotic therapy, what considerations concerning ventilatory management would be important?
17. Discuss the occurrence of pneumonia in patients with COPD.
18. What teaching considerations are of special concern for Mr. Stevens before his discharge?

Chronic Obstructive Pulmonary Disease with Pneumonia

Questions and Answers

1. Discuss the pathophysiology involved in the diagnosis of COPD.

As stated by Bucher and Melander (1999) and Stein (1998), *COPD* refers to a group of chronic diseases that obstruct airflow within the airways or the lung parenchyma. The description *chronic airflow limitation* may also be seen in the discussion of the patient with COPD. The disorders in the COPD group are as follows:

- Chronic bronchitis
- Emphysema
- Asthma

Asthma has been included in this listing, but it should be noted that with the increasing prevalence of asthma, some sources in the literature discuss asthma as a separate entity. COPD usually presents as a gradual decline in function, but an acute episode of respiratory failure can occur at any time because of the patient's lack of respiratory reserve. As described by Gawlinski and Hamwi (1999), dyspnea and hyperventilation are early signs of respiratory compromise in the patient with COPD.

Alspach (1998) and Thelan, Urden, Lough, and Stacy (1998) identified several factors in the pathogenesis of COPD:

- Tobacco use
- Air pollution
- Occupational exposure (coal miners; metal molders; workers handling stone, glass, or clay products; those who work with cotton or grain dust; firefighters; workers exposed to asbestos)
- Genetics

2. Mr. Stevens' diagnosis was chronic bronchitis. This is one of the medical diagnoses associated with COPD. Discuss chronic bronchitis and the other two medical diagnoses that belong to the COPD group.

Chronic Bronchitis

Chronic bronchitis is described as chronic cough and sputum production that is present for most days during at least 3 consecutive months for not less than 2 successive years (Heath & Mongia, 1998).

Pathophysiology.   Production of mucus increases because of the enlargement of the bronchial mucous gland and an increase in the number of goblet cells. Other changes include inflammation of the bronchial and bronchiolar walls, loss of cilia, and the presence of mucous plugs. Physiologic changes are related to the narrowed airways. Chronic bronchitis is a disease of the central airways, and approximately 80% of the measurable airway resistance is in the central airways.

Bronchography shows the degree of tapering of the airway. The tapering is nonuniform, and the airway wall surfaces and outpouchings are irregular. It is believed that these changes account for the increased airway resistance seen in bronchitis. Functionally, this resistance results in inspiratory and expiratory airflow obstruction, overinflation of the alveoli, and abnormal distribution of ventilation. The narrowed airway leads to overinflation of the alveoli with increased total lung capacity (TLC), increased residual volume (RV), and decreased vital capacity (VC) (Heath & Mongia, 1998; Stein, 1998; Madison & Irwin, 1998).

Emphysema

Emphysema is the abnormal enlargement of the air spaces distal to the terminal bronchioles, accompanied by nonuniformity in the pattern of respiratory airspace enlargement and destruction of the alveolar walls (Alspach, 1998; Stein, 1998; Thelan et al, 1998).

Genetics. One cause of emphysema is a deficiency of a serum protein called α_1-*protease inhibitor.* Patients with decreased circulatory levels of this serum protein are predisposed to early development of emphysema. Two cells are seen in the inflammatory responses in the lungs: alveolar macrophages and polymorphonuclear leukocytes (PMNs). These cells manufacture elastase, the enzyme capable of breaking down elastin. PMNs are believed to be the major source of elastase in the lung. Most people also have an elastase *inhibitor* in the lung, which allows a balance between elastase and its inhibitor. When this balance is disturbed, either by an increase in elastase or a decrease in the inhibitor, damage to the alveolar walls occurs, resulting in emphysema (Alspach, 1998; Bucher & Melander, 1999; Stein, 1998).

Pathology. Emphysema destroys the alveolar walls and enlarges the air spaces distal to the terminal bronchioles. The portion of the lung distal to the terminal bronchioles—the acinus—comprises the functional units of the lung.

The loss of airway support contributes to airway narrowing because airways collapse on expiration. This loss of alveolar wall and reduction in elastic recoil also contribute to increased lung compliance, decreased driving pressure on expiration and subsequent hyperinflation, and increased RVs. Ultimately, the surface area available for gas exchange decreases, causing alterations in diffusing capacities and ventilation-perfusion ($\dot{V}/\dot{Q}$) abnormalities. These abnormalities lead to the hypoxemia seen in emphysema.

Asthma

Asthma is a chronic disease of variable severity characterized by airway hyperactivity and airway narrowing of a reversible nature caused by bronchospasms. The bronchospasms cause air trapping, $\dot{V}/\dot{Q}$ mismatching, prolonged expiration acidosis, hypercapnia, and cough production of thick sputum. The lungs become stiff and overinflated and thus increase the workload of breathing. Intrathoracic pressure increases, thus decreasing venous return and cardiac output (Alspach, 1998; Niederman & Peters, 1998; Stein, 1998).

3. **Were Mr. Stevens' presenting symptoms among the classic signs and symptoms exhibited by patients with COPD? Compare and contrast symptoms associated with bronchitis and emphysema.**

Clinical Manifestations of Bronchitis

- Onset varies; symptoms are usually insidious.
- Cough and sputum production are present.
- Symptoms appear in patients in their 40s and 50s.
- Disability from the disease occurs in patients during their late 50s and early 60s.
- Patients have a history of frequent chest colds.
- Increased purulent sputum production is present.
- Dyspnea worsens as the disease progresses.
- Infections exacerbate the disease.

- Severe derangements in the $\dot{V}/\dot{Q}$ ratios may be seen later in the disease.
- Patients are characterized as a "blue bloaters."
- Low minute volumes are seen.
- Arterial hypoxemia and hypercapnia develop.
- Patients are usually stocky or obese.
- Central and peripheral cyanosis is seen.
- Wheezing may be present.
- Crackles (rales) may be present because of secretions.
- Pulmonary hypertension is present.
- Cor pulmonale is seen.
- Polycythemia is present.
- Hypoxemia and hypercapnia with compensated respiratory acidosis are seen.

Clinical Manifestations of Emphysema
- Signs and symptoms vary.
- Progressive expiratory flow obstruction and overinflation are seen.
- Dyspnea with exertion is seen at the beginning with dyspnea at rest as the disease progresses.
- Some patients have slow progression of disease; others rapidly become significantly disabled.
- Patients with advanced disease show enlargement of the anteroposterior diameter of the chest, dorsal kyphosis, elevated ribs, and wide costal angle (barrel chest).
- Patients have a thin physique with muscle wasting.
- Acyanotic unproductive minimal cough is seen.
- In later stages of disease, patients show signs and symptoms of right-sided ventricular failure (cor pulmonale).
- Accessory muscles are used for breathing.
- Patients may breathe through pursed lips with prolonged expiration ("pink puffers").
- Percussion shows increased resonance (hyperresonance) because of the increased lung volumes.
- Breath sounds are decreased and difficult to hear.
- Heart sounds are distant because of barrel chest.
- Expiratory wheezes may be present.
- Normal ABG values are seen in mild to moderate emphysema; in advanced emphysema, the Po_2 is commonly decreased and partial pressure of carbon dioxide (Pco_2) is increased.
- Hypoxemia is greatest while patients are sleeping.

Often patients with emphysema are seen in the intensive care unit (ICU) as a result of infection, heart failure, pulmonary embolism, pneumothorax, bronchospastic episodes, gastrointestinal tract bleeding, or metabolic abnormalities. Some patients require medical attention because they changed the dosages of their medications without the physician's knowledge. Other patients are unable to maintain their medication regimens because of coughing, nausea, or vomiting. These patients sometimes require a change in their oxygen dosage, which may also trigger acute respiratory failure (Alspach, 1998; Gawlinski & Hamwi, 1999; Stein, 1998).

Common Findings in the ICU
- Cough and fatigue
- Mental confusion
- Irritability and lethargy

- Accessory muscle use
- Tachycardia
- Hypoxia
- Crackles, wheezes, or stridor or consolidation
- Cor pulmonale
- Oxygen saturation greater than 70% (acceptable if patient has adequate cardiac output)

Because of increased pulmonary vascular pressure, patients with COPD have increased pulmonary artery systolic, diastolic, and mean pressures (Alspach, 1998; Gawlinski & Hamwi, 1999).

The usual clinical findings for COPD are as follows:

- Significant and progressive reduction in expiration of airflow as measured by the forced expiratory volume (FEV)
- Varying degrees of exertional dyspnea
- Chronic cough and sputum production
- Decreased ABG values, hypoxemia, and hypercapnia with compensated respiratory acidosis
- Polycythemia

The bottom line becomes the following:

- The degree of airflow obstruction as measured by FEV
- The patient's age at the time of diagnosis
- The degree of reversibility
- The rate of change in the FEV over time

A higher prevalence of COPD is reported in men than in women, and mortality rates are related to socioeconomic status. It is estimated that as many as 35% of patients in the ICU have COPD (Alspach, 1998; Eller et al, 1998; Madison & Irwin, 1998; Stein, 1998)

4. Why is Mr. Stevens' temperature of concern?

Carbon dioxide and oxygen consumption increase as much as 10% for each degree Fahrenheit rise in temperature; thus treatment for an elevated temperature is recommended to prevent additional strain on the respiratory system (Stein, 1998).

5. Why was a Venturi mask chosen as the route of administration for oxygen therapy?

The Venturi mask allows for precise delivery of oxygen. This is extremely important for the patient with COPD because of the "hypoxic drive." The goal of oxygen therapy is to keep the Pao_2 below 60 mm Hg and the $Paco_2$ at a level to maintain pH within normal limits (Bucher & Melander, 1999).

6. Is the organism found in Mr. Stevens' sputum cultures a common finding in patients with COPD?

In discussing pneumonia, it is common to see it discussed as community-acquired pneumonia (CAP) and hospital-acquired pneumonia (HAP). Common causes of

CAP include *S. pneumoniae, Haemophilus influenzae, Staphylococcus aureus,* anaerobic bacteria, *Moraxella catarrhalis, Klebsiella pneumoniae,* and *Legionella.* HAP is usually bacterial in origin and can include the following organisms: *Escherichia coli, K. pneumoniae,* Enterobacteriaceae, *Pseudomonas aeruginosa, S. aureus,* and *Serratia.* Pathogens may reach the lung in patients with CAP as a result of aspiration of gastric or oropharyngeal secretions into the lower respiratory tract.

One of the most common causes of bacterial pneumonia is *S. pneumoniae,* a gram-positive coccus. It is spread through droplets or airborne nuclei. The mortality rate is 50% for patients who are debilitated.

Nosocomial pneumonia is a concern for the hospitalized patient. Nosocomial pneumonia (gram-negative organisms) has been cited as one of the most commonly reported hospital-acquired infections (Gawlinski & Hamwi, 1999; Lucas, Armitage, Gross, & Yamauchi, 1999).

7. Why was Mr. Stevens given erythromycin?

Mr. Stevens' respiratory status as evidenced by his chest radiograph and his blood gas values made hospitalization necessary. However, many patients with CAP are treated as outpatients. This trend results from the growing necessity to contain medical costs and also the increasing number of effective oral antibiotics. Because of the development of antibiotic-resistant strains of bacteria, the need for continued development of new agents is still important. As stated by Lucas et al. (1999), the increasing availability of effective antibiotics has caused controversy over first-line therapy. In its current guidelines, the Infectious Diseases Society of America (IDSA) recommends a macrolide such as erythromycin, clarithromycin, or azithromycin. A newer fluoroquinolone and doxycycline were listed as the preferred agents for empiric outpatient therapy for CAP. Alternative first-line options include amoxacillin/clavulanate and some second- and third-generation cyclosporins, specifically cefuroxime. According to the IDSA, the choice for empiric therapy should be based on many patient variables, including the following:

- Severity of illness
- Antimicrobial intolerance
- Patient's age
- Comorbidities
- Concomitant medications
- Epidemiologic setting

The popularity of the macrolide erythromycin has grown because it is an excellent agent against atypical causes of CAP, which are increasingly being reported.

8. What are the contributing factors for the development of pneumonia in Mr. Stevens' case? List other contributing factors along with signs and symptoms associated with pneumonia not present in Mr. Stevens' case.

Contributing factors in Mr. Stevens' case were his frequent chest colds. Crackles were noted in the lower bases of the lung and an occasional expiratory wheeze. Mr. Stevens also had a low-grade fever for 2 to 3 days and an elevated white blood cell count, general weakness, and chills. The sputum culture showed *S. pneumoniae,* which confirmed the diagnosis of pneumonia. A chest x-ray study also revealed consolidation in the lower lung bases.

As noted by Bucher and Melander (1993), the following have been identified as contributing factors for the development of pneumonia:

- Tracheal intubation
- Decreased level of consciousness (allowing for aspiration)
- Underlying chronic lung disorder
- Endotracheal intubation (bypasses upper airway and host defense mechanisms)
- Suctioning (creates mechanical irritation or injury to the mucosa, predisposing the lungs to inoculation and colonization of bacteria)

Signs and symptoms of bacterial pneumonia include the following:

- Sudden onset, including shaking, chills, and fever of 38.9 to 40.6° C (102° to 105° F)
- Cough initially dry, becoming productive and producing sputum that is rusty in color at first and then yellow-green (rusty color from a mixture of red blood cells and inflammatory cells in infected alveoli)
- Malaise, weakness
- Headache, myalgia
- Cyanosis (depending on the degree of respiratory compromise)
- Altered mental state in elderly patients
- Coarse inspiratory rales
- Friction rub may be present
- Pleuritic chest pain
- Either lobar consolidation or scattered interstitial infiltrates seen on the chest radiograph

9. What diagnostic tests are significant in the determination of a diagnosis of pneumonia?

The following tests are necessary for the diagnosis of pneumonia:

- Vital signs
- Blood cultures
- Sputum cultures (avoid collecting saliva; may have colonization)
- Chest radiographs
- ABG values
- Electrolyte values
- Electrocardiogram
- Hemoglobin and hematocrit

Therapy is based on results obtained from Gram stain and sputum cultures (Bucher & Melander, 1999; Stein, 1998).

10. Discuss the medical management for a patient who has pneumonia.

All patients admitted to the hospital will be exposed to pathogens that make them candidates for acquiring pneumonia; prevention is the number one priority. The following criteria must be considered in the management of the patient with pneumonia (Bucher & Melander, 1999; Stein, 1998):

- Identification of risk factors and susceptible patient populations
- Aseptic technique, including handwashing and handling of respiratory equipment to prevent cross-contamination to susceptible patients
- Administration of antibiotic therapy
- Use of humidified oxygen
- Use of chest physical therapy
- Frequent turning, coughing, and deep breathing
- Assessment of airway protective mechanisms (cough, gag, and swallowing reflexes)
- Elevation of the head of the bed to decrease gastric reflux and facilitate swallowing and postural drainage
- Careful and frequent assessment of temperature, heart rate, respirations, chest sounds, respiratory effort, and use of accessory muscles with breathing; frequent chest x-ray studies
- Use of suctioning
- Assessment of patient's total volume fluid status
- Monitoring of fluid and electrolytes
- Use of bronchodilators

11. What is the goal of therapy with theophylline, and what special considerations exist with this treatment for Mr. Stevens?

Therapeutic blood levels of the theophylline compounds must be monitored closely in patients with COPD. Smokers tend to metabolize theophylline *faster* than nonsmokers, and patients with liver or cardiac disease metabolize theophylline *slower,* so dosages must be individualized.

The goal with theophylline therapy is to maintain a blood level of 10 to 20 μg/ml. Theophylline preparations have been used widely as bronchodilators for patients with COPD for more than 30 years. Theophylline treatment for patients with COPD has been analyzed by Van Andel, Reisner, Menjoge, and Witek (1999). The consensus of a multicenter study of 3720 patients with COPD was that theophylline in selected patients continues to yield a beneficial respiratory effect especially if combined with an inhaled β-agonist. The study revealed that use of inhaled corticosteroids (CCSs) for the management of COPD has gained acceptance, although their role remains undetermined. Evidence from the 3720 patients revealed that the use of inhaled CCSs is widespread in patients with COPD and that the use of theophylline is declining.

12. What is the clinical significance of the pH reading, and what is the appropriate range of partial pressure of oxygen (Po_2) values in the patient with COPD?

Normal values for the patient with COPD are as follows:

$$Pao_2 \quad <60 \text{ mm Hg}$$
$$Paco_2 \quad >50 \text{ mm Hg}$$

As stated by Stein (1998), pH is the key to diagnosis. A severely acidotic range of 0.25 or less is often given as the marker for acute respiratory failure with increases in carbon dioxide and decreases in oxygen. The goal of oxygen therapy is to keep the Pao_2 between 55 and 65 mm Hg. In this range, saturation of hemoglobin is optimal without disruption of the "hypoxic drive" stimulus. Oxygen for the patient with COPD is delivered by Venturi masks, nasal cannulas, rebreathing masks, and mechanical ventilation.

COPD increases pulmonary vascular pressures (pulmonary artery systolic and pulmonary artery diastolic), and the pulmonary artery pressure is 5 to 20 mm Hg higher than the pulmonary capillary wedge pressure. (Normally, these two readings are within 1 to 2 mm Hg of each other.) Mechanical ventilators generate falsely elevated readings, and this is especially true when positive end-expiratory pressure (PEEP) is used.

13. Why were steroids not ordered for Mr. Stevens?

The use of steroids remains controversial. Practitioners use these agents more for the care of the patient with asthma than for the management of patients with chronic bronchitis. When steroids are used, patients should be monitored for side effects of short-term therapy, such as hyperglycemia, worsening hypertension, osteoporosis, cataracts, and opportunistic infections.

Steroids such as methylprednisolone (Solu-Medrol) are used intravenously for 1 to 2 days, followed by oral prednisone in increasingly lower dosages until a maintenance dosage is reached. Aerosol delivery of steroids has not proved effective. Because COPD is not primarily a disease of airway inflammation, it is less responsive to systemic steroids. The primary benefit of the use of steroids is their antiinflammatory effect (Hafner & Ferro, 1998).

14. Were Mr. Stevens' laboratory results consistent with those expected for a patient with COPD and pneumonia?

Usual Laboratory and Diagnostic Findings

Po_2	Decreased	Hct	Often elevated
Pco_2	Normal or elevated	Cor pulmonale	Increased neck vein distension, enlarged liver, and edema; common α_1-antiprotease phenotype
Recoil of lung	Normal		

Chest X-Ray Films

Chest x-ray films usually are normal in patients who have chronic bronchitis and no complications. Classic findings seen in later stages are flattening of the diaphragm, hyperlucency, decreased vascular markings, widening of the rib spaces, and increased anteroposterior diameter (reflects hyperinflation).

ABG Levels

ABG levels may be normal in patients with mild to moderate emphysema. In advanced emphysema, the most common abnormality is decreased Po_2. Pco_2 levels may be normal or increased, especially when infection is present (Bucher & Melander, 1999; Stein, 1998).

15. What other pulmonary function tests would have assisted in the diagnosis of Mr. Stevens' COPD?

The following pulmonary function test results assist in diagnosing COPD:

- Increased RV and functional residual capacity
- Decreased VC
- Increased TLC
- Decreased diffusing capacity
- FEV_1 and ratio of FEV_1 to forced vital capacity decrease as the severity of COPD increases
- Flow-volume loop showing caved appearance

Pulmonary function tests with spirometry usually demonstrate normal findings. These may show an increased RV and a mild reduction in VC consistent with the degree of hyperinflation (Kamholz, 1999; Stein, 1999).

16. Had Mr. Stevens' condition deteriorated and not responded to the bronchodilator and antibiotic therapy, what considerations concerning ventilatory management would be important?

Ventilatory Management

Use of a ventilator allows the patient with COPD to rest and also allows deep suctioning. The problem with ventilator use with this patient population is the difficulty of weaning them from ventilator use.

Stein (1998) and Bucher and Melander (1999) state that when a patient is weaned from the ventilator, three areas must be monitored: oxygenation, carbon dioxide elimination, and mechanical efficiency. Some general guidelines for weaning that may be helpful to the clinician include the following:

- Oxygen concentration less than 50%
- PEEP less than 5 cm H_2O
- Respiratory rate less than 30 breaths/min
- Minute ventilation less than 10 L/min (volume of air patient breathes at rest)
- Low dynamic static pressures (compliance of at least 35 cm H_2O)
- Adequate ABG levels with the aforementioned guidelines

The current clinical practice for weaning is to use T-pieces or continuous positive airway pressure, alternating with full ventilator support such as synchronized intermittent mandatory ventilation or assist control. Pressure support is another mechanism for decreasing ventilator use while offering consistent internal alveoli support. The choice of weaning method will depend on the patient's underlying respiratory disorder and physical and psychologic responses to the weaning process. Patients who experience difficulty in weaning from the ventilator may benefit from techniques such as inspiratory resistance training, physical therapy, hypnosis, biofeedback, and pharmacologic support (Bucher & Melander, 1999).

17. Discuss the incidence of pneumonia in patients with COPD.

Pneumonia occurs in 10% to 40% of intubated patients, requiring mechanical ventilation for more than 24 hours, and has a mortality rate of 30% to 70%. It should be noted that changes seen on the chest radiograph can be subtle and that establishing a specific cause may be difficult. Sputum cultures may be misleading, but gram-negative, antibiotic-resistant pathogens such as *P. aeruginosa* are the most prevalent, occurring in 20% to 30% of patients who have pneumonia and are being mechanically ventilated.

Although not all cases of pneumonia require combination antibiotic therapy, pneumonia caused by *Pseudomonas, Serratia, Acinetobacter,* or *Xanthomonas* does require this approach. In these patients, either an antipseudomonal penicillin or a third-generation cephalosporin and aminoglycoside are suggested.

Pneumococcal pneumonia may take some time to resolve, with consolidation in the lungs taking up to 6 weeks to clear. A chest radiograph of the patient with pneumococcal pneumonia will reveal consolidation manifested by dullness to percussion and increased fremitus (palpable vibrations transmitted through the bronchopulmonary system to the chest wall when the patient speaks). Mortality is related more often to concomitant host disease than to the type of gram-negative organism.

Staphylococcal pneumonia has an insidious onset in the chronically ill. High fever and chills may last up to 1 week in severe cases despite the use of antibiotics. Cough with blood-tinged sputum and tachypnea with cyanosis occur early in the course of the disease. Pneumonia caused by gram-negative bacteria has a highly variable course. It may progress slowly or rapidly over a few days. Patients will have a fever, a productive cough of purulent sputum, and pleuritic chest pain.

A vaccine is available for pneumococcal pneumonia. It is recommended prophylactically for high-risk groups, including elderly patients and those with COPD, congestive heart failure, renal failure, alcoholism, cirrhosis, splenic dysfunction or splenectomy, Hodgkin's disease, myeloma, or other immunocompromised states. The vaccine can be repeated in 6 years if needed. Influenza vaccines are also available and are recommended for high-risk patient populations (Gawlinski & Hamwi, 1999; Hafner & Ferro, 1999).

18. What teaching considerations are of special concern for Mr. Stevens before his discharge?

As stated by Hafner and Ferro (1998), pulmonary function deteriorates more rapidly in smokers than in nonsmokers, and because smokers are also subject to more respiratory infections, health care personnel must be relentless in encouraging patients to stop smoking. It is common for the patient to have smoking cessation relapses. The clinician should discuss this with his or her patients and tell them that it is possible to achieve lifelong cessation, but it is common for this to take multiple attempts. Smoking cessation should be discussed at each visit, with new cessation dates set each time as necessary.

Patients with advanced pulmonary disease who stop smoking at age 65 years have an increased survival rate over those patients who continue to smoke. Other therapies that promote smoking cessation, including nicotine replacements such as gum and transdermal and intranasal formulations and bupropion (an antidepressant) should also be explored.

Other areas that need to be addressed with the patient before discharge include the following:

- Good hydration and sputum mobilization
- Prevention of and avoidance of exposure to infection

- Annual prophylactic multivalent influenza vaccines and a *S. pneumoniae* vaccine (which can be repeated after 6 years if an inadequate response is noted, such as a decline in the pneumococcal antibody titers)
- Avoidance of exposure to sudden temperature changes
- Understanding of bronchodilation therapy, normal blood levels, and diet management
- Referral to a support group

CHRONIC OBSTRUCTIVE PULMONARY DISEASE WITH PNEUMONIA

References

Alspach, J. G. (Ed.). (1998). *American Association of Critical-Care Nurses: Core curriculum for critical care nursing* (5th ed.). Philadelphia: Saunders.

Bucher, L., & Melander, S. (1999). *Critical care nursing.* Philadelphia: Saunders.

Eller, J., Ede, A., Schaberg, T., Niederman, M., Mauch, H., & Lode, H. (1998). Infective exacerbations of chronic bronchitis: relation between bacteriologic etiology and lung function. *Chest, 113*(6), 1542-1547.

Gawlinski, A., & Hamwi, D. (1999). *Acute care nurse practitioner clinical curriculum and certification review.* Philadelphia: Saunders.

Hafner, J. P., & Ferro, T. (1998). Recent developments in the management of COPD. *Hospital Medicine, 34*(1), 20-30, 32-38.

Heath, J., & Mongia, R. (1998). Chronic bronchitis: Primary care management. *American Family Physician, 57*(10), 2365-2368.

Kamholz, S. (1999). Understanding pulmonary function tests. *The Clinical Advisor, 2*(9), 30-47.

Lucas, B., Armitage, B., Gross, P., & Yamauchi, T. (1999). Respiratory infections: Which antibiotics for empiric therapy? *Patient Care, 3*(1), 76-111.

Madison, J., & Irwin, R. (1998). Chronic obstructive pulmonary disease. *The Lancet, 352*(9126), 467-473.

Niederman, M., & Peters, S. (1998). Update in pulmonary medicine. *Annals of Internal Medicine, 128*, 208-215.

Stein, J. (1998). *Internal medicine.* St Louis: Mosby.

Thelan, L., Urden, L., Lough, M., & Stacy, K. (1998). *Critical care nursing: Diagnosis and management.* St Louis: Mosby.

Van Andel, A., Reisner, A., Menjoge, S., & Witek, T. (1999). Analysis of inhaled corticosteroid and oral theophylline use among patients with stable COPD from 1987 to 1995. *Chest, 15*(3), 703-707.

CHAPTER 5

PERCUTANEOUS TRANSLUMINAL CORONARY ANGIOPLASTY AND THROMBOLYTIC THERAPY IN MYOCARDIAL INFARCTION

Alice Lowe, RN, BSN • Sheila Drake Melander, RN, DSN, ACNP-C, FCCM

CASE PRESENTATION

Mr. Smith, a 54-year-old man, began having chest pain 1 hour after supper, while he was at work. He described the pain as a "grabbing pressure" located midsternally. He rated the pain at "about 2" on a scale of 1 to 5. He stated that the pain radiated down his left arm and through to his back. He was transported to the emergency department (ED) by ambulance. On admission, Mr. Smith was pale and diaphoretic and complained of shortness of breath (SOB). He denied nausea or vomiting. In the ED, unstable angina was diagnosed and tests to rule out myocardial infarction (MI) were initiated. He had experienced chest pain for 1 hour upon arrival in the ED at 8:13 PM.

The patient reports no previous episodes of chest pain or pressure. He has smoked two packs of cigarettes daily for 25 years. His mother died of Alzheimer's disease, and his father died of cancer. He has no family history of heart disease.

On initial examination, the patient did not exhibit jugular venous distension, the carotid arteries were 2+/4 without bruits, and the point of maximum impulse was located at the fifth intercostal space, midclavicular line. Normal S_1 and S_2 sounds were auscultated with an S_3 present. No S_4 sound or murmurs were heard. There were vesicular lung sounds with scattered wheezes, but no crackles were heard. No edema was present, and bowel sounds were normal.

Diagnostic data at admission were as follows:

BP	140/90 mm Hg	Sao_2	95% with oxygen 4 L/min
HR	92 bpm and regular		per nasal cannula
Respirations	32 breaths/min	Height	173 cm
Temperature	36.9° C (98.5° F)	Weight	104 kg

The 12 lead electrocardiogram (ECG) findings at 8:15 PM were as follows:

- Normal sinus rhythm (NSR) with frequent premature ventricular contractions (PVCs) and 3 to 4 beat runs of ventricular tachycardia (VT)
- ST-segment elevation in leads I, aVL, and V_2 through V_6 (3 to 4 mm)
- ST-segment depression in leads III and aVF
- Q waves in V_2 through V_4

The chest x-ray film revealed slight cardiomegaly with mild congestive heart failure (CHF).

The echocardiogram findings were as follows:

- Trileaflet aortic valve with normal openings
- Normal mitral configuration with normal opening of mitral valve diastole and normal coaptation in systole
- Normal right atrium and right ventricle
- Thin layer pericardial effusion (mostly posterior)
- Left ventricular ejection fraction 25% to 30%
- Mild mitral valve regurgitation

Cardiac enzyme measurements were as follows at admission and on day 1:

	Admission 2013	Admission 2400	Day 1 0400
CK (U/L)	254	7357	5638
CK-MB (%)	10	>300	>300
Troponin I (ng/ml)	3.5	>50	>50

In the ED, Mr. Smith's chest pain was unrelieved after three sublingual nitroglycerin (NTG) tablets. Morphine sulfate 5 mg intravenous push (IVP) was administered, resulting in a small decrease in pain.

After evaluation of the initial laboratory results, presenting symptoms, and the ECG, the diagnosis was an extensive anterolateral MI. Mr. Smith was assessed for contraindications to thrombolytic therapy. The patient was considered a candidate for thrombolytic therapy, and administration of tissue plasminogen activator (tPA) was started immediately. An NTG drip (50 mg/250 ml in 5% dextrose in water [D5W]) was started at 20 μg/min (6 ml/hr). A heparin bolus of 8000 U was given, and a drip was begun at 10 ml/hr (1000 U/hr). Metoprolol titrate (Lopressor) 5 mg IVP was given every 5 minutes three times (total 15 mg) and an enteric-coated aspirin was administered. After the NTG and heparin drips were started, the patient's pain was relieved. He was then transferred to the coronary intensive care unit (CICU).

In the CICU, Mr. Smith's chest pain returned. He rated it as "4" on a scale of 1 to 5. His blood pressure was 96/60 mm Hg, and he began having ST-segment elevations in the anterior leads along with six to eight beat runs of VT. Three sublingual NTG tablets were given, followed by 4 mg of morphine intravenously, but the pain did not decrease. Mr. Smith was sent to the catheterization laboratory for emergency angiography and possible angioplasty.

The angiogram showed 90% blockage of the left anterior descending (LAD) artery. An emergency rescue angioplasty (percutaneous transluminal coronary angioplasty [PTCA]) was performed, but the artery continued to reocclude, so a coronary stent was inserted. While the PTCA was performed, 23,000 U of heparin and 500,000 U of urokinase were given as an intracoronary injection. Mr. Smith became hypotensive, tachycardic, pale, cool, and diaphoretic. His arterial blood oxygen saturation (Sao$_2$) dropped to 86%, and he was placed on a mechanical ventilator with a 100% nonrebreather mask. He continued having runs of VT; therefore a 100-mg bolus of lidocaine was given and a lidocaine drip (2 g/500 ml of D5W) was started at 2 mg/min. A dopamine (Intropin) infusion was started at 2 µg/kg/min and was gradually increased to 4 µg/kg/min. A dobutamine (Dobutrex) drip was started at 5 µg/kg/min. An abciximab (ReoPro) bolus of 0.25 mg/kg was administered followed by an infusion at 21 ml/hr (which will continue for 12 hours). A pulmonary artery (Swan-Ganz) catheter was placed to monitor for CHF and cardiogenic shock. An intraaortic balloon pump (IABP) was inserted in the right groin to stabilize Mr. Smith's blood pressure (BP), decrease the workload of the heart, and improve cardiac output. Upon return to the CICU, Mr. Smith was free of pain.

His vital signs and hemodynamic readings were as follows:

BP	133/59 mm Hg	RAP	10 mm Hg
HR	90 bpm	PAS	42 mm Hg
Sao$_2$	99% with 100% non-	PAD	22 mm Hg
	rebreather mask	MAP	31 mm Hg
ECG	NSR with occasional PVCs	PAWP	22 mm Hg

Findings from an ECG on the day of admission post-PTCA (11 PM) were as follows:

- NSR, T wave inverted in aVR
- ST segment elevated in leads I, aVL, and V$_2$ through V$_6$ (1 to 2 mm)

Findings from an ECG on postadmission day 1 (6:50 AM) were as follows:

- NSR, ST segment almost baseline
- Q waves in V$_2$ through V$_6$
- Inverted T waves leads V$_2$ through V$_6$
- aVR T waves now upright

Mr. Smith's lidocaine drip was discontinued the next day. The heparin drip was discontinued and the arterial line, IABP, and pulmonary artery catheter were removed on day 2. He was started on enoxaparin (Lovenox) 100 mg subcutaneously twice a day. On day 3, his dopamine, dobutamine, and NTG drip were tapered and discontinued. He was released to the cardiac progressive step-down unit on day 4. On day 6, he was released to home. He was instructed in outpatient cardiac rehabilitation, smoking cessation, and a prudent heart diet. He was sent home with prescriptions for diltiazem (Cardizem) 30 mg three times daily, captopril (Capoten) 6.25 mg three times daily, ticlopidine (Ticlid) 250 mg twice daily, metoprolol

(Lopressor) 25 mg twice daily, and NTG tablets as needed. Mr. Smith was also instructed to take an aspirin every day.

PERCUTANEOUS TRANSLUMINAL CORONARY ANGIOPLASTY AND THROMBOLYTIC THERAPY IN MYOCARDIAL INFARCTION

Questions

1. Describe angina pectoris and discuss the difference between chronic stable angina, unstable angina, and Prinzmetal's angina.
2. Define CAD and discuss associated risk factors.
3. Describe an acute myocardial infarction (AMI) and its effects on the heart and lifestyle.
4. List the symptoms of an AMI.
5. What is the significance of the following heart sounds: S_3, S_4, and a murmur?
6. What do crackles auscultated during lung sound assessment signify?
7. Discuss the use of cardiac enzymes and their normal values. What laboratory values would be indicative of an AMI for Mr. Smith?
8. What is the significance of Mr. Smith's ST-segment changes?
9. Why was an echocardiogram done?
10. What are the desired pharmacologic effects of NTG?
11. Why was Mr. Smith given an aspirin in the ED? Explain the use of abciximab (ReoPro), ticlopidine (Ticlid), and aspirin therapy for Mr. Smith.
12. Discuss the pharmacologic actions of heparin and enoxaparin (Lovenox) and the indications for use with a patient with an AMI.
13. Discuss the pharmacologic effects of morphine.
14. Describe what a β-blocker is and the rationale for Mr. Smith receiving this medication.
15. Why was Mr. Smith given lidocaine?
16. tPA is a thrombolytic agent. Discuss the effects of a thrombolytic agent and why it was used for Mr. Smith initially rather than angioplasty.
17. What are the contraindications for tPA?
18. What is a PTCA?
19. What made Mr. Smith a candidate for PTCA? What are the potential complications for a patient undergoing PTCA?
20. What is a stent and why was it used on Mr. Smith?
21. What do the readings from the pulmonary artery catheter tell the nurse about Mr. Smith?
22. What is cardiogenic shock? What symptoms did Mr. Smith exhibit?
23. What are the therapeutic effects of dopamine (Intropin) at low, moderate, and high dosages?
24. What are the therapeutic effects of dobutamine (Dobutrex)?
25. What advantage does an IABP offer Mr. Smith?
26. What significance does the IABP have in relation to the tPA and urokinase given previously?
27. Mr. Smith was sent home with a prescription for diltiazem (Cardizem). Why would a patient with heart disease be given a calcium channel blocker?
28. Why was Mr. Smith sent home with a prescription for captopril (Capoten)?

Percutaneous Transluminal Coronary Angioplasty and Thrombolytic Therapy in Myocardial Infarction

Questions and Answers

1. Describe angina pectoris and discuss the difference between chronic stable angina, unstable angina, and Prinzmetal's angina.

Angina pectoris (chest pain) is a symptom of myocardial ischemia resulting from an imbalance in the oxygen demand and the oxygen supply. "Angina is usually manifested when the coronary artery occlusion is equal to or greater than 75% of the lumen" (Becker, 1999, p. 204). Patients with angina describe a sensation of pressure, heaviness, burning, gas, or squeezing in the chest area. The pain can radiate to the neck, jaw, shoulders, arms, or hands.

Etiologic Factors for Angina Pectoris
Atherosclerotic heart disease, hypertension, aortic valve disease, anemia, arrhythmia, thyrotoxicosis, shock, CHF, and coronary artery spasm are the etiologic factors associated with angina pectoris.

Chronic Stable Angina
Chronic stable angina is a stable pattern of chest pain with the same frequency, severity, duration, and precipitating factors (exercise or exertion) that has not changed in the last 2 months (Alexander et al, 1998; Becker, 1999; Clochesy, Breu, Cardin, Whittaker, & Rudy, 1996).

Unstable Angina
Unstable angina is (1) new-onset chest pain in patients who have never had anginal symptoms before or (2) pain that is suddenly different (more intense, more frequent, brought on by less effort, or different in character) in patients who have had stable angina. The pain may be steady or it may be intermittent. It lasts longer than 15 minutes and is not relieved by NTG or rest. Unstable angina is a medical emergency. About 1 of 10 people with it develop AMI. This pain usually signifies that the patient has some CAD, and it should be evaluated. Chest pain that is not relieved with rest and NTG in 15 minutes should be evaluated in the ED (Alexander et al, 1998; Clochesy et al, 1996).

Prinzmetal's (Variant) Angina
The angina occurs without an increase in effort or stress and without warning. The pain occurs about the same time every day, commonly at bedtime or upon awakening. The pain is believed to be caused by vasospasm of the coronary artery. With Prinzmetal's angina, the ECG will show ST-segment elevations with pain and disappear when the pain is gone (Becker, 1999).

2. Define CAD and discuss associated risk factors.

CAD is subintimal deposition of atheromas in the large- and medium-sized arteries serving the heart. Atherosclerosis is the name for buildup of plaque (cholesterol, calcium, and other minerals) in the coronary arteries. Once the artery's lumen is reduced to less than 50%, it is considered significant CAD. When the blood flow is severely reduced by atherosclerosis, a clot can form as blood trickles through the narrowed vessel, causing a sudden, complete stoppage of blood flow (Alexander et al, 1998; Becker, 1999).

The following are unmodifiable risk factors for CAD:

1. *Heredity:* CAD tends to run in families. Some families have narrow coronary arteries; others have tendencies toward hyperlipidemia, hypertension, or other risk factors.
2. *Age:* CAD is more prevalent in older age groups. The incidence of AMI increases with age.
3. *Sex:* Men have a higher incidence of CAD earlier in life, but after women go through menopause (and lose the protective benefits of estrogen), the risks for CAD are about the same.
4. *Race:* White men die more often from CAD than do nonwhite men, and white women die slightly less often from CAD than do nonwhite women (Becker, 1999).
5. *Socioeconomic status:* A new report identifies low socioeconomic status as an unmodifiable risk factor. A number of mechanisms may explain this. First, risk factors for atherosclerosis, such as smoking, hypertension, obesity, and sedentary lifestyle, are higher in persons with low socioeconomic status. Second, some of these risk factors, as well as psychosocial responses to stressors, may increase exposure to CAD triggers in these groups. Finally, these groups have less access to care (Alexander et al, 1998, p. 1186).

Modifiable risk factors for CAD are as follows:

1. *Hypertension:* Systolic BP more than 160 mm Hg or diastolic greater than 95 mm Hg increases the risk of CAD two to three times.
2. *Diabetes mellitus:* Diabetic patients have a two times higher incidence of CAD than those without diabetes.
3. *Cigarette smoking:* "Smoking increases heart rate and causes vasoconstriction, thereby impairing oxygen transport by the blood and increasing myocardial oxygen demand. Smoking also facilitates atherosclerosis by making the endothelium more porous" (Becker, 1999, p. 203). Smokers have a two to six times higher risk of death from CAD than nonsmokers.
4. *Hyperlipidemia:* Hyperlipidemia is the leading risk factor responsible for atherosclerosis. Serum levels of cholesterol less than 200 mg/dl are associated with minimal risk of CAD. High levels of triglycerides (>160 mg/dl) and low-density lipoproteins (>160 mg/dl) as well as low levels of high-density lipoproteins (<35 mg/dl) contribute to CAD.

The following factors contribute to CAD:

1. *Obesity:* Morbid obesity has been shown to be positively associated with an increased risk of CAD. In addition, it also contributes to the development of hypertension and diabetes.
2. *Sedentary lifestyle:* A positive correlation exists between a sedentary lifestyle and CAD (Alexander et al, 1998; Lessig & Lessig, 1998).

3. Describe an acute myocardial infarction (AMI) and its effects on the heart and lifestyle.

An MI occurs when there is a blockage of the coronary artery that causes necrosis of the cells of an area of the heart muscle as a result of oxygen deprivation. In most patients, it is the result of severe atherosclerotic narrowing of one or more of the coronary arteries. Rarely, an MI can occur in the absence of coronary artery narrowing if there is a marked disparity between myocardial oxygen supply and demand. Cocaine abuse has been implicated as a possible cause of such a disparity (Becker, 1999). In 1996, Riegel wrote, "Infarction results from the mechanical obstruction caused by thrombosis, plaque rupture, dissection, and sometimes spasm." During an AMI, the diminished blood flow to the heart can force the myocardium to shift from aerobic to anaerobic metabolism. This results in less efficient energy production, lactic acid buildup, intracellular hypokalemia, intracellular acidosis, intracellular hypernatremia, and interference with the release of calcium from the sarcoplasmic reticulum (Braunwald, 1997).

The patient who has suffered an AMI may have an area of the heart that no longer functions or functions in a diminished capacity. The effects on the patient vary with the extent of the heart muscle affected. A severe MI can decrease the ejection fraction (amount of blood pumped from the heart with each beat) to 15% to 20% (normal, 60% to 70%), an amount that could cause disability. Patients with severely limited left ventricular (LV) function suffer from SOB and weakness with even small activities of daily living.

4. List the symptoms of an AMI.

The symptoms vary with each patient. Patients may describe the symptoms as simply "indigestion" or a burning sensation that radiates from the midchest up to the jaw. The hallmark symptom of an AMI is chest pain. The pain is typically in the middle of the chest, behind the sternum, and does not improve with NTG or rest. It usually lasts longer than 15 minutes. Other symptoms include an uncomfortable pressure, crushing, heaviness, squeezing, fullness, tightness, aching, constriction, or an oppressive feeling. The pain may radiate to the jaw, to the shoulders, through to the back, or down the arms or hands.

5. What is the significance of the following heart sounds: S_3, S_4, and a murmur?

The third heart sound, S_3, may indicate heart failure. It is an early diagnostic sound. The sound is generated from vibrations produced during rapid filling of the ventricles in patients with ventricular dysfunction and overfilled ventricles (as in CHF). It can also be a normal variant in individuals up to 30 years of age. It is a lower-frequency pitch that often can be detected best with the patient in the left lateral decubitus position and in conditions in which the venous return is increased. It is best heard at the apex with the bell of the stethoscope (VanRiper & VanRiper, 1997).

The fourth heart sound, S_4, is a low-pitched presystolic sound. It is secondary to a forceful atrial contraction into a ventricle that has decreased compliance. Chronic ischemia, ventricular hypertrophy, cardiomyopathy, and idiopathic hypertrophic subaortic stenosis are some of the conditions in which an S_4 may be heard. It can be heard best at the apex in the left lateral decubitus position with the bell (VanRiper & VanRiper, 1997).

A murmur is a turbulence in the blood flow; it can be caused by a ruptured papillary muscle, valvular disease, or mitral and aortic insufficiency. Assessment should always include auscultation of heart sounds of the patient with an MI. A patient without a murmur on admission who develops one may have ruptured the papillary muscle.

6. What do crackles auscultated during lung sound assessment signify?

Crackles signify that the heart is not handling the workload efficiently. It suggests LV failure or decreased LV compliance. "If the blood does not leave the left ventricle, the fluid will back up into the lungs and cause congestive heart failure. This can be exhibited by shortness of breath, dyspnea, or crackles on auscultation of the lung fields. If this condition is allowed to persist, then the patient may develop a productive cough of frothy, pink sputum resulting from pulmonary edema" (Becker, 1999).

7. Discuss the use of cardiac enzymes and their normal values. What laboratory values would be indicative of an AMI for Mr. Smith?

Creatine Kinase (CK) (50 to 180 U/L)
CK is an indicator of damage to the heart. It is released when a muscle is damaged. CK is an enzyme found in the heart, skeletal muscle, and brain. It consists of three isoenzymes: MM, found in the skeletal muscles; MB, found in the cardiac muscles; and BB, found in the brain tissues. Damage to any of these tissues causes the release of CK into the serum. The isoenzymes are then used to further differentiate the damaged tissue.

CK-MB (<5%)
After injury, CK and its MB isoenzymes will be released into the blood at a predictable rate. Within 4 to 8 hours, serum levels will rise above normal limits, indicating tissue destruction. A peak of 5 to 15 times the baseline is reached within 12 to 24 hours; the level will return to normal within 2 to 3 days (Becker, 1999; VanRiper & VanRiper, 1997). Because of the exclusivity of the MB isoenzymes present in the cardiac muscle, serum MB elevations greater than 3% are definitive in the diagnosis of MI. After cardiac surgery, MB elevations greater than 7% indicate MI (VanRiper & VanRiper, 1997).

Troponin (<0.3 ng/ml)
Troponin, a protein that helps regulate heart muscle contraction, can be isolated in the serum and is a sensitive indicator of MI. The troponin protein actually consists of three separate proteins: troponin I, T, and C, each with a different function. "Cardiac troponins T and I are not found in significant levels in the blood of healthy adults, so the presence of those troponins in the serum is an indication of the death of myocardial tissue" (Murphy & Berding, 1999). After MI, troponin T rises in the serum and correlates with the amount of tissue damaged. Troponin T is measurable in the serum within 3 to 5 hours of symptom onset, peaks at about 72 hours, and remains detectable in the blood for up to 14 days. The presence in the blood for up to 2 weeks provides a diagnostic advantage to patients who have delayed seeking treatment for their symptoms (Murphy & Berding, 1999; VanRiper & VanRiper, 1997). Cardiac troponin I levels begin to increase 3 hours after myocardial ischemia

occurs, peak at 14 to 18 hours, and remain elevated for 7 to 10 days (Antman et al, 1996; Murphy & Berding, 1999). A cardiac troponin I level of at least 0.4 ng/ml when a patient with unstable angina is first evaluated predicts an increased risk of short-term mortality, probably because it permits the diagnosis of non–Q wave MI that one might have overlooked by sampling only for CK-MB. With progressively higher levels of cardiac troponin I, the risk of mortality increases, presumably because the amount of myocardial necrosis increases. Measuring cardiac troponin I is therefore useful in evaluating patients with unstable angina (Antman et al, 1996).

Myoglobin (<120 µg/ml)

Myoglobin is a heme protein that is found in all striated muscle fibers, which account for about 2% of both skeletal and cardiac tissue mass. The small molecular weight of myoglobin allows it to be released rapidly from muscle tissue when the tissue is damaged. This release of myoglobin is particularly important when one is trying to determine whether cardiac muscle has been damaged. Because myoglobin escapes rapidly from damaged myocardial cells, it can be detected as soon as 2 hours after an AMI, with peak serum levels occurring in 3 to 15 hours (Murphy & Berding, 1999).

Mr. Smith's had an initial CK value of 254 U/L, CK-MB of 10%, and troponin I of 3.5 ng/ml. All of these are suggestive of AMI.

8. What is the significance of Mr. Smith's ST-segment changes?

The ST segment represents the resting phase between ventricular depolarization and repolarization. Thus it is normally neutral or isoelectric, that is, near baseline on the ECG. ST-segment shifts (elevations or depressions) associated with myocardial cell injury may be the result of an inability of the affected cells to maintain their normal intracellular polarity during the resting phase.

The T wave represents repolarization of the myocardium and is normally positive (upward deflection) in all of the 12 leads except V_1 and sometimes III and V_2. T-wave inversions may reflect ischemia or it may reflect an MI. T-wave inversion associated with AMI may persist for several days and is associated with ischemia.

Pathologic Q waves are greater than 0.04 second deep and usually greater than 0.03 second wide. Q waves normally occur in leads III and aV_F and are likely to disappear with deep inspiration or position change.

An AMI evolves in three stages:

1. *Ischemia:* Ischemia results from a temporary interruption of the myocardial blood supply. It is the least acute stage of tissue hypoxia and is often reversible with little or no permanent cell death if prompt intervention increases blood supply to the myocardium or reduces oxygen demand. Its characteristic ECG change is T-wave inversion, a result of altered tissue repolarization.

2. *Injury:* Injury to myocardial cells results from a prolonged interruption of blood flow. Its characteristic ECG change is ST-segment elevation.

3. *Necrosis:* Infarction results from an absence of blood flow to myocardial tissue, leading to necrosis. The ECG shows pathologic Q waves, reflecting abnormal depolarization in damaged tissue or absent depolarization of scar tissue.

Inferior MI (Leads II, II, and aVF)

The right coronary artery supplies the inferior myocardium and lower third of the interventricular septum. Infarction of these surfaces is best reflected in the inferior leads. Because the infarcted tissue on the inferior surface no longer depolarizes, opposing forces become dominant, and current traveling away from the positive pole is visible as a new Q wave.

Anterior MI (Leads V_1 through V_6)

The LAD supplies the anterior ventricular myocardium and upper two thirds of the septum. Infarction in this area is best seen in leads V_1 through V_6. The result is smaller or absent R waves. Loss of R waves in V_2 through V_4 indicates necrosis of the anteroseptal surface; loss of R waves in V_2 through V_6 indicates extensive anterior or anterolateral infarction.

Lateral MI (Leads I, aVL, V_5, and V6)

The circumflex artery and the diagonal branches of the LAD supply the lateral myocardium. Infarction in this area is best seen in leads I, aVL, and V_5 and V_6.

Posterior MI (Leads V_1 and V_2)

The mid and posterior marginal branches of the circumflex artery supply the posterior wall of the heart. The process of infarction here can sometimes be seen in leads V_1 and V_2 as ST-segment depression, reversal of the T-wave polarity, or initial R-wave upswing that is wider than normal.

On Mr. Smith's ECG, the elevations in leads I, aV_L, and V_1 through V_6 signify that anterolateral injury is present. The Q waves in leads V_1 through V_4 could be from a previous MI or could represent some necrosis in the anterior portion of the myocardium. The ST-segment depression in leads III and aV_F signifies reciprocal changes of the damage in the anterior leads (Bucher & Melander, 1999).

9. Why was an echocardiogram done?

Echocardiograms use ultrasound waves to obtain and display images of cardiac structures. This test is performed to rule out aortic valvular disease, idiopathic hypertrophic subaortic stenosis, or other structural malformations. It can also help determine the extent to which LV wall motion has been affected and to estimate ejection fraction (Becker, 1999).

10. What are the desired pharmacologic effects of NTG?

Nitrates decrease the myocardial oxygen demand in patients with fixed obstructive CAD and coronary vasospasm. NTG is a vasodilator that increases venous capacitance. It relaxes vascular smooth muscle, thereby reducing blood pressure by generalized vasodilation. Both of these actions lower peripheral resistance against which the heart must pump, decreasing preload. Decreases in preload lead to an increase in cardiac output. Nitrates also decrease systemic arterial pressure and afterload, which may result in hypotension. The combined effects reduce the preload on the heart and help relieve chest pain (Clochesy et al, 1996; LeFever-Kee & Hayes, 1997; Lessig & Lessig, 1998).

11. **Why was Mr. Smith given an aspirin in the ED? Explain the use of abciximab (ReoPro), ticlopidine (Ticlid), and aspirin therapy for Mr. Smith.**

Antiplatelet therapy, specifically aspirin, is now standard therapy for unstable angina and treatment after an MI. The American Heart Association (1999) recommends the use of aspirin in patients who have experienced an MI, unstable angina, ischemic stroke, or transient ischemic attacks. The primary mechanism accounting for the benefit is believed to be related to irreversible inhibition of the cyclooxygenase pathway in platelets, blocking formation of thromboxane A_2 and thromboxane A_2–induced platelet aggregation. This inhibition is complete with small doses of aspirin. It is strongly recommended that all patients with AMI receive nonenteric-coated aspirin, 160 to 325 mg, to chew and swallow as soon as possible after the clinical impression of evolving AMI is formed, and whether or not thrombolytic therapy is to be given. The dose should be repeated daily by mouth indefinitely (Cairns, Theroux, Lewis, Ezekowitz, & Sutton, 1998). The adverse effects of aspirin are related to bleeding, particularly gastrointestinal.

Ticlopidine (Ticlid) is given in 250-mg doses twice a day. It is also an antiplatelet agent, but unlike aspirin, it does not block cyclooxygenase but interferes with the platelet activation mechanism mediated by adenosine diphosphate (ADP) and with transformation of the fibrinogen receptor glycoprotein IIb/IIIa into its high-affinity state. It can be associated with diarrhea, rash, reversible neutropenia, thrombocytopenia, and liver function abnormalities. It takes approximately 2 weeks of treatment before the full benefit of ticlopidine is achieved (Alexander et al, 1998; Cairns et al, 1998; Clochesy et al, 1996).

Abciximab (ReoPro) is a platelet glycoprotein IIb/IIIa receptor inhibitor with proven efficacy in the management of ischemic coronary syndromes (Casserly et al, 1998). Abciximab is started during the PTCA and is most often used as adjunctive therapy to intracoronary stent implantation (Hasdai et al, 1998). It is administered as an intravenous bolus of 0.25 mg/kg followed by an infusion at a rate of 10 µg/min for 12 hours. This regimen results in greater than 80% receptor occupancy and inhibition of platelet aggregation induced by ADP. The drug can be found on platelets as long as 15 days after its discontinuation (Cairns et al, 1998).

Eptifibatide (Integrilin) is another antiplatelet agent. It works by preventing the binding of fibrinogen, von Willebrand factor, and other adhesive ligands to glycoproteins IIb/IIa. The recommended regimen consists of a bolus ranging from 90 to 250 µg/kg followed by an infusion at rates of 0.5 to 3 µg/kg/min. It is recommended for use in patients with acute coronary syndrome, including patients who are to be managed medically and those undergoing PTCA. It has been shown to decrease the rate of a combined endpoint of death, new MI, or need for urgent intervention (Key Pharmaceuticals, 1998).

There is a striking reduction in adverse outcomes in patients treated with inhibitors of the platelet glycoprotein IIb/IIIa receptor as an adjunct to angioplasty and combined with thrombolytic therapy (GUSTO IIb, 1997).

12. **Discuss the pharmacologic actions of heparin and enoxaparin (Lovenox) and the indications for use with a patient with an AMI.**

During an AMI, there is a hypercoagulability that leads to blood cells "sticking together." This can increase the closure of arteries and lead to a more severe MI. The anticoagulant effects of heparin and enoxaparin (Lovenox) keep the blood thinner and prevent clotting. This can help the blood travel arteries that are very narrow with atherosclerosis.

Heparin is an anticoagulant. It inhibits activated factors IS, S, SI, and XII, which are involved in the conversion of prothrombin to thrombin, thereby reducing clot formation. At low dosages, it prevents the conversion of prothrombin to thrombin. At higher dosages, it neutralizes thrombin, preventing the conversion of fibrinogen to fibrin and thus thrombus formation and extension of existing thrombi. Heparin must be titrated for effect using activated partial thromboplastin times (aPTT). Heparin and aspirin are used together to prevent the formation of thrombus (Gurfinkel, Fareed, Antman, Cohen, & Mautner, 1998). "It is recommended that all patients who have received tPA or reteplase should receive heparin" (Cairns et al, 1998).

Enoxaparin is a new low-molecular-weight heparin (LMWH). The pharmacologic properties of LMWHs include a binding affinity for antithrombin III, antifactor IIa activity, excellent bioavailability, minimal protein binding, predictable anticoagulant response, and clinical tolerance by patients. Enoxaparin is given subcutaneously, usually at 1 mg/kg every 12 hours. The emerging role of LMWHs is to offer efficacy plus safety for the treatment of acute coronary problems and in treatment for patients who received coronary stents. This new pharmacologic antithrombic approach offers a significant reduction in rehospitalization rate, interventions, and medical costs (Gurfinkel et al, 1998; Zidar, 1998). Enoxaparin has the benefit of being therapeutic at the onset of administration; whereas heparin must be titrated to the aPTT for a therapeutic effect. It may take several hours to get the aPTT to the desired level.

13. Discuss the pharmacologic effects of morphine.

Catecholamines are released in response to the pain and anxiety associated with an MI. This causes an increase in heart rate and blood pressure and vasoconstriction. All of these increase the workload on the heart. Morphine can relieve anxiety, thereby reducing the catecholamine release and easing the workload on the heart. Morphine also exerts mild hemodynamic effects by increasing the venous capacitance and by reducing systemic vascular resistance. The result of both effects is a reduction in myocardial oxygen demand.

14. Describe what a β-blocker is and the rationale for Mr. Smith receiving this medication.

A β-blocker acts by blocking the β-adrenergic responses to catecholamine stimulation. It can decrease heart rate, blood pressure, contractility, and myocardial oxygen demand. This sudden decrease in workload will increase the cardiac output and lessen the severity of the MI. β-Blockers can interrupt evolving infarcts, limit infarct size, and decrease the incidence of ventricular arrhythmias by decreasing oxygen demand. They increase diastolic filling time and increase exercise tolerance. β-Blockers are contraindicated in patients with heart failure, hypotension, bradycardia, heart block, and bronchial asthma (Alexander et al, 1998; Clochesy et al, 1996; Lessig & Lessig, 1998). For AMI, metoprolol titrate (Lopressor) 5 mg is given intravenously every 2 to 5 minutes for three doses (total 15 mg). After each bolus, vital signs must be assessed for 2 to 5 minutes. The boluses are stopped if the heart rate decreases to less than 60 bpm or systolic blood pressure drops to less than 100 mm Hg (LeFever-Kee & Hayes, 1997).

15. Why was Mr. Smith given lidocaine?

One of the adverse effects of a decrease in myocardial blood flow is arrhythmias. Arrhythmias can be life-threatening. Tachycardias increase the oxygen demand and decrease coronary perfusion. Bradycardias can result in CHF. Heart blocks decrease coronary and systemic perfusion and can contribute to cardiogenic shock. When myocardial blood supply or oxygen decreases, myocardial tissue becomes irritable and can trigger VT. Reperfusion arrhythmias (especially PVCs) can result when the blood supply is restored after tPA or PTCA. They are so common that they are considered signs of successful reperfusion.

Previously, lidocaine was used as a preventive treatment in all MI patients. It is no longer recommended as prophylactic treatment for AMIs. However, in Mr. Smith's case, he began having VT after the PTCA restored blood supply to the myocardium (reperfusion arrhythmia). A reperfusion arrhythmia is considered a good sign, but the arrhythmias still need to be treated, especially VT. Therefore he was given a 100-mg bolus of lidocaine and a drip at 2 mg/min. Toxic effects of lidocaine include drowsiness, slurred speech, hallucinations, and seizures. These effects are potentiated in elderly patients and those with renal failure (Bucher & Melander, 1999).

16. tPA is a thrombolytic agent. Discuss the effects of a thrombolytic agent and why it was used for Mr. Smith initially rather than angioplasty.

Not only are the coronary arteries closed by plaque, but the plaque also causes turbulence in them and slows the blood flow. This can cause a clot to form at that site, completely closing the artery. tPA is a human protein manufactured by genetic engineering. "Tissue plasminogen activator is one of several drugs now approved for use in certain patients having a heart attack. These drugs have the ability to dissolve the blood clots that are responsible for causing the majority of all heart attacks. Studies have shown that tPA and other thrombolytic agents can reduce the amount of damage to the heart muscle as well as the number of heart attack deaths if administered soon (within a few hours) after symptoms begin" (American Heart Association, 1999). The desired effect of tPA is to break up the clots that have formed in the coronary arteries. "It is strongly recommended that all patients with AMI be considered for anticoagulant therapy" (Cairns et al, 1998). tPA is given as a 15-mg bolus, then 0.75 mg/kg (maximum of 50 mg) over 30 minutes, followed by 0.5 mg/kg (maximum of 35 mg) over 60 minutes for a total of 100 mg over 90 minutes (Lessig & Lessig, 1998). Signs of reperfusion include pain relief, reperfusion arrhythmias (accelerated idioventricular rhythm, ventricular ectopy, and bradycardia), and ST-segment resolution. The side effects of tPA are related to its systemic action that breaks up any clots in the body. This is why there is a long list of contraindications for tPA.

Reteplase is a third-generation thrombolytic agent. It has a half-life of 13 to 16 minutes. Because of its short half-life, it can be given as a 10-U double-bolus injection (30 minutes apart). No dosing adjustment is necessary for weight, and no formation of antibodies has been detected. Reteplase is just beginning to be used in major hospitals in the United States (Kline-Rogers, Martin, & Smith, 1999).

There has been controversy about whether direct angioplasty is better than therapy with tPA. Direct angioplasty became an attractive alternative in 1993 when three small, randomized trials concluded that the technique saved an estimated 40 lives per 1000 patients treated, a huge clinical advantage. However, these trials were performed at "selected hospitals with a lot of experience, involved few patients, and except in one case, used thrombolytic regimens that are suboptimal by today's standards" (GUSTO IIb, 1997; Twombly, 1997). Initially, the Duke study was designed to include as many patients as possible for a lengthier period. It looked at the outcomes of 1138 patients who were given either the clot-busting drug tPA or direct angioplasty in 57 hospitals in 9 countries as part of a substudy of the GUSTO IIb clinical trial. It concluded that direct angioplasty had a "small to moderate" clinical advantage over thrombolytic drug therapy 1 month after treatment. Those same patients have now been followed for 6 months, and researchers have found that the advantage has diminished. The rate of death or second heart attack was not statistically different between the two therapies (Aversano, 1998). The Myocardial Infarction Triage and Intervention (MITI) Project Registry is the largest study published to date comparing primary angioplasty with thrombolytic therapy in AMI patients. There was no difference between in-hospital or 3-year mortality rates for patients treated with primary angioplasty and those treated with thrombolytic therapy, even after controlling for differences in baseline characteristics known to affect mortality (Aversano, 1998).

At present, physicians deciding which therapy to offer a patient who is eligible for either treatment should return to fundamentals established in multiple large studies. The rapid restoration of brisk antegrade coronary flow is critical in reducing mortality. If a skilled cardiologist is readily available and the patient can be treated rapidly, angioplasty may be preferable. In most situations, however, thrombolytic therapy should still be regarded as an excellent strategy of reperfusion. The important point is not to delay restoration of myocardial reperfusion in suitable candidates with either of the two attractive alternatives (GUSTO IIb, 1997).

Mr. Smith was admitted late in the evening (8 PM) with severe chest pain and was already showing signs of cardiogenic shock. Therefore, because the catheterization laboratory was closed for the evening, it was better time management to treat Mr. Smith with tPA. Unfortunately, tPA was not completely successful in restoring the blood supply to the myocardium, and he needed angioplasty later that evening.

17. What are the contraindications for tPA?

Contraindications for tPA include the following (Bucher & Melander, 1999):

- Active internal bleeding
- Intracranial neoplasm or recent head injury
- Prolonged, traumatic cardiopulmonary resuscitation
- Suspicion of aortic dissection
- Pregnancy
- History of hemorrhagic, cerebrovascular accident, or recent nonhemorrhagic cerebrovascular accident

- Recorded blood pressure greater than 200/120 mm Hg
- Trauma or surgery, that is, a potential bleeding source, within the previous 2 weeks
- Allergy to streptokinase or anisoylated plasminogen streptokinase activator complex if being considered

18. What is a PTCA?

A PTCA is an effective revascularization procedure used to increase the diameter of coronary arteries that have been stenosed by CAD and therefore to increase coronary blood flow (Lessig & Lessig, 1998). The PTCA is performed in the catheterization laboratory. Using fluoroscopy, the cardiologist inserts a catheter through the femoral or radial artery and guides it through the ascending aorta and into the ostium of the right or left coronary artery. A balloon-tipped catheter is passed into the area of blockage and the balloon is inflated for 30 to 129 seconds. This occludes the blood flow to the area of the heart supplied by this artery, and the patient may experience chest pain for the few seconds after the balloon is inflated. The balloon compresses the plaque against the artery lumina and also stretches the lumina of the artery to allow improved blood flow. The balloon may need to be deflated and reinflated several times to decrease the obstruction and open the clogged blood vessel (Becker, 1999; Clochesy et al, 1996; Lessig & Lessig, 1998). Progression of coronary atherosclerosis remains a significant problem after PTCA, requiring patients to make ongoing modifications in their risk factors for coronary disease and lifestyle. Research has supported the reduction in risks for CAD by positive lifestyle modifications and by drug interventions (e.g., lipid- and blood pressure–lowering therapy, and aspirin therapy). Most patients need comprehensive risk factor modification plans. When patients are educated regarding lifestyle changes, achieving balance seems to be the most realistic, attainable, and satisfying approach to use (Gulanick, Bliley, Perino, & Keough, 1998).

19. What made Mr. Smith a candidate for PTCA? What are the potential complications for a patient undergoing PTCA?

The indications for PTCA are as follows:

- Unstable or chronic angina
- AMI and post-AMI
- Postoperative angina after coronary artery bypass grafting

The ideal patient has single- or double-vessel disease with at least 50% stenosis; a lesion that is discrete; preferably proximal, noncalcific, concentric blockage located away from bifurcations; and the potential to survive emergency surgery if the procedure is complicated or fails. PTCA is contraindicated in patients with left main CAD, especially if the patient is not considered a good surgical risk, in patients with variant angina, in patients with vessels stenosed at the orifice by the aortic wall, and in patients with critical valvular disease (Clochesy et al, 1996; Lessig & Lessig, 1998).

Complications of PTCA include the following:

- Acute coronary occlusion, necessitating emergency surgery
- Dissection of the artery

- Reaction to contrast medium
- Bleeding or hematoma at the insertion site; retroperitoneal bleeding
- Decrease in peripheral pulses distal to the insertion site
- Vasovagal reaction at time of sheath removal
- Pseudoaneurysm of artery
- Restenosis of artery within 6 months (30% to 40%)
- A clot breaking loose and migrating to other areas causing a stroke or MI

Mr. Smith was a candidate for a PTCA because he continued to experience pain after the thrombolytic therapy. Because of his continued pain, we can assume the atherosclerotic changes had caused blockage of a coronary artery. tPA is a "clot buster" and can be very successful in restoring adequate blood supply to the heart; however, sometimes it is not enough, and the patient continues to experience chest pain as the artery remains occluded. PTCA allows the cardiologist to compress the plaque and so that blood flow resumes.

20.   What is a stent and why was it used on Mr. Smith?

A stent is a small, circular, stainless steel tube that fits on the end of the balloon-tipped catheter and is inserted into a coronary artery just after PTCA to prevent reocclusion or to help repair a dissection. Stents are also used after restenosis in patients who had undergone previous angioplasties. Evidence has shown that there is a benefit of stenting in patients in whom there was renarrowing of a coronary vessel after balloon angioplasty (Erbel et al, 1998; Topol, 1998). Holmes (1999) states, "Coronary stenting has revolutionized the practice of interventional cardiology and has arguably been as large an incremental step as the initial introduction of percutaneous transluminal coronary angioplasty." To place a stent, the guidewire with the balloon is withdrawn, and another guidewire with the stent and balloon is placed at the occlusion. Inflating the balloon causes the stent to expand and embeds it into the lumen of the artery. After the balloon is deflated and removed, the stent remains in place, keeping the artery open. Placing a stent requires that the patient had been receiving anticoagulant therapy for 6 to 8 weeks. Zidar (1998) states, "This trial (ENTICES) has demonstrated that the combination of enoxaparin (Lovenox), ticlopidine (Ticlid), and aspirin after elective stenting is a well-tolerated and effective treatment strategy to decrease ischemic complications and hemorrhagic vascular complications."

21.   What do the readings from the pulmonary artery catheter tell the nurse about Mr. Smith?

Heart function is optimal when there is a balance between myocardial oxygen demand and myocardial oxygen supply. "Cardiac output is a function of heart rate and stoke volume. If the volume ejected decreases, the heart rate will increase as a compensatory mechanism to maintain the same cardiac output. If the heart rate is unable to maintain the same level of cardiac output, blood pressure will drop" (Becker, 1999). The determinants of cardiac output are preload, afterload, contractility, and heart rate. Therapy can be implemented to affect each of the determinants of cardiac output to achieve optimum heart function (Clochesy et al, 1996).

Preload

Preload is defined as the volume of pressure generated at end-diastole. LV preload is recorded as the pulmonary artery wedge pressure (PAWP). A normal PAWP is between 6 and 12 mm Hg. The PAWP can be used to monitor the relative extent of pulmonary congestion. A PAWP of 18 to 20 mm Hg is considered moderate congestion, and a PAWP of greater than 30 mm Hg is acute pulmonary edema. Right ventricular preload is recorded as the central venous pressure or the right atrial pressure and the normal is 2 to 7 mm Hg.

Afterload

Afterload is defined as the impedance to the ejection of blood from the ventricle. It is the resistance that the ventricle must overcome to eject blood in a forward direction. The two determinants of afterload are (1) the volume and mass of blood ejected from the ventricle and (2) the compliance and total cross section of the vascular space into which the blood is ejected.

Right ventricle afterload is recorded as peripheral vascular resistance (PVR). The normal PVR is 150 to 250 dynes/sec/cm^{-5}. LV afterload is systemic vascular resistance, the normal of which is 800 to 1500 dynes/sec/cm^{-5} (Clochesy et al, 1996).

Medications that decrease the systemic vascular resistance (SVR) include nitroprusside, hydralazine, and captopril. Dobutamine may also be used to decrease the SVR by increasing the cardiac output. Medications that increase the SVR include dopamine, epinephrine, norepinephrine, and phenylephrine (Clochesy et al, 1996; Lessig & Lessig, 1998).

Ranges of normal values for hemodynamic parameters are as follows (Clochesy et al, 1996):

RAP	1-7 mm Hg	PAWP	6-12 mm Hg
RVP		MAP	70-105 mm Hg
Systolic	15-25 mm Hg	SVR	800-1500 dynes/sec/cm^{-5}
Diastolic	0-8 mm Hg	PVR	150-250 dynes/sec/cm^{-5}
PAP		CO	4-8 L/min
Systolic	15-25 mm Hg	CI	2.5-4.5 L/min/m^2
Diastolic	8-15 mm Hg	SV	60-130 ml/beat

22. What is cardiogenic shock? What symptoms did Mr. Smith exhibit?

Cardiogenic shock is when the body's needs for oxygen are not met for a prolonged period. The body begins to compensate for the decreased oxygen supply by increasing the heart rate, stroke volume, and contractility. However, as the condition continues, these compensatory measures result in cardiac decompensation. The patient begins to show signs of shock: low blood pressure, increased or decreased heart rate, and decreased oxygen saturation. Auscultation of rales signifies that the patient is developing CHF or pulmonary edema. The patient may have a decreased level of consciousness, diaphoresis, nausea, and vomiting. This condition is critical and must be addressed immediately.

Mr. Smith's had an S_3 with wheezes on auscultation and his chest radiograph showed some CHF before angioplasty. After PTCA, his pulmonary artery systolic pressure was 42 mm Hg, his pulmonary artery diastolic pressure was 22 mm Hg, and his Sao_2 dropped to 86%, requiring mechanical ventilation with a 100% nonrebreather mask. All of these represent moderate congestion of the lungs. He became hypotensive, tachycardic, pale, cool, and diaphoretic. These are typical signs of cardiogenic shock. After the PTCA, a IABP was placed to help decrease the workload of the heart and ease the cardiogenic shock. Therapy with dobutamine (Dobutrex) was started to increase his blood pressure and cardiac output.

23. What are the therapeutic effects of dopamine (Intropin) at low, moderate, and high dosages.

Dopamine has α- and β-adrenergic effects as well as dopaminergic effects. At low dosages of 1 to 2 μg/kg/min, it increases renal and mesenteric blood flow. At moderate dosages of 2 to 10 μg/kg/min, its positive inotropic effects increase cardiac output, blood pressure, and cerebral blood flow. At dosages greater than 10 μg/kg/min, dopamine exhibits pure α stimulation, causing peripheral vasoconstriction (with increased SVR and afterload) and loss of renal and mesenteric dilation. Dopamine is indicated to treat hypotension in shock states not caused by hypovolemia (LeFever-Key & Hayes, 1997; Lessig & Lessig, 1998).

24. What are the therapeutic effects of dobutamine (Dobutrex)?

Dobutamine (Dobutrex) stimulates β-receptors in the heart. It is a direct-acting positive inotropic agent. It increases stroke volume and cardiac output by increasing contractility and decreasing SVR (Lessig & Lessig, 1998).

Cardiogenic shock can be the result of a "stunned myocardium," a situation in which the heart does not work very well because the muscle is still in a state of shock from the decreased blood supply during the MI. Dobutamine can increase the cardiac output and stroke volume by increasing the heart's contractility, thereby decreasing the workload of the heart.

25. What advantage does an IABP offer Mr. Smith?

The purpose of the IABP is to decrease myocardial oxygen demand by decreasing myocardial workload, to increase coronary perfusion, and to decrease afterload. An IABP can prevent cardiogenic shock, limit infarct size, and limit myocardial ischemia (Lessig & Lessig, 1998). For Mr. Smith, the IABP was used because of cardiogenic shock after an AMI and refractory chest pain after administration of tPA.

To place an IABP, a balloon catheter is inserted via the femoral artery into the descending thoracic aorta. The inflation and deflation of the balloon are synchronized with the patient's ECG. The balloon is inflated during diastole, which augments diastolic pressure and increases coronary blood flow and myocardial oxygen supply. The result is improved myocardial contractility. The balloon is deflated just before systole, creating a vacuum effect. This helps the ventricle empty its contents more fully, reducing the LV end-diastolic pressure. In addition, deflation in systole reduces the afterload for the left ventricle, decreasing its myocardial oxygen requirements (Clochesy et al, 1996; Lessig & Lessig, 1998).

26. What significance does the IABP have in relation to the tPA and urokinase given previously?

Potential complications associated with the use of an IABP are (1) ischemia of the limb distal to the insertion site, (2) dissection of the aorta, (3) thrombocytopenia, (4) septicemia, and (5) infection at the insertion site (Lessig & Lessig, 1998). A common complication of IABP therapy is bleeding of the insertion site. The patient usually receives heparin (except after coronary artery bypass graft surgery) during the course of treatment with IABP, and this potentiates the bleeding.

Mr. Smith, who has received tPA and urokinase, has an extremely high risk of bleeding at the insertion site of the IABP. The insertion site, pulses in the left radial artery, peripheral pulses, urine output, and level of consciousness need to be checked every 15 minutes for the first 2 hours, then every 30 minutes for 2 hours, and then at least hourly.

27. Mr. Smith was sent home with a prescription for diltiazem (Cardizem). Why would a patient with heart disease be given a calcium channel blocker?

Calcium channel blockers decrease the entry of calcium into smooth muscle and dilate coronary arteries and peripheral arterioles. Vasodilation of the coronary arteries provides an increase in coronary blood flow and oxygen supply. Arteriolar vasodilation in peripheral circulation produces a reduction in afterload and reduces myocardial oxygen demand. This decreases systemic blood pressure, total peripheral resistance, and afterload of the heart. Platelet aggregation may be inhibited and bleeding prolonged (Alexander et al, 1998: Clochesy et al, 1996; Freeman-Clark, Queener, & Burke-Karb, 1997). Examples of calcium channel blockers include diltiazem (Cardizem), nifedipine (Procardia), and verapamil (Calan).

28. Why was Mr. Smith sent home with a prescription for captopril (Capoten)?

Captopril (Capoten) is an angiotensin-converting enzyme (ACE) inhibitor. ACE inhibitors block the conversion of angiotensin I to angiotensin II. Angiotensin II is a potent vasoconstrictor. The goal is to decrease the patient's blood pressure and afterload without causing an increase in heart rate or a change in cardiac output. Studies have shown that patients who exhibit LV dysfunction have improved mortality and morbidity rates from major cardiovascular events when these drugs are used (Becker, 1999). ACE inhibitors are continued for 4 to 6 weeks after MI.

PERCUTANEOUS TRANSLUMINAL CORONARY ANGIOPLASTY AND THROMBOLYTIC THERAPY

References

Alexander, R. W., Schlant, R. C., Fuster, V., O'Rourke, R. A., Roberts, R., & Sonnenblick, E. H. (1998). *Hurst's the heart* (9th ed.). St Louis: McGraw-Hill Health Professions Division.

American Heart Association. (1999). *Your heart* [WWW document]. URL http://www.americanheart.org/catalog/Heart_catpage16.html.

Antman, E. M., Tanasijevic, M. J., Thompson, B., Schactman, M., McCabe, C. H., Cannon, C. P., Fischer, G. A., Fung, A. Y., Thompson, C., Wybenga, D., & Braunwald, E. (1996). Cardiac-specific troponin I levels to predict the risk of mortality in patients with acute coronary syndromes. *New England Journal of Medicine, 335*, 1342-1349.

Aversano, T. (1998, September). Primary angioplasty in the treatment of acute myocardial infarction. In R. D. Bahr (Chair), *The strategy of chest pain units (in emergency departments) in the war against heart attacks: Proceedings of the First Maryland Chest Pain Center Research Conference*, Dearborn, MI [WWW document]. URL www.aspen.newc.com/chestpain/clinicalinformation/maryland/aversano.html.

Becker, D. (1999). Coronary artery disease. In L. Bucher & S. Melander (Eds.), *Critical care nursing* (pp. 201-225). Philadelphia: Saunders.

Braunwald, E. (Ed.). (1997). *Heart disease: A textbook of cardiovascular medicine* (5th ed., Vols. 1 and 2). Philadelphia: Saunders.

Bucher, L., & Melander, S. (Eds.). (1999). *Critical care nursing*. Philadelphia: Saunders.

Cairns, J. A., Theroux, P., Lewis, H. D., Jr. Ezekowitz, M., Meade, T. W., & Sutton, G. C. (1998). Antithrombic agents in coronary artery disease. *Chest, 114*(Suppl. 5), 611-628.

Casserly, I. P., Hasdai, D., Berger, P. B., Holmes, D. R., Jr. Schwartz, R. S., & Bell, M. R. (1998). Usefulness of abciximab for treatment of early coronary artery stent thrombosis. *The American Journal of Cardiology, 82*, 981-984.

Clochesy, J. M., Breu, C., Cardin, S., Whittaker, A. A., & Rudy, E. B. (Eds.). (1996). *Critical care nursing* (2nd ed.). Philadelphia: Saunders.

Erbel, R., Haude, M., Hopp, H. W., Franzen, D., Rupprecht, H. J., Heublein, B., Fischer, K., DeJaegere, P., Serruys, P., Rutsch, W., & Probst, P. (1998). Coronary-artery stenting compared with balloon angioplasty for restenosis after initial balloon angioplasty. *The New England Journal of Medicine. 339*, 1672-1678.

Freeman-Clark, J. B., Queener, S. F., & Burke-Karb, V. (1997). *Pharmacologic basis of nursing practice* (5th ed.). St Louis: Mosby.

Gulanick, M., Bliley, A., Perino, B., & Keough, V. (1998). Recovery patterns and lifestyle changes after coronary angioplasty: The patient's perspective. *Heart & Lung, 27*, 253-262.

Gurfinkel, E., Fareed, J., Antman, E., Cohen, M., & Mautner, B. (1998). Rationale for the management of coronary syndromes with low-molecular-weight heparins. *The American Journal of Cardiology, 82*, 151-181.

Global Use of Strategies to Open Occluded Coronary Arteries in Acute Coronary syndromes (GUSTO IIb). (1997). A clinical trial comparing primary coronary angioplasty with tissue plasminogen activator for acute myocardial infarction. *New England Journal of Medicine, 336*, 1621-1627.

Hasdai, D., Rihal, C. S., Bell, M. R., Berger, P. B., Grill, D. E., Garratt, K. N., & Holmes, D. R., Jr. (1998). Abciximab administration and outcome after intracoronary stent implantation. *The American Journal of Cardiology, 82*, 705-709.

Holmes, D. R., Jr. (1999, January). Coronary stenting: a revolution in cardiology. *Cardiology Today.*

Key Pharmaceuticals, Inc. (1998). Product information: Integrilin. Kenilworth, NJ.

Kline-Rogers, E., Martin, J. S., & Smith, D. D. (1999). New era of reperfusion in acute myocardial infarction. *Critical Care Nurse, 19* (1), 21-31.

LeFever-Kee, J., & Hayes, E. R. (1997). *A pocket companion for pharmacology. A nursing process approach* (2nd ed.). Philadelphia: Saunders.

Lessig, M. L., & Lessig, P. M. (1998). The cardiovascular system. In J. G. Alspach (Ed.). *American Association of Critical-Care Nurses: Core curriculum for critical care nursing* (5th ed.). Philadelphia: Saunders.

Murphy, M. J., & Berding, C. B. (1999). Use of measurements of myoglobin and cardiac troponins in the diagnosis of acute myocardial infarction. *Critical Care Nurse, 19*(1), 58-66.

Riegel, B. (1996). Myocardial infarction. In J. M. Clochesy, C. Brew, S. Cardin, A. A. Whittaker, E. B. Rudy (Eds.). *Critical care nursing* (2nd ed.). Philadelphia: Saunders.

Tcheng, J. E. (1996). Glycoprotein IIb/IIIa receptor inhibitors: putting the EPIC, IMPACT II, RESTORE, and EPILOG trials into perspective. *American Journal of Cardiology, 78,* 35-40.

Topol, E. J. (1998). Coronary-artery stentsógauging, gorging, and gouging. *New England Journal of Medicine. 339,* 1702-1703.

Twombly, R. (1997, November 10). Study reversal: Direct angioplasty isn't better than clot-busting drugs for treating heart attacks [WWW document]. *Duke Medical Center News,* URL http://news.mc.duke.edu/.

VanRiper, S., & VanRiper, J. (1997). *Cardiac diagnostic tests. A guide for nurses.* Philadelphia: Saunders.

Zidar, J. P. (1998). Low-molecular-weight heparins in coronary stenting (the ENTICES trial). *The American Journal of Cardiology. 82*(Suppl. 5B), 29-32.

CHAPTER 6

CORONARY ARTERY BYPASS GRAFT

Karen L. Jones, RNC, BSN, MSN • Sheila Drake Melander, RN, DSN, ACNP-C, FCCM

CASE PRESENTATION

Mr. Howard, a 57-year-old man, had a 3-month history of progressive typical anginal chest pain. He reported that the symptoms first occurred with heavy exertion and involved what he described as a "heaviness" in his chest. The symptoms were promptly relieved with rest. Over the past weeks, he had been experiencing increasingly frequent episodes of chest pain and diaphoresis. The episodes had become more prolonged, and he had experienced one episode of pain occurring at rest after a heavy meal. Mr. Howard was moderately obese and had a 20-year history of hypertension, which was being treated. Other risk factors in Mr. Howard's history include hypercholesterolemia (350 mg/dl), which he was attempting to treat with dietary modifications, and a 30-year, two-packs-a-day smoking history, which continued up to the present time. Mr. Howard previously had surgery for a bilateral inguinal hernia repair, cholecystectomy, and arthroscopic surgery on his left knee. He also gave a history of problems with gastric reflux and was currently taking cimetidine (Tagamet).

Mr. Howard was evaluated by his family physician after a prolonged episode of chest pain. The results of an electrocardiogram (ECG) were unremarkable; however, in view of the progression of his symptoms, he was referred to a cardiologist. Mr. Howard underwent a stress treadmill examination with a thallium scan. The stress test was terminated after 3.2 minutes because he developed anterior chest pain. This pain was promptly relieved with administration of sublingual nitroglycerin. The thallium scan revealed two areas of reversible defects in the anterior wall of the left ventricle. The decision was made to proceed with cardiac catheterization to further delineate the extent of disease. Cardiac catheterization revealed the following:

- Severe triple-vessel coronary artery disease was found with significant left main stenosis of 70%.
- The left anterior descending coronary artery (LAD) had 99% obstruction.
- The right coronary artery (RCA) had 90% (dominant) obstruction.
- The first obtuse marginal ramus (OM1) had 80% obstruction.

- The mitral and aortic valves both appeared normal and were without significant stenosis or regurgitation.
- The left ventricular end-diastolic pressure (LVEDP) was 7 mm Hg before injection and 14 mm Hg after dye injection. The left ventricular ejection fraction was estimated to be within the normal range at 55%.
- Mild to moderate hypokinesia was seen in the anterior wall.
- The left internal mammary artery was found to be of good caliber and available for a conduit.

Because of the critical stenosis of the left main coronary artery and the presence of severe triple-vessel disease, angioplasty was ruled out. Urgent coronary artery revascularization was scheduled for the next morning, with bypass grafts proposed to the LAD, diagonal artery, RCA, circumflex coronary artery, and OM1. Immediately after the catheterization, Mr. Howard developed severe (rated as a 9 on a 1 to 10 pain scale) anterior chest pain with radiation to the left arm. He became diaphoretic, and his systolic blood pressure fell to 90 mm Hg. He was given intravenous (IV) nitroglycerin and an infusion of dobutamine (Dobutrex) (3 µg/kg/min) to stabilize his condition. Because of the left main artery stenosis, an intraaortic balloon pump (IABP) was inserted via the left femoral artery. Excellent augmentation was obtained with a 2:1 setting, and all pain was relieved. The next morning, cardiac surgery was performed, using the left internal mammary artery to bypass the LAD, with separate saphenous vein grafts placed to the LAD, diagonal artery, OM1, and RCA. Atrial and ventricular pacing wires were placed. The IABP was left in place and functioned before and after the bypass. The surgery was uneventful, and Mr. Howard was admitted to the open-heart recovery area 4 hours after initiation of anesthesia.

On Mr. Howard's admission to the open-heart recovery area, the following data were obtained:

BP	110/70 mm Hg (via arterial line)	PAP	25/8/18 mm Hg (systolic, diastolic, MAP)
HR	110 bpm (sinus tachycardia)	PCWP	7 mm Hg
		Cardiac index	2.3 L/min/m² (cardiac output: 4.2 L/min)
Respirations	10 breaths/min (ventilation with IMV 10)	SVR	1500 dyne/sec/cm^{-5}
Temperature	35.1° C (95.2° F)		

A chest x-ray film confirmed correct placement of the pulmonary artery (Swan-Ganz) catheter, endotracheal tube, and nasogastric tube.

The following laboratory data were obtained:

Hgb	10.3 g/dl	Glucose	220 mg/dl
Hct	31%	K$^+$	3.2 mmol/L

The following ventilator settings were used:

IMV	10	Fio$_2$	90%
V$_T$	1000 ml	PEEP	5 cm

Arterial blood gas measurements showed the following:

pH	7.38	HCO_3^-	16 mmol/L
Po_2	96 mm Hg	Sao_2	96%
Pco_2	24 mm Hg		

The following lines were placed:

- Right radial arterial line
- Pulmonary artery (Swan-Ganz) catheter in the right subclavian vein
- Endotracheal tube (oral)
- Nasogastric tube via the left nares to low continuous suction
- Peripheral IV line via no. 19 angiocatheter in left forearm
- Chest tube in mediastinum, which drained 150 ml since placement
- Foley catheter
- IABP

Mr. Howard's urinary output values were as follows:

- Produced 300 ml of urine during bypass
- Produced 250 ml since termination of bypass

The following drugs were given via drip:

- Dobutamine (Dobutrex) 5 µg/min
- Nitroglycerin 15 µg/min

CORONARY ARTERY BYPASS GRAFT

Questions

1. Discuss the pathophysiology of coronary artery atherosclerosis. Include a discussion of risk factors associated with the development of this disease. How does Mr. Howard fit the profile of the "typical" patient who has coronary artery bypass graft (CABG) surgery?
2. Explain the purpose of thallium scanning and include a discussion of Mr. Howard's findings and how these led to the decision to proceed with cardiac catheterization.
3. What are the indications for CABG surgery? Why was angioplasty not considered as an option for Mr. Howard? What would be the relative risk of CABG surgery for Mr. Howard?
4. Discuss the significance of left main coronary artery stenosis.
5. Mr. Howard requested that the surgeon perform the "new" minimally invasive surgery. Discuss minimally invasive direct coronary artery bypass graft (MIDCABG) surgery and its applicability to Mr. Howard's case.
6. Discuss the mode of action of the IABP and the reason for its use in this case.
7. Compare and contrast the use of the internal mammary artery and saphenous vein as conduits in CABG surgery. What are the relative benefits and concerns associated with each?

8. Explain the purpose of the pulmonary artery (Swan-Ganz) catheter in Mr. Howard. Include in the discussion normally expected parameters. What are the potential complications associated with its use?

9. Describe the reason for use of dobutamine (Dobutrex) and nitroglycerin (Tridil) in Mr. Howard. How do each of these drugs affect volume, preload, contractility, and afterload? Discuss the parameters used in titrating these drugs.

10. Analyze the hemodynamic findings as presented and discuss therapy adjustments that might be necessary.

11. Based on the arterial blood gas results, are the ventilator settings correct? If not, what alterations would you recommend and why? What complications might be expected as a consequence of Mr. Howard's history of smoking?

12. Describe the cardiopulmonary bypass machine, and discuss myocardial protection during surgery. What are the potential complications associated with the bypass machine?

13. What is the expected postoperative chest tube drainage in a patient after CABG surgery? Discuss autotransfusion as it relates to patients undergoing CABG surgery.

14. List appropriate nursing diagnoses that might be used in planning care for the patient after CABG surgery.

15. Discuss lifestyle modifications that might be necessary after CABG surgery. What is the importance of a cardiac rehabilitation program in the recovery of the patient?

CORONARY ARTERY BYPASS GRAFT

Questions and Answers

1. Discuss the pathophysiology of coronary artery atherosclerosis. Include a discussion of risk factors associated with the development of this disease. How does Mr. Howard fit the profile of the "typical" patient who has coronary artery bypass graft (CABG) surgery?

Atherosclerosis produces a hardening of the arteries or thickening of the arterial walls. Atherosclerosis generally is characterized by lipid deposits that can progress to partial or total obstruction of the lumen wall. Coronary arteries are particularly susceptible to atherosclerosis, which is most commonly seen in patients with a history of smoking, sedentary lifestyle, and high-fat diets. The exact cause is still unknown. There are basically two theories with widespread acceptance: the response to injury theory and the thrombogenic theory. The atherosclerotic lesion or plaque consists of an elevated area of fatty streaks, which are muscle cells filled with lipids and secondary deposits of calcium salts and blood products. An elevated level (>200 mg) of cholesterol is associated with an increased risk for development of coronary artery disease (Bucher & Melander, 1999; National Institutes of Health, 1989).

Risk factors can be divided into two categories: modifiable and nonmodifiable. Nonmodifiable risk factors are uncontrollable and include age older than 55 years, gender (men have a greater incidence than women until menopause), family history of coronary artery disease, and race (African Americans have a higher incidence than whites). Modifiable risk factors are controllable and include hypertension (blood pressure >140/90 mm Hg), smoking, hyperlipidemia (increased low-density lipoprotein levels), obesity, stress, diabetes, and sedentary lifestyle (Bucher & Melander, 1999; Castelli, Garrison, Wilson, Abbott, Kalousdian, & Kannel, 1986).

Mr. Howard's history fits the "typical" profile of a patient who has CABG surgery. He is moderately obese and has a 20-year history of hypertension. He also has hypercholesterolemia with a laboratory value of 350 mg/dl, which he states he is attempting to modify through his diet. Mr. Howard also has a 30-year, two-packs-a-day smoking history and a family history positive for coronary atherosclerosis.

2. Explain the purpose of thallium scanning and include a discussion of Mr. Howard's findings and how these led to the decision to proceed with cardiac catheterization.

Thallium-201 is the radioactive isotope used in conjunction with either a treadmill stress ECG or bicycle ergometer to differentiate between ischemia and infarction. Thallium scanning will reveal wall motor defects and evaluate heart pump performance during increased oxygen demand. When the thallium is injected during peak exercise, normal myocardium will have greater activity than abnormal myocardium; thus cold spots indicate decreased or absent blood flow. Ischemia is indicated by thallium scan results that are abnormal during exercise but that return to normal 4 hours after exercise. If the scan results indicate infarction, they will remain abnormal even after the patient has rested. If a patient has normal results from a thallium stress study, there may be no need for a cardiac catheterization (Julian, Cowan, & McLenachan, 1998, pp. 79-80).

Mr. Howard's stress thallium scan was terminated after 3.2 minutes because he developed anterior chest pain. The scan revealed two areas of reversible defects in the anterior wall of the left ventricle. Because of the test results, it was necessary to proceed with the cardiac catheterization for further evaluation of cardiac disease.

3. What are the indications for CABG surgery? Why was angioplasty not considered an option for Mr. Howard? What would be the relative risk of CABG surgery in Mr. Howard?

The following indicators for CABG surgery were stated by Gray and Matloff (1990, p. 15), Clochesy, Breu, Cardin, Whittaker and Rudy (1996, p. 386), and Alexander (1998, p. 1473):

- Chronic stable angina refractory to medical therapy
- Significant left main coronary occlusion (>50%)
- Triple-vessel coronary artery disease
- Left ventricular dysfunction or proximal LAD disease
- Unstable angina
- Left ventricular failure (congestive heart failure or cardiogenic shock)
- Critical triple-vessel disease after thrombolytic therapy
- Postinfarction angina with multivessel disease
- Acute left ventricular aneurysm in patients with nonmechanical cardiogenic shock, if the patient's condition is stabilized

- Mechanical defects such as ventricular septal defects, mitral regurgitation (intermittent and persistent), and cardiac rupture with tamponade

Mr. Howard's diagnosis was severe triple-vessel disease with significant left main stenosis, both of which indicate the need for CABG surgery and rule out the need for angioplasty.

4. Discuss the significance of left main coronary artery stenosis.

The left main coronary artery supplies the apex, part of the lateral wall, the anterior wall, and two thirds of the septum. Because of the amount of myocardium that depends on blood supply from the left main coronary artery, significant stenosis of this artery or the proximal LAD places the myocardium at increased risk for myocardial infarction. Prompt surgical intervention in patients with left main coronary artery disease has been effective in increasing their 3-year survival rates to 85% or 90% compared with medical treatment rates of 65% to 69% (Braunwald, 1992, p. 245; CASS, 1984; Willerson & Cohm, 1995, p. 403).

5. Mr. Howard requested that the surgeon perform the "new" minimally invasive surgery. Discuss minimally invasive direct coronary artery bypass graft (MIDCABG) surgery and its applicability to Mr. Howard's case.

The MIDCABG is a relatively new type of heart surgery done to bypass blockages in one or two coronary arteries. The procedure is most often used when the LAD needs to be bypassed. An obstruction in the right descending coronary artery may also be bypassed with this type of surgery. Obstructions in coronary arteries on the inferior and posterior portions of the heart are not amenable to this type of surgery. Approximately 10% of patients requiring coronary artery bypass grafting will be candidates for this type of surgery (Weinschelbaum et al, 1998). The major advantages are the smaller chest incision and the lack of use of the bypass machine (Calafiore, Teodori, & DiGiammarco, 1997). Both of these advantages translate into shorter lengths of stay in the hospital and fewer complications for most patients. There is a quicker return to normal activities and less morbidity associated with the surgery (Arom, Emery, Nicoloff, Flavin, & Emery, 1997; Magover, Benckart, Landreneau, Sakert, & Magovern, 1998; Subramanian, McCabe, & Geller, 1997).

For Mr. Howard, an MIDCABG is not the appropriate operation because of the complexity of his disease and the need for multiple bypass grafts.

6. Discuss the mode of action of the IABP and the reason for its use in this case.

The IABP is used to increase coronary artery perfusion and support failing coronary circulation. Indications for use of the IABP include the following:

1. Left ventricular failure after cardiac surgery
2. Unstable angina refractory to medications
3. Recurrent angina

4. Complications of acute myocardial infarction include the following (Bojar, 1992, p. 427):
    a. Cardiogenic shock
    b. Papillary muscle dysfunction
    c. Ventricular septal defect
    d. Refractory ventricular arrhythmias

The IABP inflates during diastole and deflates before systole. Balloon inflation is timed by using the dicrotic notch, which denotes the closure of the aortic valve. The inflation forces blood forward and backward simultaneously to increase coronary perfusion and decrease afterload. The forward flow increases perfusion to the organs and the periphery, whereas the backward flow forces an increased amount of blood into the coronary arteries. The sudden deflation reduces the pressure in the aorta and decreases afterload, which lessens the workload of the heart (Julian et al, 1998, p. 386).

The IABP was used in Mr. Howard after the catheterization, when he developed severe chest pain and his systolic pressure dropped to 90 mm Hg. Because of Mr. Howard's severe left main coronary artery stenosis, the IABP did assist in increasing coronary artery perfusion, decreasing his afterload, and lessening the workload of the heart. Once the IABP was in place, all pain was relieved.

7. **Compare and contrast the use of the internal mammary artery and saphenous vein as conduits in CABG surgery. What are the relative benefits and concerns associated with each?**

The conduits, or vessels, most commonly used today are the saphenous vein and the internal mammary (or internal thoracic) artery. Both conduits have been used successfully in surgical revascularization individually and in combination when multiple graft sites were necessary. The patency rate for saphenous vein grafts at 1 year is 98% but falls to 81% at 10 years. Advantages for use of the saphenous vein include technical ease, decreased harvest time, and flexibility of the vein.

The internal mammary artery is viewed by many as the graft of choice for bypass of the LAD (Loop et al, 1986; Lytle et al, 1994; Willerson & Cohm, 1995, p. 689). Use of both internal mammary arteries in younger patients enhances revascularization results and increases survival rates and graft longevity (Dougenis & Brown, 1998). As reported by Loop et al. (1986) and Grover, Johnson, Marshall, and Hammemeister (1994), the patency rate of the internal mammary artery at 10 years is 96%. The absence of valves minimizes luminal turbulence, which reduces the risk of occlusion by thrombosis. Angiography has validated the ability of the internal mammary artery to dilate in response to increased demand (Bojar, 1992, p. 124). Limitations include increased time needed for harvesting of the graft, increased bleeding, and increased postoperative chest wall discomfort. The internal mammary artery may not be suitable as a conduit because of small size, inadequate flow, or damage incurred during harvesting. In patients who have undergone chest wall irradiation, its use may also be limited. The internal mammary artery may be used as pedicle or as a free graft (Bojar, 1992, pp. 124-125).

8. **Explain the purpose of the pulmonary artery (Swan-Ganz) catheter in Mr. Howard. Include in the discussion normally expected parameters. What are the potential complications associated with its use?**

Postoperative hemodynamic monitoring is needed for patients after CABG surgery so that vascular tone (preload and afterload), myocardial contractility, cardiac output, and volume or fluid balance may be monitored at the bedside. This is accomplished through use of a pulmonary artery (Swan-Ganz) catheter. Postoperatively, patients may exhibit a low cardiac output because of preexisting heart disease or prolonged time on the cardiopulmonary bypass machine. In most patients, reduced preload is the cause of the reduced cardiac output. In addition, high systemic vascular resistance or increased afterload from vasoconstriction can result in patients with decreased cardiac output. Through use of the pulmonary artery (Swan-Ganz) catheter parameters can be assessed, and early intervention can be pursued to correct any postoperative problems (Bojar, 1994, pp. 137-142; Willerson & Cohm, 1995, p. 355).

The balloon-tipped pulmonary artery (Swan-Ganz) catheter allows for measurements of the following: (1) right atrial pressure (RAP) or central venous pressure (CVP) through use of the proximal port, which represents the right ventricular end-diastolic pressure and reflects venous return to the right side of the heart, and (2) CVP, which indicates pressure from the great veins and also the RAP and is used to monitor right ventricle function, central venous return, and blood volume.

Normal values for CVP vary from person to person; therefore it is important to monitor the trend in CVP along with the clinical picture. In general, values of 2 to 8 cm H_2O are considered within normal limits. The pulmonary artery (Swan-Ganz) catheter also measures (1) right ventricle pressures (RVP), (2) pulmonary artery pressures (PAP), and (3) pulmonary capillary wedge pressures (PCWP), which are measured through the distal port. Pulmonary artery systolic pressure represents pressures that are produced by the right ventricle. The pulmonary artery diastolic pressure reflects LVEDP and is used as a measure of diastolic filling and left ventricular function or preload. The PCWP reflects the left atrial pressures and is used in the assessment of left ventricular filling pressure (LVEDP). Left atrial pressure (LAP) measurement is achieved through percutaneous insertion of a catheter directly into the left atrium during cardiac surgery and brought out of the chest wall to be connected to pressure monitoring devices. This provides a continuous display of left atrium pressures, which can be used instead of inflating the balloon on the Swan-Ganz catheter to obtain a PCWP. LAP is the most accurate measurement of left ventricular preload and in the normal heart is the same as the LVEDP. Increased levels may be caused by decreased contractility, tachyarrhythmias, fluid overload, and mitral stenosis or regurgitation. Decreased levels may be caused by hypovolemia, indicating hemorrhage postoperatively (Alspach, 1998). See Table 6-1.

TABLE 6-1	Normal Hemodynamic Readings			
CVP		3 cm H_2O		
LAP		2 mm Hg		
	RAP	RVP	PAP	PCWP
Systolic	20-30 mm Hg	20-30 mm Hg		
Diastolic	1-5 mm Hg	10-20 mm Hg		
Mean arterial	2-6 mm Hg	2-6 mm Hg	10-15 mm Hg	4-12 mm Hg

9.   **Describe the reason for use of dobutamine (Dobutrex) and nitroglycerin (Tridil) in Mr. Howard. How do each of these drugs affect volume, preload, contractility, and afterload? Discuss the parameters used in titrating these drugs.**

Dobutamine (Dobutrex) is a synthetic catecholamine with mostly a β_1 effect. Dobutamine is more effective than dopamine for increasing myocardial contractility. It increases stroke volume and cardiac output by increasing contractility; it also decreases systemic vascular resistance and reduces the PCWP. Dobutamine is very effective in the treatment of heart failure, especially for patients who are hypotensive and cannot tolerate vasodilator therapy. Dobutamine does not have the renal vasodilating effect of dopamine, except indirectly as an effect of increased cardiac output. At low dosages, dobutamine can decrease blood pressure, especially if the patient is volume depleted. A major advantage of dobutamine is its effect of reducing the PCWP or left ventricular preload, which is especially important in patients after surgery. Many physicians combine this drug with dopamine to maximize the renal blood flow and reduce the PCWP. An arterial line should be used to assess blood pressure. Dobutamine should be infused via a volumetric infusion pump. The normal dosage is 2.5 to 20 μg/kg/min, which should be titrated on the basis of hemodynamic parameters (Opie, 1997, pp. 161-162).

Nitroglycerin (Tridil) is a nitrate and a direct smooth muscle relaxant. This drug produces smooth muscle relaxation, which causes decreased peripheral vascular resistance. Hypotension may occur as a result of peripheral vasodilation. Patients may complain of headaches from the cerebral vasodilation. This pooling of blood in the systemic circulation decreases venous return and decreases preload. It is indicated for left ventricular failure, hypertension, angina pectoris, and congestive heart failure; it is also indicated after cardiac surgery. Patients should have an arterial line so that continuous blood pressure readings may be obtained. Nitroglycerin should be infused via a volumetric infusion pump for accuracy and safety. Usually, the IV infusion is started at 5 μg/min and titrated to the lowest amount that produces the desired effect. This drug should not be stopped suddenly but instead should be tapered by reducing the flow rate 5 to 10 μg every 15 minutes. During the tapering process, the patient should be constantly observed for return of ischemic symptoms or hypertension (Opie, 1997, pp. 31-40).

10.   **Analyze the hemodynamic findings as presented and discuss therapy adjustments that might be necessary.**

The hemodynamic parameters that would be of concern are the increased heart rate at 110 bpm, blood pressure of 110/70 mm Hg, PCWP of 7 mm Hg, cardiac index of 2.3 L/min/m² body surface area, systemic vascular resistance of 1500 dyne/sec/cm^{-5}, and temperature of 35.1° C (95.2° F). These data indicate that the patient is "dry" and cold. When the patient begins to warm up after surgery, the vasodilation coupled with volume depletion could possibly cause the patient to "bottom out" hemodynamically. Administration of plasma expanders, such as albumin, and possibly an increase in the rate of IV fluids should be instituted at this time.

11.   **Based on the arterial blood gas results, are the ventilator settings correct? If not, what alterations would you recommend and why? What complications might be expected as a consequence of Mr. Howard's smoking history?**

Mr. Howard's pH is slightly acidotic even though it is currently within normal limits. His Pco_2 value is a little low, as is his HCO_3^-; to prevent hyperventilation, incrementally increasing the positive end-expiratory pressure (PEEP) to 7.5 cm H_2O, and to 10 cm H_2O if needed, while monitoring the blood pressure, would improve Mr. Howard's ventilation. According to the successful use of the PEEP, the fraction of inspired oxygen may be decreased from 90% to 80%. Arterial blood gas measurements should be obtained in 1 hour to evaluate the patient's response to these changes.

Mr. Howard's extensive history of smoking may increase the difficulty level of weaning Mr. Howard from the ventilator postoperatively. He could develop increased secretions, which could alter oxygen exchange. Close monitoring of Mr. Howard's arterial blood gas results, vital signs, and airway secretions may be necessary.

12. **Describe the cardiopulmonary bypass machine and discuss myocardial protection during surgery. What are the potential complications associated with the bypass machine?**

The cardiopulmonary bypass machine provides a mechanism to divert the patient's blood from the arrested heart's right atrium through a membrane or a bubble oxygenator. Once in the oxygenator, carbon dioxide is given off and oxygen is bound to hemoglobin through diffusion. Once arterialized with oxygen, the blood is returned to the systemic circulation through the aorta. This diversion creates a bloodless, motionless area in which to operate. The patient is systemically given heparin before initiation of the bypass pump to prevent clotting within the bypass circuit (Clochesy et al, 1996).

Myocardium protection during bypass surgery has been a concern from inception of this surgery. Experience has shown that the key to myocardium preservation is continuous myocardial hypothermia. This decreases the need for oxygen. A balance must be struck between heat escaping and heat entering the tissues, especially during cross-clamping of the aorta. To prevent tissue injuries from warm venous blood entering the heart chambers, cold cardioplegia and topical cooling measures are used. Intermittent infusion of cardioplegic solution approximately every 20 to 30 minutes after the initial dose for diastolic arrest is necessary for the maintenance of myocardial hypothermia and cardioplegic arrest. Whether a cooling jacket, topical measures, or cardioplegia is used, myocardial hypothermic temperatures should remain between 12 and 20° C below normal to provide adequate protection (Clochesy et al, 1996; Gray & Matloff, 1990). Potential complications from the use of the cardiopulmonary bypass are outlined as probable causes and effects in Table 6-2.

13. **What is the expected postoperative chest tube drainage in a patients after CABG surgery? Discuss autotransfusion as it relates to patients undergoing CABG surgery.**

Bojar (1994) states that more than 300 to 400 ml of chest tube drainage during the first 2 hours after bypass surgery would be reason to reenter the chest to assess the situation. Normal chest tube drainage should be no more than 100 to 150 ml/hr. One of the dangers of increased bleeding is cardiac tamponade.

TABLE 6-2 Potential Complications of Cardiopulmonary Bypass	
Causes	Effects
Third space losses, postoperative diuresis, sudden vasodilation (drugs, rewarming)	Intravascular fluid deficit (hypotension)
Decreased plasma protein concentration, increased capillary permeability	Third space losses (weight gain, edema) and subsequent relative hypovolemia
Hypothermia, increased systemic vascular resistance, prolonged cardiopulmonary bypass pump time, preexisting heart disease, inadequate myocardial protection	Myocardial depression (decreased cardiac output)
Systemic heparinization, mechanical trauma to platelets, depressed release of clotting factors from liver as a result of hypothermia	Coagulopathy (bleeding)
Decreased surfactant production, pulmonary microemboli, interstitial fluid accumulation in the lungs	Pulmonary dysfunction (decreased lung mechanics and impaired gas exchange)
Red blood cell damage in pump circuit	Hemolysis (hemoglobinuria)
Decreased insulin release, stimulation of glycogenolysis	Hyperglycemia (rise in serum glucose)
Intracellular shifts during bypass, postoperative diuresis secondary to hemodilution	Hypokalemia and hypomagnesemia
Inadequate cerebral perfusion, microemboli to the brain	Neurologic dysfunction
Catecholamine release and systemic hypothermia causing vasoconstriction	Hypertension

Data from Thelan, L., Urden, L., Lough, M., & Stacy, K. (1998). *Critical care nursing: Diagnosis and management* (3rd ed.). St Louis: Mosby.

Autotransfusion is a mechanism in which the patient's own blood can be collected, filtered, and reinfused to minimize complications from using blood from donors or the blood bank system. Heparin or regional anticoagulants such as citrate phosphate dextrose or acid phosphate dextrose are added to the autotransfusion collection system. The blood may then be reinfused to the patient as whole blood or packed red blood cells. Potential complications are coagulation problems, air embolism, hemolysis, cardiac tamponade, and sepsis. Autotransfusion is a common procedure after open-heart surgery and is accomplished through use of mediastinal drainage systems. When these systems are used as autotransfusion mechanisms, it is necessary to remove all air and add a filter that will remove all clots before the blood is returned to the patient (Hartshorn, Lamborn, & Noll, 1993).

14. **List appropriate nursing diagnoses that might be used in planning care for the patient after CABG surgery.**

Nursing diagnoses for the patient after CABG surgery include the following (Bucher & Melander, 1999; Gordon, 1987; Vaca, Daake, & Lambrechts, 1997):

- Decreased cardiac output
- Ineffective airway clearance

- Ineffective breathing pattern
- Impaired gas exchange
- Altered tissue perfusion
- Activity intolerance
- Self-care deficit
- Altered body temperature, hypothermia
- Acute pain
- Altered sensory-perceptual deficit
- Altered thought processes
- Anxiety
- Fear
- Powerlessness
- Self-concept disturbance
- High risk for sexual dysfunction
- Fluid volume deficit
- High risk for fluid volume overload
- High risk for infection
- Impaired swallowing
- Impaired tissue integrity
- Altered oral mucous membranes
- High risk for constipation

15. Discuss lifestyle modifications that might be necessary after CABG surgery. What is the importance of a cardiac rehabilitation program in the recovery of the patient?

Patients who have had CABG surgery must maintain the regimen of care prescribed by their physicians after they leave the hospital. Nurses in the critical care unit begin instructing the patient in the regimen, and this process continues in the step-down units until the patient is discharged. Compliance is stressed in the areas of diet, exercise, medications, stress reduction, control of hypertension, and smoking cessation. As stated by Rankin, Hennein, and Keith (1994), risk modification and continued medical therapy are necessary after CABG surgery because atherosclerotic involvement of saphenous vein grafts is a long-term major complication. Lipid abnormalities must be treated through drug administration or diet to reduce the chance of reoperation for coronary artery disease.

Spouses or significant others should be included in all teaching sessions when possible. Patients and families should be linked to a support group, if possible. Cardiac rehabilitation must continue after discharge because it provides a built-in support group to assist in the maintenance of new lifestyle modifications. Often, rehabilitation facilities provide support groups for spouses of patients who had CABG surgery to emphasize food preparation (low-fat, low-cholesterol, low-sodium diets) or exercise. Spousal support groups can be effective in dealing with fears and concerns of the group members. Continuing cardiac rehabilitation once the patient is discharged from the hospital is the key to recovery after CABG surgery (Clochesy et al, 1996). Gray and Matloff (1990) state that participation in an inexpensive rehabilitation program involving simple calisthenics and graduated walking has been shown to significantly increase employment rates after surgery.

CORONARY ARTERY BYPASS GRAFT

References

Alexander, R. W., Schlant, R. C., Fuster, V., O'Rourke, R. A., Roberts, R., & Sonnenblick, E. H. (1998). *Hurst's the heart* (9th ed.). St Louis: McGraw-Hill Health Professions Division.

Alspach, J. G. (Ed.) (1991). *American Association of Critical-Care Nurses: Core curriculum for critical care nursing* (4th ed.). Philadelphia: Saunders.

Arom, K., Emery, R., Nicoloff, D., Flavin, T., & Emery, A. (1997). Minimally invasive direct coronary artery bypass grafting: Experimental and clinical experiences. *Annals of Thoracic Surgery, 63* (6, Suppl):548-552.

Bojar, R. (1992). *Adult cardiac surgery.* London: Blackwell.

Bojar, R. (1994). *Manual of perioperative care in cardiac and thoracic surgery.* London: Blackwell.

Bucher, L., & Melander, S. (Eds.). (1999). *Critical care nursing.* Philadelphia: Saunders.

Braunwald, E. (1992). *Heart disease* (4th ed.). Philadelphia: Saunders Company.

Calafiore, A., Teodori, G., & DiGiammarco, G. (1997). Minimally invasive coronary artery bypass grafting on a beating heart. *Annals of Thoracic Surgery, 63*: 572-575.

CASS Principle Investigators. (1984). Myocardial infarction and mortality in the coronary artery surgery study (CASS) randomized trial. *New England Journal of Medicine, 310*(12), 750-758.

Castelli, W. P., Garrison, R. J., Wilson, P. W., Abbott, R. D., Kalousdian, S., & Kannel, W. B. (1986). Incidence of coronary heart disease and lipoprotein cholesterol levels: The Framingham study. *JAMA, 256*(20), 2835-2838.

Clochesy, J., Breu, C., Cardin, S., Whittaker, A. & Rudy, E. (Eds.). (1996). *Critical care nursing* (2nd ed.). Philadelphia: Saunders.

Dougenis, D., & Brown, A. (1998). Internal mammary artery vs. saphenous vein grafts: Which is better? *Heart 80*, 9-13.

Gordon, M. (1987). *Nursing diagnosis: Process and application.* New York: McGraw-Hill.

Gray, R., & Matloff, J. (1990). *Medical management of the cardiac surgical patient.* Baltimore: Williams & Wilkins.

Grover, F., Johnson, R., Marshall, G., & Hammemeister, K. (1994). Impact of mammary grafts on coronary artery bypass operative mortality and morbidity. *Annals of Thoracic Surgery, 57*(3), 559-568.

Hartshorn, J., Lamborn, M., & Noll, M. (1993). *Introduction to critical care nursing.* Philadelphia: Saunders.

Julian, D., Cowan, J., & McLenachan, J. (1998). *Cardiology* (7th ed.). New York: Saunders.

Loop, F., Lytle, B., Cosgrove, D., Stewart, R., Goormastic, M., Williams, G., Golding, L., Taylor, P., & Sheldon, W. (1986). Influence of the internal mammary artery graft on 10 year survival and other cardiac events. *New England Journal of Medicine, 314*, 1-6.

Lytle, B., McElroy, D., McCarthy, P., Loop, F., Taylor, P., Goormastic, M., Stewart, R., & Cosgrove, D. (1994). Influence of arterial coronary artery bypass grafts on the mortality in coronary reoperations. *Journal of Thoracic Cardiovascular Surgery, 107*(3), 875-882.

Magover, J., Benckart, D., Landreneau, R., Sakert, T., & Magovern, G. (1998). Morbidity, cost, and six month outcome of minimally invasive direct coronary artery bypass grafting. *Annals of Thoracic Surgery, 66*(4), 1224-1229.

National Institutes of Health. (1989). *Report of the expert panel on the detection, evaluation, and treatment of high blood cholesterol in adults* (NIH Publication No. 89-2925). Bethesda, MD: Author.

Opie, L. (1997). *Drugs for the heart.* Philadelphia: Saunders.

Rankin, J., Hennein, H., & Keith, F. (1994). The heart: 1. Acquired disease.In *Current surgical diagnosis and treatment*. Norwalk, CT: Appleton & Lange.

Subramanian, V., McCabe, J., & Geller, C. (1997). Minimally invasive direct coronary artery bypass grafting: Two year clinical experience. *Annals of Thoracic Surgery, 64*(6), 1648-1653.

Thelan, L., Urden, L., Lough, M., & Stacy, K. (1998). *Critical care nursing: Diagnosis and management* (3rd ed.). St. Louis: Mosby–Year Book.

Vaca, K., Daake, C., & Lambrechts, D. (1997). Nursing care of patients undergoing thoracoscopic minimally invasive bypass grafting. *American Journal of Critical Care, 6*(4), 281-286.

Weinschelbaum, E., Rodriguez, C., Cabello, M., DosSantos, A., Machain, A., Bertolotti, O., & Fraguas, H. (1998). Left anterior descending coronary artery bypass grafting through minimal thoracotomy. *Annals of Thoracic Surgery, 66*(3), 1008-1011.

Willerson, J., & Cohm, J. (1995). *Cardiovascular medicine*. New York: Churchill Livingstone.

CHAPTER *7*

CARDIAC SHOCK IN ANTERIOR WALL MYOCARDIAL INFARCTION

Debra L. Harmon, RN, MSN, CCRN

CASE PRESENTATION

Mrs. Adams, a 50-year-old woman, came to the emergency department at 6:30 AM with a 2-hour history of crushing substernal chest pain radiating to the jaw, back, and subxiphoid area. She was mildly diaphoretic and slightly short of breath, and she complained of nausea. Her lungs had bibasilar crackles on auscultation. Heart sounds revealed the presence of an S_3 heart sound without murmurs. The initial chest x-ray film showed no abnormalities. Her initial vital signs were as follows:

BP	156/98 mm Hg	Respirations	30 breaths/min
HR	124 bpm	Temperature	37° C (98.6° F)

Mrs. Adams had a history of stable angina for an undetermined period of time. However, she revealed that for the past 3 weeks, she had experienced substernal pain radiating to the back every hour. Chest pain was relieved with sublingual nitroglycerin (NTG). There was a family history of a brother dying from a myocardial infarction (MI) and a sister with a history of three MIs. Mrs. Adams had a 30-year history of cigarette smoking and continued to smoke one pack of cigarettes a day. She has been taking the following medications:

- Aspirin 81 mg qd
- Propranolol hydrochloride (Inderal) 80 mg qd
- Isosorbide mononitrate (Imdur SR) 30 mg qd
- Diltiazem (Cardizem CD) 120 mg qd

Upon arrival at the emergency department, intravenous (IV) NTG 50 mg in 250 ml of dextrose 5% in water (D5W) was started and titrated to Mrs. Adams's pain level and blood pressure. Mrs. Adams was also given morphine sulfate 2 mg via slow IV push, and oxygen at 6 L through a nasal cannula was started. The initial 12-lead electrocardiogram (ECG) revealed early Q waves and massive

ST-segment elevation in leads V_1 to V_4. Initial baseline laboratory data results were as follows:

WBCs	13.9 mm^3	Myoglobin	120 ng/L
Glucose	117 mg/dl	K$^+$	4 mmol/L
Hgb	14 g/dl	Troponin T	0.0 µg/L
BUN	6 mmol/L	Cl$^-$	103 mmol/L
Hct	41.8%	CK-MB	1.8%
Creatinine	0.9 mg/dl	CO$_2$	24 mmol/L
Na$^+$	141 mmol/L	Troponin I	0.0 µg/L

Mrs. Adams was assessed and confirmed to be a candidate for thrombolytic therapy. A tissue plasminogen activator (tPA) bolus and infusion were given, and a weight-based heparin drip of 25,000 U/250 ml of D5W was started at 1200 U/hr. She was then transferred to the cardiac intensive care unit (CICU) at 8:30 AM.

Once the tPA infusion was complete, Mrs. Adams experienced pain relief and occasional premature ventricular contractions (PVCs). An echocardiogram revealed dyskinesia with the entire septum, apex, and anterior wall. The ejection fraction (EF) was 20%.

At 12:30 PM (6 hours later), enzyme and arterial blood gas levels were determined:

Myoglobin	150 ng/L	P$_{CO_2}$	52.1 mm Hg
pH	7.261	Troponin I	5.2 µg/L
CK-MB	36%	HCO$_3^-$	22.4 mmol/L

Mrs. Adams was then given 60% oxygen via face mask, and her vital signs were as follows:

BP	140/100 mm Hg
HR	130 bpm
Respirations	34 breaths/min

Day 1

The next morning, Mrs. Adams continued to complain of shortness of breath and restlessness with level 2 chest pain. Rales were auscultated throughout all lung fields. A chest x-ray film revealed increasing congestive heart failure (CHF) with pulmonary edema. Vital signs were as follows:

BP	100/60 mm Hg	Respirations	36 breaths/min
HR	128 bpm	Urine output	20 ml/hr for past 2 hr

Mrs. Adams was given dopamine (Intropin) at 5 µg/kg/min and dobutamine (Dobutrex) at 5 µg/kg/min. She was also given 40 mg of furosemide (Lasix) intravenously. The NTG drip was continued at the same rate as that when she was admitted to the CICU. Morning enzyme levels were as follows:

Myoglobin	63 ng/L	Troponin I	5.0 µg/L
CK-MB	24%	Troponin T	0.2 µg/L

A morning 12-lead ECG revealed resolution of the ST-segment elevation but development of a new left bundle-branch block (LBBB). Mrs. Adams was given another 40 mg of furosemide intravenously. The dopamine drip was continued with the order to titrate to maintain systolic blood pressure of 100 mm Hg, and the dobutamine drip was continued at 5 µg/kg/min. Because Mrs. Adams continued to complain of chest pain despite the NTG drip, placement of an intraaortic balloon catheter (IABP) and a pulmonary artery catheter was done in the catheterization laboratory.

After her return to the CICU, Mrs. Adams' vital signs and hemodynamic values were as follows:

BP	90/60 mm Hg	CO	2.5 L/min
PCWP	22 mm Hg	Respirations	30 breaths/min
SVR	1800 dynes/sec/cm^{-5}	CI	1.5 L/min/m^2
HR	130 bpm		

The IABP was timed at 1 to 1. Mrs. Adams continued to receive dopamine 6 µg/kg/min (to maintain blood pressure) and dobutamine 5 µg/kg/min. The NTG drip was decreased to 1 µg/kg/min to reduce afterload. The urine output had increased to 150 ml/hr, and the patient was breathing easier and was less restless and more alert.

Day 2

The morning of the second day of her hospital stay, Mrs. Adams' vital signs and hemodynamic values were as follows:

BP	100/60 mm Hg	CO	3 L/min
PCWP	18 mm Hg	Respirations	28 breaths/min
SVR	1420 dynes/sec/cm^{-5}	CI	2 L/min/m^2
HR	110 bpm		

Her cardiac enzyme levels continued to return to normal, and the transient LBBB was gone. Urine output was 100 ml/hr, and the drips remained unchanged.

Day 3

The morning of the third day, Mrs. Adams was free of pain and had unlabored respirations. Oxygen was decreased to 4 L/min through a nasal cannula. Vital signs and hemodynamic values were as follows:

BP	1000/60 mm Hg	CO	4 L/min
PCWP	14 mm Hg	Respirations	24 breaths/min
SVR	1250 dynes/sec/cm^{-5}	CI	2.1 L/min/m^2
HR	110 bpm		

The IABP settings were reduced to 2 to 1. The dopamine drip was decreased to 3 μg/kg/min, the dobutamine drip was reduced to 2 μg/kg/min, and the NTG drip was discontinued.

Day 5

By the morning of the fifth day, the vasoactive drips and the IABP were discontinued. Hemodynamic values were within normal range for Mrs. Adams, and her vital signs were as follows:

BP	110/60 mm Hg
HR	83 bpm
Respirations	22 breaths/min

Mrs. Adams was scheduled for an afternoon cardiac catheterization for follow-up after thrombolysis and her brief episode of cardiogenic shock.

CARDIOGENIC SHOCK IN ANTERIOR WALL MYOCARDIAL INFARCTION

Questions

1. What is the clinical presentation of a patient having an acute myocardial infarction (AMI)? Identify Mrs. Adams' clinical presentation to the emergency department.
2. How is a diagnosis of AMI determined? Identify the results for Mrs. Adams that confirmed the diagnosis of AMI.
3. What are the treatment goals for a patient with an AMI?
4. Discuss the role of thrombolytic therapy in a patient with AMI. Include indications and contraindications for use of thrombolytics.
5. Discuss the role of nitrates and β-blockers in the patient with AMI.
6. What are complications are commonly seen after a MI? What are the most common complications seen with an anterior wall MI?
7. What significant 12-lead ECG changes are sometimes seen following an anterior AMI? What 12-lead changes occurred with Mrs. Adams?
8. Define cardiogenic shock and why it occurs after an anterior MI. What is the prognosis for the patient with cardiogenic shock?
9. What are the hemodynamic parameters seen in the patient with cardiogenic shock in comparison to normal hemodynamic parameters?
10. Discuss the goals of pharmacologic management in cardiogenic shock. Which medications were used for Mrs. Adams?
11. What types of mechanical support devices can be used for patients in cardiogenic shock and why? Which type was used for Mrs. Adams? Identify any specific nursing responsibilities for the device chosen for Mrs. Adams.
12. What are the nursing diagnoses for the patient in cardiogenic shock after an anterior MI?

CARDIOGENIC SHOCK IN ANTERIOR WALL MYOCARDIAL INFARCTION

Questions and Answers

1. **What is the clinical presentation of a patient having an acute myocardial infarction (AMI)? Identify Mrs. Adams' clinical presentation to the emergency department.**

The clinical presentation of patients experiencing an AMI is established from a variety of physical findings that are influenced by the severity and location of the infarct. Chest pain is the most common physical finding of an acute coronary syndrome or AMI and occurs in approximately 70% to 80% of patients (American Heart Association [AHA], 1997). The pain is usually described as "substernal and as crushing, heavy, constricting, or oppressive discomfort," as stated by the AHA (1997, pp. 9-4). The chest pain may also radiate down the ulnar aspect of the left hand or involve the neck, jaw, teeth, shoulders, and intrascapular region. The pain may be confused with indigestion, but this is less commonly seen. In the Framingham study follow-up, 20% to 60% of first infarcts in men and 50% in women were symptomless or unrecognized (AHA, 1997). Furthermore, about half of these symptomless infarcts were truly silent, with the other 50% presenting with atypical chest pain.

According to Bucher (1999) and Lessig and Lessig (1998), patients experiencing an AMI are usually extremely uncomfortable, restless, anxious, and agitated. ECG patterns of patients with AMI may reveal symptomatic or nonsymptomatic bradycardia, tachyarrhythmias, ventricular ectopy, and/or atrioventricular blocks. Other cardiovascular findings include normotension or hypotension; additional heart sounds, consisting of S_3, S_4, new murmurs, and/or pericardial friction rubs; and signs of CHF, including shortness of breath, frothy sputum, jugular venous distension, peripheral edema, and auscultated crackles in lung fields. Urine output and peripheral pulses may be diminished as a result of decreased cardiac output (CO). Gastrointestinal symptoms may include nausea and vomiting, which are more common with female patients. Finally, the patient's integumentary assessment may reveal pallor and diaphoresis.

Mrs. Adams' Clinical Presentation

Mrs. Adams clinical presentation included 1 hour of substernal, crushing chest pain that radiated to the jaw, back, and subxiphoid area. Mrs. Adams was also diaphoretic and short of breath and complained of nausea. Heart sounds revealed the presence of an S_3.

2. **How is a diagnosis of AMI determined? Identify the results for Mrs. Adams that confirmed her diagnosis of AMI.**

Criteria established by the World Health Organization (WHO) to diagnose AMI are recognized by health care providers as the foundation of rapid treatment of AMI (Murphy & Berding, 1999). Two of the three following criteria must be met for a confirmed diagnosis of AMI:

1. ST-segment changes or new, pathologic Q waves must be present on the patient's ECG.

2. The patient must have a clinical presentation of reported chest pain characteristic of AMI.

3. The patient must have abnormally elevated serum levels of cardiac enzymes such as creatine kinase myocardial band (CK-MB), an isoenzyme of CK.

The initial and serial ECGs are the most useful tools for diagnosis of an AMI (Bucher, 1999). A baseline 12-lead ECG should be done as early as possible and continuous ECG monitoring should be initiated once chest pain develops to track changes in the evolution of the AMI. ECG changes associated with an AMI include patterns of ST-segment and T-wave abnormalities and the development of pathologic Q waves in the area of infarct. However, these ECG changes are not always present immediately on a 12-lead ECG. Bucher (1999) stated that as many as 50% of patients with chest pain who are actually having an AMI have normal or nondiagnostic 12-lead ECGs initially. Therefore normal results from an ECG alone do not rule out the possibility of cardiac dysfunction.

The clinical presentation, as described in question 1, helps establish the diagnosis of AMI. Although chest pain characteristics vary from person to person, it is a significant finding in the process of diagnosing an AMI.

Various cardiac serologic markers can be additional resources for early evaluation and diagnosing of an AMI. CK-MB has been the standard enzyme for AMI diagnosis for several years. Although CK-MB is the dominant isoenzyme of creatine kinase in the heart and is highly specific for myocardial tissue, timing of peak levels and return to normal levels limit the window of opportunity for diagnostic use (Brogan et al, 1997). The recent identification of three new markers—myoglobin, troponin I, and troponin T—has provided more sensitive indicators for diagnosing an AMI (Murphy & Berding, 1999). A comparison of the four markers is provided in Table 7-1 (Plaut, 1998). Although the CK-MB is the most specific and sensitive indicator after the first 3 hours of the onset of an AMI, myoglobin rises faster (30 minutes to 2 hours) and is more sensitive for AMIs with very early onset of symptoms (Murphy & Berding, 1999). The CK-MB returns to normal levels in 48 to 72 hours after elevation, whereas the cardiac troponins provide a longer diagnostic window by remaining sensitive for up to 15 days. The cardiac troponins would be better indicators of myocardial damage for those patients seen with chest pain for longer than 48 hours. Furthermore, CK-MB may be the best indicator for reinfarction that occurs between 48 hours and 7 days after initial chest pain because of its time window of normal and peak levels.

Although not part of the WHO diagnostic criteria, the echocardiogram is often used to confirm the infarction. Echocardiograms enable the physician to determine the extent of the MI by showing wall motion irregularities, structural damage, and EF (Kim, Adams, & Hendel, 1997).

TABLE 7-1 Acute Myocardial Infarction Serum Markers

Marker	Time Appears	Peak Time	Return to Normal
Myoglobin	0.5-2 hr	5-12 hr	18-30 hr
Troponin I	3-6 hr	14-20 hr	5-15 days
Troponin T	3-6 hr	10-24 hr	10-15 days
CK-MB	3-8 hr	9-30 hr	2-3 days

Modified from Plaut (1998).

CK-MB, creatine kinase myocardial band.

Note: These values depend on both the analytical method and the cutoff used.

Mrs. Adams' Diagnostic Results That Confirmed the AMI Diagnosis

Mrs. Adams' 12-lead ECG showed Q waves in leads V_1 to V_4, indicating an anterior wall MI. The baseline results indicated only elevated myoglobin with the other cardiac enzyme levels within the normal range. By the sixth hour enzyme, CK-MB, troponin I, and troponin T levels were elevated abnormally, indicative of extensive damage to the myocardium. The echocardiogram revealed a significantly reduced EF of 20% and dyskinesia affecting the entire septum, apex, and anterior wall.

3. **What are the treatment goals for a patient with an AMI?**

"Minutes means myocardium" is a saying often used by the AHA (1997) in regard to treating an AMI. The time to treatment is critical to patient outcomes. The closer the treatment is to the onset of AMI symptoms, the more optimistic the outcomes. Treatment strategies are focused on preserving the myocardium and reducing mortality and morbidity (AHA, 1997; Bucher, 1999). The goals for a patient with AMI are to limit the size of the infarct, support the heart during the shock, relieve pain, and manage arrhythmias. Other goals include providing education concerning the diagnosis and necessary lifestyle changes needed to prevent another infarct in the future.

4. **Discuss the role of thrombolytic therapy in a patient with AMI. Include indications and contraindications for use of thrombolytics.**

Thrombolytics are the most effective treatment for limiting infarct size according to the AHA (1997) and Bucher (1999). Eight percent to 90% of AMIs are the result of a thrombus or embolus. Dissolution of clots with thrombolytics has affected coronary artery reperfusion. Thrombolytic therapy and early reperfusion have become a standard of care for treatment of AMIs.

Thrombolytic therapy should be initiated within 6 hours of symptom onset for the greatest benefit. The earlier therapy is initiated, the lower the mortality. An additional selection criterion is ECG evidence of ST-segment elevation of 1 mm or more in two contiguous leads. Thrombolytics appear to be most effective in patients younger than 75 years who are experiencing their first anterior wall MI. Absolute contraindications include active hemorrhage (except menses), history of a hemorrhagic stroke, known intracranial neoplasm, and suspected aortic dissection. Relative contraindications include severe uncontrolled hypertension, current use of anticoagulants, pregnancy or recent delivery, recent trauma or major surgery (2 to 4 weeks), active peptic ulcer, and prolonged cardiopulmonary resuscitation longer than 10 minutes (AHA, 1997; Bucher, 1999).

Concurrent therapies recommended with thrombolytic therapy are oral aspirin 165 to 325 mg daily and intravenous weight-based heparin (AHA, 1997). The benefit of aspirin is a significant reduction in early mortality associated with AMI. The benefits of heparin are early coronary artery reperfusion and reduction of coronary artery reocclusion from clots.

Reperfusion Strategies Used for Mrs. Adams

Mrs. Adams received thrombolytic therapy in the form of tPA. She had experienced pain for approximately 2 hours and was only 50 years of age. Mrs. Adams had no obvious contraindications. Therapy with IV heparin was started concurrently with the tPA. She did not have any side effects from the thrombolysis except for reperfusion arrhythmias, which are expected.

5. Discuss the role of nitrates and β-blockers in the patient with AMI.

Nitrates are recommended for treating patients with AMI. NTG dilates the large coronary arteries, prevents vasospasm, and increases coronary collateral blood flow to the ischemic myocardium (AHA, 1997). Bucher (1999) suggests that NTG may trigger antiplatelet effects, reduce infarct size, and improve ventricular remodeling. Sublingual NTG decreases left ventricular filling pressure without significantly lowering systemic vascular resistance (SVR). IV NTG reduces both left ventricular filling pressure and SVR, which may result in hypotension. NTG must be administered cautiously because a 10% reduction in blood pressure may cause compromised coronary artery perfusion and aggravate myocardial ischemia (AHA, 1997).

β-Blocker therapy within 12 hours of onset of infarction has been confirmed to decrease infarct size, prevent extension of the infarct, and reduce mortality from AMI (AHA, 1997; Bucher, 1999). When β-blockers are started with thrombolytics, reinfarction rates and recurrent ischemia are reduced. IV metoprolol (Lopressor) or atenolol (Tenormin) should be started within 2 hours of infarct presentation for optimal effectiveness. β-Blockers are contraindicated in patients with bradyarrhythmias, hypotension, moderate to severe CHF, and certain pulmonary disorders such as severe chronic obstructive pulmonary disease and asthma.

Nitrate and β-Blocker Use for Mrs. Adams

Mrs. Adams received IV NTG for control of chest pain before the initiation of thrombolysis. She had been receiving propranolol 80 mg daily at home before this admission and was not given further β-blockade because of her pulmonary status during cardiogenic shock.

6. What complications are commonly seen after a MI? What are the most common complications seen with an anterior wall MI?

Complications after an AMI include the following, in order of occurrence: arrhythmias, heart failure, infarct expansion, left ventricular mural thrombus, pericarditis, cardiogenic shock, left ventricular aneurysm, and other structural defects (Bucher, 1999).

Specific complications of an anterior AMI include tachyarrhythmias (sinus tachycardia, atrial fibrillation, atrial flutter, paroxysmal supraventricular tachycardia, ventricular tachycardia, and ventricular fibrillation), left ventricular dysfunction, CHF, ventricular aneurysm, and other structural defects (Bucher, 1999).

A study conducted in 1997 attempted to predict early complications in patients with AMI by calculating the score of the ST segment in the admission ECG (Gwechenberger et al, 1997). Each patient enrolled in the study had a confirmed anterior or inferior AMI and was a candidate for thrombolysis. *Early complications* were defined as acute CHF or severe rhythm disturbances within 24 hours after thrombolysis. A finding seen in those who developed evidence of complications was that the sum of ST-segment elevations was significantly higher compared with that of patients without complications. The conclusions of the study revealed that the ST-segment score (the sum of all significant ST-segment elevations on the 12-lead

ECG greater than 1 mm from baseline) was useful in predicting the probability of early complications in patients with AMI after thrombolysis. This study may have an important effect on the further treatment of patients with AMI receiving thrombolysis.

Mrs. Adams' Complications

Mrs. Adams experienced several life-threatening complications after her anterior AMI. She developed heart failure, as was noted by her dyspnea, crackles in all lung fields, and chest x-ray film that depicted pulmonary edema. She developed cardiogenic shock and a new LBBB the first day after her anterior AMI.

7. What significant 12-lead ECG changes are sometimes seen following an anterior AMI? What 12-lead changes occurred with Mrs. Adams?

Most anterior AMIs are related to an occlusion of the left anterior descending (LAD) coronary artery. The LAD supplies blood to a large area of the left ventricle and almost all of the bundle of His and bundle branches of the ventricular conduction system. One of the most common ECG complications following an anterior AMI is the development of a LBBB (Bucher, 1999). A patient with LBBB has an increased risk for death from left ventricular failure, ventricular tachycardia, or ventricular fibrillation. However, early recognition and treatment can reduce mortality. Use of prophylactic temporary transvenous pacing followed by thrombolysis is the guideline recommended by the American College of Cardiology and the AHA for new LBBB after AMI.

Other arrhythmias commonly seen with an anterior wall MI include sinus tachycardia, PVCs, premature atrial contractions, atrial tachycardia, atrial flutter, and atrial fibrillation. Intraventricular conduction disturbances include right and left bundle branch blocks, and Mobitz II block progressing to complete atrioventricular block often occurs (Bucher, 1999).

Many of the aforementioned arrhythmias can prove fatal after an AMI in patients with CHF. A meta-analysis published in 1997 reviewed data from 6500 patients in randomized trials on the effects of prophylactic amiodarone on mortality after AMI and with CHF (Connolly, 1997). The data support prophylactic use of amiodarone and confirm an overall reduction in the rate of arrhythmia/sudden death in high-risk patients with recent AMI and CHF by 13% in total mortality. Prophylactic amiodarone may be a reasonable treatment for high-risk patients after an AMI.

Mrs. Adams' 12-Lead ECG Changes

Mrs. Adams experienced several rhythm disturbances during thrombolysis, which were expected. However, she did develop a transient LBBB with cardiogenic shock on her first day after the anterior AMI. The LBBB resolved without intervention by the third day.

8. Define cardiogenic shock and why it occurs after an anterior MI. What is the prognosis for the patient with cardiogenic shock?

Cardiogenic shock is defined by Jones and Bucher (1999) as "low cardiac output and hypotension with clinical signs of inadequate blood flow to the tissues" (pp. 47-49). Cardiogenic shock occurs when the heart cannot maintain enough CO to meet the body's demands. The most common cause is MI, but other cardiac disorders such as end-stage cardiomyopathy, valvular heart disease, cardiopulmonary bypass, and cardiac tamponade may be the precipitating events. Clinical manifestations of cardiogenic shock include cool and clammy skin, alterations in level of consciousness, decreased peripheral pulses, and a low urinary output.

Cardiogenic shock often follows a massive anterior AMI because of the link to the destruction of 40% or more of the left ventricle. The pathophysiologic process involved in cardiogenic shock is a self-perpetuating vicious cycle. Loss of cardiac muscle leads to decreased pumping ability of the ventricles and reduced stroke volume that causes a decreased CO. The decreased CO perpetuates a decrease in blood pressure and coronary perfusion, which causes progressive myocardial ischemia and cellular dysfunction. The incidence of cardiogenic shock after an anterior MI is 6% to 20% with a mortality rate of 75% to 90% (Jones & Bucher, 1999; Lessig & Lessig, 1999).

The prognosis of patients with an anterior wall MI is significantly worse than that of patients with an inferior wall MI (Jones & Bucher, 1999). Patients with an anterior wall MI usually have a blockage in the LAD that generally involves greater myocardial damage than those with inferior wall infarction. Because the left ventricle is involved, the likelihood of heart failure or cardiogenic shock is much greater with an anterior wall MI.

9. **What are the hemodynamic parameters seen in the patient with cardiogenic shock in comparison to normal hemodynamic parameters?**

Hemodynamic parameters are severely altered in the patient with cardiogenic shock. CO and cardiac index (CI) are dramatically lowered. Tachycardia occurs as the body attempts to compensate for the drop in systolic blood pressure. The pulmonary artery catheter readings show an increase in the central venous pressure, the pulmonary capillary wedge pressure (PCWP), and SVR, reflecting an increase in preload and afterload (Jones & Bucher, 1999).

In the assessment of the severity of cardiogenic shock, the CI is an effective parameter to provide hemodynamic information. A CI of less than 1.8 L/min/m² is indicative of cardiogenic shock. Clinical manifestations of hypoperfusion (as listed in answer 8) are observed when the CI is between 1.8 and 2.2 L/min/m². The body attempts to compensate for these changes by way of the sympathetic nervous system's release of epinephrine and norepinephrine. However, the results only cause the heart rate to increase and cause further peripheral vasoconstriction. Thus the complex activated mechanisms of cardiogenic shock dominate and normalization of the hemodynamic parameters is nearly impossible (Jones & Bucher, 1999).

Mrs. Adams' Hemodynamic Parameters
It is important to note that Mrs. Adams did not have a pulmonary artery catheter (PAC) placed initially because of thrombolysis. However, when she continued to have chest pain, a PAC was placed while she was in the catheterization laboratory. Mrs. Adams showed hemodynamic changes consistent with cardiogenic shock.

10. **Discuss the goals of pharmacologic management in cardiogenic shock. Which medications were used for Mrs. Adams?**

In cardiogenic shock, the goal is to decrease the preload and afterload while optimizing myocardial contraction. This presents a challenge pharmacologically. The use of multiple intravenous medications and drips in varying doses may need to be tailored for each individual with cardiogenic shock. The three main categories of drugs used for cardiogenic shock are diuretics, inotropes, and vasoactive medications. Although these pharmacologic agents may not alter mortality rates in some patients with cardiogenic shock, they will assist in maintaining vital organ perfusion while other interventions are used in an attempt to salvage the myocardium (AHA, 1997).

Diuretics

Even when patients have hypotension, a diuretic may be needed for fluid removal from the intravascular spaces. A loop diuretic, such as furosemide (Lasix), in small amounts may provide enough diuresis to allow myocardial fibers to stretch more efficiently (Jones & Bucher, 1999). The better the myocardial stretch, the better the CO and blood pressure. Even small improvements such as this can make a major difference in the progression and resolution of cardiogenic shock.

Inotropes

Inotropes (positive) are used to increase the contractility of the heart. These include dobutamine (Dobutrex), dopamine (Intropin), and amrinone (Inocor).

Dobutamine stimulates β-adrenergic receptors, which leads to an improved CI, improved oxygen delivery, and reduced pulmonary artery pressure (PAP), PCWP, SVR, and pulmonary vascular resistance (Jones & Bucher, 1999). Unless the patient is hypotensive, dobutamine is the inotrope preferred for use in cardiogenic shock. An additional advantage of dobutamine is augmentation of diastolic coronary blood flow and collateral flow to ischemic areas of the heart. Dobutamine has minimal effects on myocardial oxygen demand and produces a better balance between oxygen supply and demand than other inotropes (AHA, 1997). Conventional dosing of dobutamine from 2 to 20 µg/kg/min produces optimal increases in myocardial contractility with very little increase in heart rate. At higher dosages (>20 µg/kg/min), tachycardia may result.

Dopamine is the agent of choice if hypotension is present (Jones & Bucher, 1999). However, dopamine effects are dose dependent. At low dosages (1 to 2 µg/kg/min), renal and mesenteric perfusion is increased while heart rate and blood pressure remain unaffected. In midrange dosages (2 to 10 µg/kg/min), dopamine stimulates both β_1- and α-adrenergic receptors, which increases CO and improves myocardial contractility. Dopamine will also produce a mild increase in the SVR and preload in midrange doses. At a dosage range above 10 µg/kg/min, peripheral arterial and venous vasoconstriction occur, causing a significant increase in afterload and preload. Dopamine is usually given when hemodynamically significant hypotension occurs in the absence of hypovolemia. A disadvantage of dopamine is that cardiac workload increases without significantly increasing coronary blood flow (AHA, 1997). Even a therapeutic or midrange dosage of dopamine can stimulate β_1-receptors and increase heart rate, consuming myocardial oxygen supply. The preferred inotropic therapy is the combination of dopamine and dobutamine at moderate dosages.

Amrinone (Inocor) is a third inotrope that improves CO and PAP with little increase in myocardial workload (Jones & Bucher, 1999). However, amrinone works differently. It is a phosphodiesterase inhibitor that increases myocardial contractility without involving the sympathetic nervous system. It must be noted that although amrinone has been studied extensively in patients with congestive cardiomyopathy, its efficacy for ischemic heart problems such as cardiogenic shock has not been validated and should be used with caution (AHA, 1997). The optimal dosing range is 2 to 15 µg/kg/min.

Vasoactive Agents

Vasoactive drugs such as sodium nitroprusside (Nipride) and nitroglycerin (Tridil) are given to improve the pumping action of the heart by decreasing both preload and afterload (SVR) (Jones & Bucher, 1999). Although nitroglycerin is not as strong of a vasodilator as sodium nitroprusside, it dilates coronary arteries, reduces coronary artery vasospasms, and increases coronary collateral blood flow to ischemic myocardium (AHA, 1997). In small doses, vasoactive agents can assist the failing heart in cardiogenic shock by reducing the workload of the heart.

Mrs. Adams' Medications While in Cardiogenic Shock

Mrs. Adams was given dopamine and dobutamine at midrange dosages during cardiogenic shock for inotropic purposes. Her NTG drip was reduced to 1 µg/kg/min for afterload purposes, once her chest pain was relieved by the insertion of the IABP. The vasoactive drips were withdrawn by day 3.

11. **What types of mechanical support devices can be used for patients in cardiogenic shock and why? Which type was used for Mrs. Adams? Identify any specific nursing responsibilities for the device chosen for Mrs. Adams.**

The patient in cardiogenic shock may require the use of IABP counterpulsation. The purpose of the IABP is twofold. First, the balloon inflates during ventricular diastole, which results in increased coronary artery perfusion. Second, deflation of the balloon occurs during ventricular systole, which decreases afterload or the workload of the heart. Jones and Bucher (1999) and Zaacks, Kelly, Klein, Parrillo, and Liebson (1997) state that 75% of patients who receive IABP therapy demonstrate clinical improvements in their condition.

Other mechanical support devices used include ventricular assist devices (VADs) and extracorporeal membrane oxygenation (ECMO). Types of VADs include centrifugal, pneumatic, pulsatile, and electrical pulsatile. VADs may be implanted for extended periods and are used as a bridge to cardiac transplantation. The mechanical support device, ECMO, is used in children but is poorly tolerated in adults over long periods. Major complications such as biventricular failure, bleeding, and infection occur with VADs and ECMO. However, these mechanical devices can be a successful means of supporting patients experiencing cardiac failure who would otherwise die (Jones & Bucher, 1999).

Mrs. Adams' Mechanical Support Devices

Mrs. Adams required placement of an IABP because of unrelieved chest pain and development of cardiogenic shock. She tolerated the balloon pump well, and her hemodynamic values improved to allow weaning by day 3.

Specific Nursing Responsibilities with an IABP

Lessig and Lessig (1998) identify specific nursing responsibilities when caring for a patient with an IABP:

- Maintain appropriate timing of IABP inflation and deflation by monitoring heart rate, heart rhythm, and mean arterial pressure every 15 minutes. Irregular arrhythmias and tachyarrhythmias will decrease IABP effectiveness. Maintenance of mean arterial pressure at 90 mm Hg may be supported with inotropic agents as needed.

- Assess pulses in both feet (dorsalis pedis and posterior tibial) with a Doppler every hour and mark the location heard. Note the presence, quality, and any change from baseline assessment.
- Monitor the IABP insertion site every hour, noting any oozing or increase in bleeding/hematoma.
- Monitor for migration of the IABP catheter by assessing the left radial pulse versus the right radial pulse every 2 hours and urinary output every hour. If the left radial pulse is absent or decreased, the left subclavian artery may be occluded by the catheter. If urinary output decreases to less than 30 ml/hr, the renal arteries may be occluded by the catheter. Daily and as-needed chest x-ray films are crucial to check placement of the IABP catheter.
- Secure and check all IABP connections from the site of insertion to the connection with the external machine every hour. The patient will require education regarding the importance of keeping the affected extremity straight. This may also require a soft restraint on the extremity and maintenance of the head of the bed at 30 degrees or lower. All of these precautionary measures can prevent inadvertent IABP catheter migration.
- Monitor for IABP malfunction via external machine alarms. Most IABP machines fill, time, and troubleshoot automatically. However, if the IABP catheter is placed on standby for longer than 5 minutes, it must be programmed or be manually inflated/deflated slightly to prevent thrombus formation and possible occurrence of emboli.

12. What are the nursing diagnoses for the patient in cardiogenic shock after an anterior AMI?

Nursing diagnoses for patients in cardiogenic shock after an anterior AMI include the following (Jones & Bucher, 1999; Lessig & Lessig, 1998):

- Decreased cardiac output
- Fluid volume excess
- Altered renal, cerebral, cardiopulmonary, and peripheral tissue perfusion
- Altered comfort: pain related to myocardial ischemia during AMI
- Impaired gas exchange
- Altered nutrition, less than body requirements
- Ineffective individual and family coping related to anxiety and fear of death and the critical care environment

CARDIAC SHOCK IN ANTERIOR WALL MYOCARDIAL INFARCTION

References

American Heart Association (1997). The acute coronary syndromes, including acute myocardial infarction. In Cummins, R. (Ed.). *Advanced cardiac life support* (pp. 9-1 to 9-41). Dallas: Author.

Brogan, G., Bock, J., McCuskey, C., Hollander, J., Thode, H., Gawad, Y., & Jackowski, G. (1997). Evaluation of cardiac status CK-MB/myoglobin device for rapid ruling out of acute myocardial infarction. *Clinics in Laboratory Medicine, 17,* 655-669.

Bucher, L. (1999). Acute myocardial infarction. In Bucher, L., & Melander, S. (Eds.). *Critical care nursing* (pp. 227-257). Philadelphia: WB Saunders.

Connolly, S. (1997). Effect of prophylactic amiodarone on mortality after acute myocardial infarction and in congestive heart failure: meta-analysis of individual data from 6500 patients in randomised trials. *The Lancet, 350,* 1417-1424.

Gwechenberger, M., Schreiber, W., Kittler, H., Binder, M., Hohenberger, B., Laggner, A., & Hirschl, M. (1997). Prediction of early complications in patients with acute myocardial infarction by calculation of the st score. *Annals of Emergency Medicine, 30,* 563-570.

Jones, K., & Bucher, L. (1999). Shock. In Bucher, L., & Melander, S. (Eds.). *Critical care nursing* (pp. 1010-1035). Philadelphia: Saunders.

Kim, S., Adams, S., & Hendel, R. (1997). Role of nuclear cardiology in the evaluation of acute coronary syndromes. *Annals of Emergency Medicine, 30,* 210-218.

Lessig, M. L., & Lessig, P. (1998). The cardiovascular system. In Alspach, J. (Ed.). *American Association of Critical-Care Nurses: Core curriculum for critical care nurses* (5th ed., pp. 137-337). Philadelphia: WB Saunders.

Murphy, M., & Berding, C. (1999). Use of measurements of myoglobin and cardiac troponins in the diagnosis of acute myocardial infarction. *Critical Care Nurse, 19*(1), 58-65.

Plaut, D. (1998). Serum markers of cardiac cell damage. *American Medical Technologists Events CE Supplement, 15,* 210-215.

Zaacks, S., Kelly, R., Klein, L., Parrillo, J., & Liebson, P. (1997). Intra-aortic balloon counterpulsation: Which patient will benefit? *The Journal of Critical Illness, 12,* 424-435.

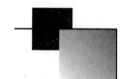

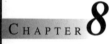

CHAPTER 8

NON–Q-WAVE MYOCARDIAL INFARCTION

Sheila Drake Melander, RN, DSN, ACNP-C, FCCM •
Amy Reese Ramirez, RN, BSN, MSW, MSN, FNP

CASE PRESENTATION

Mrs. Jarvis is a 70-year-old, 87.8-kg (194-lb) African-American woman with a history of insulin-dependent diabetes mellitus, hypertension, atherosclerotic peripheral vascular disease, cancer of the breast and uterus, and congestive heart failure. Mrs. Jarvis was seen at an outlying hospital with a complaint of chest pain and shortness of breath. Further questioning revealed that she had been having more frequent episodes of chest pain for the past week accompanied by shortness of breath.

The initial orders were as follows:

- >2 L of oxygen through a nasal cannula
- Intravenous (IV) line of normal saline started at a keep-open rate
- Cardiac monitor, which showed a normal sinus rhythm without ectopy
- 12-lead electrocardiogram (ECG)
- Immediate measurement of cardiac enzymes; repeat every 6 hours for 24 hours

Her diagnostic data on admission were as follows:

BP	190/94 mm Hg	CK	216 U/L
HR	106 bpm	CK-MB	5.6%
Respirations	32 breaths/min	LDH	400 U/L
CI	2.2 L/min/m²	AST (SGOT)	25 U/L
Troponin I	1.5 mg/L	Myoglobin	95 ng/L

The ECG revealed ST-segment elevation in leads V_2 and V_3.

Mrs. Jarvis was given one sublingual nitroglycerin (NTG) tablet, which resolved her pain. She was admitted to the coronary care unit with the order to "rule out myocardial infarction (MI)."

Her serial cardiac enzyme levels continued to rise; values from the third set of cardiac enzyme measurements were the following:

CK	350 U/L	LDH	680 U/L
CK-MB	5.8%	AST (SGOT)	52 U/L
Troponin I	5.3 μg/L	CI	1.8 L/min/m²
Myoglobin	125 ng/L		

Day 2

Mrs. Jarvis had recurrent pain that was not eased with three NTG tablets, diaphoresis, and profound shortness of breath requiring intubation. An ECG demonstrated no change from the previous tracings. Mrs. Jarvis was then taken to the cardiac catheterization laboratory. Cardiac catheterization revealed the following:

- Ejection fraction of 35%
- 90% obstruction of the left anterior descending coronary artery
- 90% to 95% obstruction of the circumflex artery
- 80% obstruction of the right coronary artery

An intraaortic balloon pump was placed for control of Mrs. Jarvis's refractory chest pain, and a dopamine infusion of 3 µg/kg/min was started. NTG at 1.5 µg/ml and heparin at 800 U/hr were continued. At this time, Mrs. Jarvis was transferred to another facility with the diagnosis of non–Q-wave MI and three-vessel disease with the need for emergency bypass surgery. Mrs. Jarvis subsequently underwent bypass surgery on day 3 and has done very well since that time.

NON–Q-WAVE MYOCARDIAL INFARCTION

Questions

1. What are the differences between a non–Q-wave MI and a transmural MI?
2. What methods are used in the diagnosis of non–Q-wave MIs?
3. Describe the characteristics of patients with the diagnosis of non–Q-wave MI.
4. Which pharmacologic agents may be used in the treatment of a non–Q-wave MI?
5. What are the current recommendations for the use of percutaneous transluminal coronary angioplasty (PTCA) and coronary artery bypass graft (CABG) surgery in the patient with a non–Q-wave MI?
6. Discuss extension of a non–Q-wave MI, including the time frame of occurrence and possible outcomes.
7. What are some nursing concerns for the patient with a non–Q-wave MI?
8. What are some nursing actions required for patients taking β-blockers (metoprolol and atenolol)?
9. What are nursing implications for patients receiving thrombolytic therapy?
10. Develop a list of appropriate nursing diagnoses for the care of the patient with a non–Q-wave MI.

NON–Q-WAVE MYOCARDIAL INFARCTION

Questions and Answers

1. What are the differences between a non–Q-wave MI and a transmural MI?

The terminology used to classify non–Q-wave and transmural MIs has been debated. Traditionally, the classification of a Q-wave MI indicated the involvement of all three layers of the heart muscle; therefore it was labeled a transmural or full-thickness MI. When no abnormal Q waves were present, the area of necrosis was thought to be confined to the subendocardium; therefore this was termed a nontransmural or partial-thickness MI. Research has found that classifying MIs as transmural or nontransmural is imprecise (Bucher & Melander, 1999). Bucher and Melander (1999) state that pathologic Q waves can be found in nontransmural infarctions, and normal Q waves can be located in transmural infarctions. Based on this information, the terms *Q-wave MI* and *non–Q-wave MI* are the most appropriate.

Pathologic Q waves must be wider (=0.04 second in duration) and deeper (at least one fourth of the height of the QRS complex) than normal (Bucher & Melander, 1999). Q waves may appear immediately or within the first few days after symptom onset. The pathophysiology of a non–Q-wave MI appears to be similar to that of unstable angina except for the greater incidence and extent of thrombus formation and coronary artery occlusion with non–Q-wave MIs (Liebson & Klein, 1997). Compared with Q-wave infarctions, non–Q-wave MIs generally are associated with smaller areas of necrosis, lower levels of cardiac enzymes, and fewer incidences of congestive heart failure. Comparatively, Q-wave infarctions present with greater loss of heart tissue, creating a greater risk of ventricular dysfunction (Bucher & Melander, 1999).

2. What methods are used in the diagnosis of non–Q-wave MIs?

The diagnosis of a non–Q-wave MI has been based on the presence of at least two of the following criteria: (1) typical chest pain lasting at least 30 minutes, (2) elevation of two serum cardiac enzyme levels to more than 1.5 times the normal limit, and (3) the presence of ST-segment or T-wave changes on the ECG with no development of Q/QS waves (Haim et al, 1998b). ECG changes associated with a non–Q-wave MI are usually ST-segment elevation, ST-segment depression, and deep T-wave inversion.

The three major enzymes released into the blood at abnormal levels are creatinine phosphokinase, lactate dehydrogenase (LDH), and troponin. In the past, creatinine kinase (CK) levels and LDH levels were the main diagnostic markers for myocardial injury. However, these markers peak a few days after MI (CK in 12 to 24 hours; LDH in 3 to 6 days). The elevation in an isoenzyme of CK, CK-MB, is often relied on as a definitive diagnostic finding when a patient has nonspecific ECG changes or atypical signs and symptoms. CK-MB is diagnostic of MI at elevations higher than 3% (Bucher & Melander, 1999). However, CK-MB levels also do not increase until 4 to 8 hours after the ischemic event, returning to normal within 48 to 72 hours. This creates a limited window of opportunity for diagnostic use.

More recently, troponin I and myoglobin have supplemented and, in some cases, replaced these more traditional enzyme markers (Murphy & Berding, 1999). Troponin I is only found in myocardial cells, making it the only biomarker that is 100% specific for myocardial necrosis. Cardiac troponin levels begin to increase 3 hours after myocardial ischemia, peak at 14 to 18 hours, and remain elevated for 5 to 7 days, providing a longer diagnostic window. The upper reference level generally accepted as indicative of acute myocardial infarction (AMI) is a serum level of cardiac troponin I of at least 1.5 to 3.1 µg/L (Murphy & Berding, 1999). Myoglobin, a heme protein found in all striated muscle fibers, is rapidly released from damaged muscle tissue. Because of this rapid escape, myoglobin can be detected as soon as 2 hours after an MI, with peak serum levels occurring in 3 to 15 hours. Because both cardiac and skeletal muscles contain myoglobin, cardiac bypass surgery as well as many non–cardiac-related conditions such as strenuous exercise, renal failure, and intramuscular injections can elevate serum levels. Therefore Murphy and Berding (1999) suggest that myoglobin is most helpful when used in conjunction with other cardiac markers in the rapid determination of MI.

3. **Describe the characteristics of patients with the diagnosis of non–Q-wave MI.**

Patients with a non–Q-wave MI present with elevated cardiac enzyme levels (CK-MB, troponin, and myoglobin), no Q wave on an ECG, and nonspecific ST-segment and T-wave ECG changes. Diagnostic findings of ST-segment depression and an anterior infarct location are associated with a greater risk for clinical events after discharge from the hospital (Evanoski, 1997; Liebson & Klein, 1997). Women are seen more often with single-vessel disease and non–Q-wave infarcts, whereas, men more often have triple-vessel disease and a Q-wave infarct (Evanoski, 1997). In the Thrombolysis in Myocardial Infarction (TIMI) IIIB trial, men and women with a non–Q-wave MI were evaluated to determine gender differences in characteristics and outcome (Hochman et al, 1997). Compared with men, women who have non–Q-wave MIs are older, are less often white, have higher incidences of diabetes and hypertension, and are already taking cardiac medications. However, coronary angiography showed less severe coronary artery disease in women than in men. The 42-day rate of death and MI in TIMI IIIB subjects was similar for women and men (7.4% versus 7.5%). The overall outcome of a non–Q-wave MI was found to be related to severity of the illness and not to gender.

The following are clinical characteristics of patients with a non–Q-wave MI (Liebson & Klein, 1997):

- Lower in-hospital mortality rate
- One-year postdischarge mortality rates comparable to those for Q-wave MIs
- Less extensive infarction (therefore better ejection fractions)
- Higher incidence of reinfarction and recurrent angina

4. **Which pharmacologic agents may be used in the treatment of a non–Q-wave MI?**

The classification of Q-wave or non–Q-wave infarction has less prognostic meaning and should guide therapy to a lesser degree than clinical markers of risk, such as heart failure, recurrent chest pain, late ventricular arrhythmias, and persistent ST-segment depression (Rakel, 1999). Therefore initial care of the patient with a non–Q-wave MI includes the same regimen of care as that for the patient with a Q-wave MI: oxygen, cardiac monitoring, cardiac enzyme monitoring, and arrhythmia management. Recent studies report a decreased rate of in-hospital complications and death in patients with non–Q-wave MIs in the 1990s compared with the 1980s (Hiam et al, 1998b). These mortality rate reductions have been associated with the use of newer therapeutic modalities, including thrombolytics, aspirin, β-blockers, and angiotensin-converting enzyme inhibitors. They have also been attributed to the improved survival of these patients.

Aspirin and low-dose heparin (enoxaparin) should be administered on admission after a non–Q-wave MI to decrease further thrombus formation (Futterman & Lemberg, 1999; Mark et al, 1998). In the ESSENCE trial (Efficacy and Safety of Subcutaneous Enoxaparin in Non–Q-Wave Coronary Events), enoxaparin reduced the 30-day incidence of death, myocardial infarction, and recurrent angina compared with IV unfractionated heparin in patients with non–Q-wave MIs. Aspirin and heparin block only one of the pathways involved in platelet activation, leaving other thrombotic pathways unchecked (COR Therapeutics, 1998; Mark et al, 1998). Platelet receptor glycoprotein (GP) IIb-IIIa has been identified as the final common pathway to platelet aggregation. In recent randomized clinical trials, eptifibatide, a platelet GP IIb-IIIa inhibitor, has been found to be a valuable addition to the therapeutic approach for the treatment of non–Q-wave MIs. When given in combination with aspirin and heparin, eptifibatide has been found to help reduce ischemic complications, including MI and death (COR Therapeutics, 1998; Mark et al, 1998).

Diltiazem administration is recommended for patients who have non–Q-wave MI but no evidence of pulmonary congestion to prevent recurrent nonfatal AMI (Liebson & Klein, 1997). β-Blockers have been found to reduce mortality by 40% in patients with a non–Q-wave MI (Gottlieb, McCarter, & Vogel, 1998). Symptom-limiting stress testing using ECG and thallium-201 imaging are now recommended before discharge or in the early postdischarge period to determine the extent of cardiac damage (Liebson & Klein, 1997).

5. What are the current recommendations for the use of percutaneous transluminal coronary angioplasty (PTCA) and coronary artery bypass graft (CABG) surgery in the patient with a non–Q-wave MI?

The use of invasive therapy in the patient with a non–Q-wave MI remains controversial. The Veterans Affairs Non–Q Wave Infarction Strategies In-Hospital Study concluded that most patients with a non–Q-wave MI do not benefit from routine, early invasive management consisting of coronary angiography and revascularization (Boden et al, 1998). The TIMI IIIB study also reported that early surgical intervention did not result in any significant improvement in patient outcome over medical therapy (Cohen, 1998). However, Hiam et al. (1998b) reported that invasive procedures such as PTCA and CABG surgery were being used more frequently in the 1990s than in the 1980s and were associated with decreased mortality rates and more favorable outcomes in patients with non–Q-wave MIs. Currently, CABG surgery is recommended for patients who remain symptomatic after thrombolytic therapy or angioplasty or who have major multivessel disease. For patients who are eligible for thrombolytic therapy, the role of PTCA is now controversial (Bucher & Melander, 1999). More studies are needed to determine the benefits of PTCA and CABG revascularization in the patient with a non–Q-wave MI.

6. Discuss extension of a non–Q-wave MI, including the time frame of occurrence and possible outcomes.

Hospital mortality is higher for patients with a Q-wave MI than for those with a non–Q-wave MI. However, after discharge, nonfatal reinfarction and mortality rates in patients with non–Q-wave and Q-wave MIs are comparable (Behar et al, 1996).

Although patients with non–Q-wave MIs show less extensive infarction as well as lower in-hospital mortality rates, studies find that those with non–Q-wave MIs to have higher incidences of reinfarction and recurrent angina, presumably because of the large degree of jeopardized myocardium (Boden et al, 1998; Liebson & Klein, 1997). Haim, Benderley, Hod, Reicher-Reiss, Goldbourt, and Beher (1998a) evaluated the prognosis for patients with a first non–Q-wave MI according to their ECG on admission. For patients with ST-segment elevation, hospital and 1-year mortality rates were 15% and 21%, respectively. For patients with ST-segment depression, hospital mortality rates were 17% and 27%, respectively. These rates were significantly higher than for patients with no ST-segment changes (3% and 10%, respectively). The cumulative 5-year mortality was highest among patients with ST-segment depression (51%) compared with patients with ST-segment elevation (34%) and no ST-segment deviation (21%). Overall, these findings show that patients with a first non–Q-wave MI with ST-segment elevation and depression on admission have similar hospital and 1-year mortality risks, but the long-term mortality risk is higher among patients with ST-segment depression (Liebson & Klein, 1997).

7. What are some nursing concerns for the patient with a non–Q-wave MI?

Nursing concerns for the patient experiencing a non–Q-wave MI are as follows:

- Patients must continually be assessed for any signs of chest pain or chest tightness, which could signal reinfarction or the development of unstable angina.
- Cardiac enzyme levels must be monitored closely and changes reported to the physician immediately.
- All regimens of care such as thrombolytic therapy and antithrombolytic medications should be explained to the patient.
- Before the patient is discharged with any prescribed medications, all possible side effects should be explained thoroughly.
- Cardiac rehabilitation should begin while the patient is still in the cardiac intensive care unit and should continue after discharge by a multidisciplinary cardiac rehabilitation team (Bucher & Melander, 1999).

8. What are some nursing actions required for patients receiving β-blockers (metoprolol and atenolol)?

Nursing actions required for patients receiving IV or oral β-blockers include the following:

- Administer the IV dose slowly.
- Monitor the patient for symptomatic bradycardia, hypotension, and signs and symptoms of congestive heart failure and heart block.
- Instruct the patient to slowly change from a sitting or lying position to a standing position to avoid orthostatic hypotension.
- Monitor the patient for possible interactive effects with other medications, such as an additive effect on blood pressure in patients receiving other hypotensive medications.

- Consider the need for a reduced dosage in elderly patients and in patients with hepatic or renal impairment.
- Avoid abrupt cessation of drug, which may precipitate chest pain, ventricular arrhythmias, or AMI (Bucher & Melander, 1999).

9. What are the nursing implications for patients receiving thrombolytic therapy?

Nursing implications for patients receiving thrombolytic therapy include the following:

- Monitor the patient for potential bleeding risks before initiating thrombolytic therapy.
- Monitor the patient for physical signs of bleeding, including ecchymosis and petechiae; bleeding gums; blood in stool, urine, emesis, nasogastric drainage, or sputum; bleeding from the IV site; decreased blood pressure and increased heart rate; cool and clammy skin; and changes in mentation.
- Monitor the patient for subjective signs of bleeding, including anxiety and palpitations.
- Observe for signs of reperfusion, including resolution of chest pain, early peaking of CK-MB enzyme levels, reperfusion arrhythmias, and normalization of the ST segments.
- Monitor venipuncture sites, incisions, and drains for bleeding every 15 to 60 minutes.
- Keep the patient in bed with the side rails up to avoid injury.
- Avoid unnecessary handling of the patient to decrease potential tissue damage that causes large hematomas.
- Assess the patient's neurologic status at least once a shift and more often if intracranial bleeding is suspected.
- Monitor for adverse reactions, including severe spontaneous hemorrhage, hypotension, arrhythmias, edema, nausea or vomiting, and hypersensitivity reactions (Bucher & Melander, 1999).

10. Develop a list of appropriate nursing diagnoses for the care of the patient with a non–Q-wave MI.

Nursing diagnoses for the patient with a non–Q-wave MI include the following:

- Pain (acute) related to decreased coronary blood flow that causes myocardial injury and necrosis
- Altered myocardial tissue perfusion secondary to coronary artery disease
- Decreased cardiac output related to ischemic or infarcted myocardium
- Activity intolerance related to cardiac disease and dysfunction
- Anxiety related to threat of death, change in health status and body image, and threat to socioeconomic status
- Knowledge deficit related to new diagnosis, medications, or treatment regimens (Alspach, 1998)

NON–Q-WAVE MYOCARDIAL INFARCTION

References

Alspach, J. G. (Ed.). (1998). *American Association of Critical-Care Nurses: Core curriculum for critical care nursing* (5th ed.). Philadelphia: Saunders.

Behar, S., Hiam, M., Hod, H., Kornowski, R., Reicher-Reiss, H., Zion, M., Kaplinsky, E., Abinader, E., Palant, A., Kishon, Y., Reisin, L., Zahavi, I., & Goldbourt, U. (1996). Long-term prognosis of patients after a Q wave compared with a non-Q wave first acute myocardial infarction. Data from the SPRINT Registry *European Heart Journal, 17,* 1532-1537.

Boden, W, O'Rourke, R., Crawford, M., Blaustein, A., Deedwania, P., Zoble, R., Wexler, L., Klieger, R., Pepine, C., Ferry, D., Chow, B., & Lavori, P. (1998). Outcomes in patients with acute non-Q wave myocardial infarction randomly assigned to an invasive as compared with a conservative management strategy. *The New England Journal of Medicine, 338,* 1785-1792.

Bucher, L., & Melander, S. (Eds.). (1999). *Critical care nursing.* Philadelphia: WB Saunders.

Cohen, M. (1998). Approaches to the treatment of unstable angina and non-Q wave myocardial infarction. *Canadian Journal of Cardiology, 14*(Suppl. E), 11E-14E.

COR Therapeutics, Inc. and Key Pharmaceuticals, Inc. (1998). *Treatment pathways and clinical care plan templates for the management of unstable angina and non-Q-wave myocardial infarction.* San Francisco, CA and Kenilworth, NJ.

Evanoski, C. A. (1997). Myocardial infarction: The number one killer of women. *Critical Care Clinics of North America, 9,* 489-495.

Futterman, L. G. & Lamberg, L. (1999). Low-molecular-weight heparin: An antithrombotic agent whose time has come. *American Journal of Critical Care, 8,* 520-523.

Gottlieb, S. S., McCarter, R. J., & Vogel, R. A. (1998). Effect of beta-blockade on mortality among high-risk and low-risk patients after myocardial infarction. *The New England Journal of Medicine, 339,* 489-497.

Haim, M., Benderley, M., Hod, H., Reicher-Reiss, H., Goldbourt, U., & Behar, S. (1998a). The outcome of patients with a first non-Q wave acute myocardial infarction presenting with ST segment depression, ST segment elevation, or no ST deviations on the admission electrocardiogram. *International Journal of Cardiology, 67,* 39-46.

Haim, M., Gottlieb, S., Boyko, V., Reicher-Reiss, H., Hod, H., Kaplinsky, E., Mandelzweig, L., Goldbourt, U., & Behar, S. (1998b). Prognosis of patients with a first non-Q-wave myocardial infarction before and in the reperfusion era. *American Heart Journal, 136,* 245-251.

Hochman, J., McCabe, C., Stone, P., Becker, R., Cannon, C. DeFeo Fraulini, T., Thompson, B., Steingart, R., Knatterud, G., & Braunwald E. (1997). Outcomes and profile of women and men presenting with acute coronary syndromes: A report from TIMI IIIB. TIMI Investigators. Thrombolysis in Myocardial Infarction. *Journal of the American College of Cardiology, 30,* 141-148.

Liebson, P. R. & Klein, L. W. (1997). The non-Q wave myocardial infarction revisited: 10 years later. *Progressive Cardiovascular Disease, 39,* 399-444.

Mark, D., Cowper, P., Berkowitz S., Davidson Ray, L., DeLong, E., Turpie, A., Califf, R., Weatherly, B., & Cohen, M. (1998). Economic assessment of low-molecular weight heparin (enoxaparin) versus unfractionated heparin in acute coronary syndrome patients: Result from the ESSENCE randomized trial. Efficacy and Safety of Subcutaneous Enoxaparin in Non-Q wave Coronary Events [unstable angina or non-Q-wave myocardial infarction]. *Circulation, 97,* 1702-1707.

Murphy, M. J. & Berding, C. B. (1999). Use of measurements of myoglobin and cardiac troponins in the diagnosis of acute myocardial infarction. *Critical Care Nurse, 19,* 58-65.

Rakel, R. E. (Ed.). (1999). *Conn's current therapy.* Philadelphia: WB Saunders.

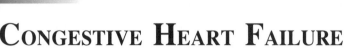

CONGESTIVE HEART FAILURE

Joan E. King, RN, PhD, ACNP

CASE PRESENTATION

John Arnold, age 80 years, was admitted to the hospital after visiting his primary physician with complaints of having experienced general malaise for 3 to 4 days, shortness of breath, and abdominal pain. Initial assessment revealed bibasilar crackles, an audible S_3, and tachycardia. Mr. Arnold also informed the nurse of occasional epigastric pain, which he attributed to his "ulcer acting up."

Mr. Arnold's history includes diabetes for more than 30 years, peptic ulcer, and hypertension and coronary artery disease (past examinations indicated an 80% blockage of the left anterior descending coronary artery and 60% blockage of the right coronary artery). Following are his diagnostic data on admission:

BP	150/72 mm Hg	Hgb	11.8 g/dl
HR	102-123 bpm and irregular	Hct	36.2%
Respirations	24-32 breaths/min	AST (SGOT)	134 U/L
Temperature	37.3° C (99.2° F) (tympanic)	Cl⁻	102 mmol/L
Height	175 cm (5 ft 10 in)	BUN	17 mg/dl
Weight	79 kg (175 lb)*	Glucose	332 mg/dl
Urine	Yellow and cloudy	Creatinine	1.2 mg/dl
Na⁺	135 mmol/L	LDH	705 U/L
K⁺	4.2 mmol/L	CK	587 U/L

*Mr. Arnold stated that his weight had increased approximately 3 kg (6 lb) during the last 3 days

A chest x-ray film showed mild congestive heart failure (CHF) superimposed on chronic obstructive pulmonary disease (COPD) and chronic pulmonary parenchymal changes.

An electrocardiogram (ECG) revealed atrial fibrillation with a ventricular response of 112, no Q waves or ST-segment or T-wave changes.

Shortly after admission, Mr. Arnold's skin became cool and clammy. Respirations were labored, and he complained of abdominal pain. Upon physical examination, Mr. Arnold was found to be diaphoretic and gasping for air, with jugular venous distension and a positive hepatojugular reflux and diminished bowel sounds. Bilateral crackles were present with an expiratory wheeze. Audible crackles were also heard with respirations. Mr. Arnold was placed in a high-Fowler position, and oxygen therapy of 4 L/min was initiated. It was noted that urinary output had been less than 30 ml/hr since admission.

Within 30 minutes, Mr. Arnold showed further decompensation as he developed pulmonary edema. He was immediately transferred to the cardiac care unit (CCU) for aggressive diuretic therapy. Creatinine kinase myocardial band (CK-MB), an isoenzyme of CK, was confirmed at this time to be 4%.

Routine CCU orders were initiated, and the plan of care was briefly explained to Mr. Arnold. His heart monitor showed atrial fibrillation with a rapid ventricular response of 130. Furosemide (Lasix) 100 mg intravenously (IV) and digoxin 0.5 mg IV were administered. A Swan-Ganz catheter was inserted to monitor his hemodynamic parameters. His overall condition continued to deteriorate, and dobutamine (Dobutrex) 1 g in 250 ml of normal saline solution at 5 µg/kg/min was begun. Additional diagnostic data include the following:

BP	190/100 mm Hg	CI	2.34 L/min/m^2
HR	130 bpm	HCO$_3^-$	24 mmol/L
Respirations	42 breaths/min	pH	7.46
PAP	50/22 mm Hg	Paco$_2$	31 mm Hg
PCWP	24 mm Hg	Pao$_2$	80 mm Hg
CO	4.64 L/min	Sao$_2$	96% (with 4 L of oxygen
CVP	19 cm H$_2$O		by nasal cannula)
SVR	1810 dynes/sec/cm^{-5}		

At this point, Mr. Arnold's dobutamine drip was increased to 10 µg/kg/min. Administration of nitroprusside (Nipride) was initiated and titrated at 0.3 µg/kg/min. A dopamine drip was ordered to be on standby. An additional 200 mg of furosemide was administered IV, and a significant improvement in urinary output was obtained.

Within a short time, Mr. Arnold said that he found it "easier to breathe." Hemodynamic and laboratory results were as follows:

BP	140/90 mm Hg	CI	2.8 L/min/m^2
HR	109 bpm	HCO$_3^-$	25 mmol/L
Respirations	24 breaths/min	pH	7.43
PAP	30/10 mm Hg	Paco$_2$	36 mm Hg
PCWP	12 mm Hg	Pao$_2$	89 mm Hg
CO	5.5 L/min	Sao$_2$	98% (with 2 L oxygen by
CVP	8 cm H$_2$O		nasal cannula)
SVR	1340 dynes/sec/cm^{-5}		

Over the next 2 days, Mr. Arnold's dobutamine and nitroprusside drips were discontinued, and he was given furosemide 160 mg twice daily., captopril 25 mg every 6 hours, and digoxin 0.125 mg daily. In addition, Mr. Arnold was given nitroglycerin ointment 5 cm every 6 hours and potassium supplement 20 mEq every 12 hours. The heart monitor showed normal sinus rhythm, and an echocardiogram indicated an ejection fraction of 30%. The patient was transferred to the medical-surgical floor, and discharge planning, including patient and family teaching, was begun. Mr. Arnold was evidently discharged 2 days later and was scheduled to be followed in the cardiology clinic 1 week after discharge.

Congestive Heart Failure

Questions

1. Discuss the pathophysiology of CHF.
2. Discuss the various classifications of CHF.
3. Discuss Mr. Arnold's signs and symptoms that were consistent with CHF.
4. Describe Mr. Arnold's predisposing risk factors for CHF.
5. List the nursing diagnoses appropriate for Mr. Arnold's care.
6. Briefly define the following terms: cardiac output, cardiac index, central venous pressure, preload, afterload, pulmonary artery pressure, and pulmonary artery occlusive pressure.
7. Describe the benefits of using a pulmonary artery catheter during CHF.
8. Briefly describe the pathophysiology of pulmonary edema.
9. List the pharmacologic agents used in Mr. Arnold's care and explain their importance to his treatment.
10. Discuss long-term management of a patient with CHF.
11. Discuss new drug therapies for CHF that are on the horizon.

Congestive Heart Failure

Questions and Answers

1. Discuss the pathophysiology of CHF.

CHF is the inability for the heart to pump enough blood to meet the body's demands. The amount of blood pumped per minute is the cardiac output (CO). *CO* is also defined as the product of the stroke volume times the heart rate. There are numerous causes of CHF, including myocardial infarction, ischemic heart disease, arrhythmias, hypertension, cardiomyopathy, and valvular dysfunction. Regardless of the cause, when the CO drops, compensatory mechanisms are activated. Initially, the sympathetic nervous system (SNS) is stimulated, and the heart rate increases as well as force of contraction. SNS stimulation also produces vasoconstriction and hence increases afterload or systemic vascular resistance (SVR). The body's goal in increasing the SVR or afterload is to increase venous return to the heart. By increasing the venous return, the body is attempting to increase the preload, or the volume of blood that is present in the left ventricle right at the end of diastole. The preload is also called the left ventricular end-diastolic pressure. The Frank-Starling law states that up to a point, the greater the preload, the greater the CO. However, after a critical point, increasing the preload will cause a decline in the CO. Physiologically, this is attributed to the myocardial fibers providing the best CO when they are maximally stretched, but overstretching the fibers reduces the force of contract and subsequently reduces CO. These four compensatory mechanisms (increase in heart rate [HR], increase in force of contraction, increase in SVR, and increase in preload) are all initial attempts by the body to increase the CO. At first, these compensatory mechanisms are beneficial but at the expense of an increase in myocardial oxygen consumption.

In addition to SNS stimulation to increase CO, the kidneys play a vital role in both the compensatory process and the further development of CHF. When the CO drops, renal perfusion decreases, activating the renin-angiotensin system (RAS). The RAS activates the release of angiotensin II and aldosterone. The increased secretion of aldosterone leads to sodium retention. As the serum sodium level increases, secretion of antidiuretic hormone (ADH) is also stimulated, thus causing the kidneys to reabsorb more water. This combination of increase in sodium and water retention leads to a further increase in preload. The RAS also results in the formation of angiotensin II. Angiotensin II is a powerful vasoconstrictor that attempts to increase the venous return to increase the preload. Aldosterone, ADH, and angiotensin II all work to try to increase the preload with the hope that an increase in preload will increase the CO. However, as previously stated, according to the Frank-Starling law, increasing the preload beyond the optimal point actually reduces the CO. In addition, just as SNS stimulation increases the SVR and hence the afterload, angiotensin II also contributes to an increase in the afterload and an increase in the heart's workload.

In both acute and chronic CHF, these compensatory mechanisms become counterproductive. Increasing the preload, HR, and SVR begins to increase the workload on the heart, to increase myocardial oxygen consumption, and to decrease the CO. Current research has led to a further understanding of the dynamics of chronic CHF. Over time, not only is the CO reduced because of the increase in preload and afterload, but prolonged SNS stimulation and angiotensin II and aldosterone secretion cause direct changes in the myocardial fibers and myocytes. This results in a phenomenon known as *remodeling,* which leads to a decrease in cardiac function (Albert, 1998; Michael & Parnell, 1998; Mosar, 1998).

When either the right or left ventricle can no longer handle the preload it receives, fluid begins to back up. When the left ventricle fails as a pump, fluid is backed up into the pulmonary bed, producing signs and symptoms such as shortness of breath, dyspnea on exertion, orthopnea, and as in Mr. Arnold's case, pulmonary edema. When the right ventricle fails, fluid is backed up into the systemic circulation, producing signs and symptoms such as elevated central venous pressure (CVP), elevated jugular venous distension, hepatomegaly, ascites, anorexia, and peripheral edema (Table 9-1).

2. Discuss the various classifications of CHF.

CHF can be classified in a number of different ways. Often, CHF is defined as left ventricular failure (LVF), right ventricular failure (RVF), or a combined failure. As previously stated, when the left ventricle fails initially, there is both a decrease in CO and a backup of fluid in the pulmonary bed. Signs and symptoms of LVF are rales or crackles, shortness of breath, dyspnea on exertion, orthopnea, paroxysmal nocturnal dyspnea, and pulmonary edema. As in the case presentation, hemodynamic changes seen with LVF are reduced CO, elevated SVR, and elevated pulmonary capillary wedge pressure.

When the right ventricle fails, the blood backs up into the systemic circulation, producing elevated jugular venous distension, elevated CVP, hepatomegaly, ascites, anorexia, and pedal edema. Often and especially with chronic CHF, the patient will have signs and symptoms of both right-sided and left-sided heart failure.

Another classification of CHF is systolic versus diastolic heart failure. *Systolic heart failure* refers to the heart's inability to contract effectively. It is usually defined as an ejection fraction less than 35% to 40% (Albert, 1998; Konstam, Dracup, & Baker, 1996). Common causes of systolic dysfunction are coronary artery disease,

Table *9-1*	Signs and Symptoms of Left- and Right-Sided Heart Failure	
Left-Sided Heart Failure		**Right-Sided Heart Failure**
Capillary refill >3 sec		Hepatomegaly
Orthopnea		Splenomegaly
Dyspnea, dyspnea on exertion		Dependent pitting edema
Nocturnal dyspnea		Venous distension
Cough with frothy sputum (pulmonary edema)		Hepatojugular reflux >1 cm
Tachypnea		Oliguria
Diaphoresis		Arrhythmias
Basilar crackles, rhonchi		Elevated central venous, right atrial, and right ventricular pressure
Cyanosis		
Hypoxia, respiratory acidosis		Narrowing pulse pressure
Elevated pulmonary artery pressures		Kussmaul's sign
Elevated pulmonary artery occlusive pressures		Murmur of tricuspid insufficiency
Audible S_3 and S_4 heart sounds		Audible S_3 and S_4 heart sounds
Nocturia		Fatigue, weakness
Mental confusion		Abdominal pain
Weight gain		Anorexia
Fatigue, weakness, lethargy		Chest radiograph shows enlarged right atrium and right ventricle
Murmur of mitral insufficiency		
Chest radiograph shows enlarged left ventricle, left atrium and the presence of pleural effusion		Ascites
		Weight gain
Narrowing pulse pressure		
Pulsus alternans		

hypertension, and idiopathic dilated cardiomyopathy (American College of Cardiology/American Heart Association Task Force, 1995). Diastolic heart failure implies that the heart can contract effectively, but the ventricle has an increased resistance to filling during diastole, thus reducing the stroke volume. *Diastolic failure* is usually defined as a ejection fraction of greater than 40%. Diastolic heart failure may be caused by cardiomyopathy (hypertrophic or restrictive), hypertrophy of the ventricle caused by hypertension, constrictive pericarditis, or impaired ventricular relaxation (Goldman & Braunwald, 1998, p. 319). As with right- and left-sided heart failure, it is possible to have combined diastolic and systolic dysfunction. To distinguish between diastolic and systolic heart failure, the clinician should use an echocardiogram to document the ejection fraction (Konstam et al, 1996, p. 89).

Documentation of systolic versus diastolic dysfunction is important because of the treatment ramifications. The cornerstone of therapy for systolic dysfunction is a diuretic plus an angiotensin-converting enzyme (ACE) inhibitor. If the patient remains symptomatic, digoxin is also part of the treatment plan for systolic dysfunction. However, it is recommended for patients who have a diastolic dysfunction that diuretics and digoxin be avoided because they may contribute to reduced diastolic filling. β-Blockers or calcium channel blockers may be used with patients experiencing diastolic dysfunction. The focus of β-blocker therapy is to reduce the heart rate and hence increase diastolic filling time. Calcium channel blockers may be used to promote relaxation of the myocardium during diastole to increase the left ventricular end-diastolic volume (Beattie & Pike, 1996).

3. Discuss Mr. Arnold's signs and symptoms that were consistent with CHF.

On initial assessment, Mr. Arnold complained of fatigue and shortness of breath. Physical findings revealed bibasilar crackles, an audible S_3, and tachycardia. These signs and symptoms indicate left-sided heart failure. Mr. Arnold's fatigue is related to his decreased CO. As his CO decreased, his SNS was activated and he became tachycardic. His heart also was in atrial fibrillation with a rapid ventricular response, which may have been either the cause or the result of his CHF (Shapiro & Brundage, 2000). An audible S_3 indicates impaired filling during diastole. Mr. Arnold's increase in weight and his reduced urinary output represent activation of the RAS and the subsequent release of aldosterone and ADH. Mr. Arnold's abdominal pain and positive hepatojugular reflux result from his right-sided heart failure with an increase in hepatic engorgement. His hypoactive bowel sounds indicate a decrease gastric motility.

As Mr. Arnold's condition worsened, he became diaphoretic as a result of reduced CO and an increase in SNS stimulation. Hemodynamic changes included elevated blood pressure caused by SNS stimulation and elevated pulmonary artery pressures and pulmonary capillary wedge pressure caused by a backup of fluid into the pulmonary bed. The backup of fluid into the pulmonary bed also contributed to his labored respirations, dyspnea, and adventitious breath sounds. According to Goldman and Braunwald (1998), the development of rales correlates to a pulmonary capillary pressure of about 25 mm Hg. Elevated jugular venous distension and the presence of a hepatojugular reflux indicated right-sided heart failure as well. In addition, Mr. Arnold's SVR was elevated as a result of SNS stimulation and release of angiotensin II, and his cardiac index was reduced because of the combined failure of both his right and left ventricles. Mr. Arnold's ejection fraction of 30% indicated that his failure was systolic in nature as the result of his ventricles failing to contract effectively.

4. Describe Mr. Arnold's predisposing risk factors for CHF.

Goldman and Braunwald (1998), stated that 1% to 2% of the Western population has heart failure, and approximately 4.8 million people in the United States have CHF (Michael & Parnell, 1998, p. 172). Mr. Arnold's predisposing risk factors for developing CHF include his history of diabetes, his hypertension, and his coronary artery disease. Diabetes contributes to the development of coronary artery disease as the result of vascular changes. The existence of hypertension, which increases the workload on the heart, and documented blockages in the left and right coronary arteries indicate a potential for myocardial dysfunction resulting from ischemia and possible infarction. Also as previously stated, Mr. Arnold's atrial fibrillation could have been the result of his CHF or an initial cause of his CHF. In either event, the presence of his atrial fibrillation with a rapid ventricular response contributed to the reduced CO secondary to a loss of atrial kick and a decreased diastolic filling time.

Other predisposing factors that Mr. Arnold should be assessed for are (1) possible noncompliance with his antihypertensive therapy, (2) the possibility for either hypothyroidism or hyperthyroidism, and (3) a possible history of heavy alcohol intake. According to Goldman and Braunwald (1998), an intake of two drinks per day may be sufficient to exacerbate an already dysfunctional heart and lead to the development of CHF (p. 314).

5. List the nursing diagnoses appropriate for Mr. Arnold's care.

According to Kotecki (1999), the following are appropriate nursing diagnoses for the patient with CHF:

- Decreased cardiac output related to ventricular damage, ischemia, and restriction
- Impaired gas exchange related to increase in pulmonary interstitial fluid secondary to decreased cardiac output
- Altered tissue perfusion, myocardial related to imbalance between oxygen supply and demand
- Fluid and electrolyte imbalance related to decreased cardiac output and aldosterone and ADH secretion and medication regimen
- Ineffective breathing pattern related to imbalance between oxygen supply and demand.
- Fatigue related to imbalance between oxygen supply and oxygen demand
- Anxiety related to uncertain outcome
- Knowledge deficit related to new diagnosis and new medication regimen
- Ineffective coping related to health care demands of a newly diagnosed chronic illness

6. Briefly define the following terms: cardiac output, cardiac index, central venous pressure, preload, afterload, stroke volume, pulmonary artery pressure, and pulmonary artery occlusive pressure.

Cardiac output (CO) is the amount of blood ejected from the heart per minute. It is the product of the stroke volume times heart rate (SV × HR). The normal CO is 4 to 8 L/min (Morelli, 1999).

Cardiac index (CI) is the cardiac output divided by the body surface area. It takes into account the patient's size or body surface area, and hence provides a more realistic indicator of cardiac function. The normal cardiac index is 2.5 to 4 L/min (Morelli, 1999).

Central venous pressure (CVP) is the pressure in the right atrium. It reflects the pressure in the right side of the heart; thus as the pressure in the right ventricle increases with right ventricular failure, the CVP will increase. The normal CVP is 2 to 8 mm Hg (Morelli, 1999).

Preload is the volume of blood in the ventricle at the end of diastole. It is also called the *left ventricular end-diastolic pressure*. Clinically, the preload is measured as the pulmonary artery occlusive pressure or the "wedge" pressure.

Afterload is the amount of work or resistance the ventricles must overcome to eject a given stroke volume. It is also referred to as *systemic vascular resistance* (SVR). The formula to determine the SVR is [(MAP – CVP)/CO] × 80. The normal SVR is between 800 and 1200 dynes/sec/cm^{-5} (MAP is mean arterial pressure).

Stroke volume (SV) is the amount of blood ejected per beat. The formula for determining the stroke volume is CO/HR. The normal stroke volume is 60 to 80 ml/beat.

Pulmonary artery pressure (PAP) is the systolic and diastolic pressure within the pulmonary bed, in addition to the mean pulmonary pressure. The normal values are as follows (Morelli, 1999):

- Systolic PAP: 15 to 30 mm Hg
- Diastolic PAP: 8 to 15 mm Hg
- Mean PAP: 10 to 20 mm Hg

Pulmonary artery occlusive pressure (PAOP) is the pressure in the pulmonary artery upon inflation of the balloon tip in a pulmonary artery catheter. The pulmonary arterial occlusive pressure reflects the preload or the left ventricular end-diastolic pressure. It is also called the *wedge pressure*. The normal pulmonary artery occlusive pressure is 8 to 15 mm Hg (Morelli, 1999).

7. Describe the benefits of using a pulmonary artery catheter during CHF.

As stated previously, when the left and right ventricles begin to fail, fluid backs up into the pulmonary and systemic beds, respectively. Although signs and symptoms of CHF are important in determining a patient's status, they are often not accurate enough to help monitor the patient during critical phases of treatment. The pulmonary artery catheter can provide more accurate data to determine the CO and CI, the PAOP, the PAPs, and the CVP. As stated in question 1, according to the Frank-Starling law, the greater the preload, the greater the CO up to a point. By using the pulmonary artery catheter and measuring the CO/CI and the PAOP simultaneously, one can plot the Frank-Starling curve and determine the appropriate preload for the most optimal CO. This allows the clinician to titrate intravenous fluid administration, use of diuretics, use of ACE inhibitors, and vasopressor therapy to provide the most optimal CO for a given patient.

8. Briefly describe the pathophysiology of pulmonary edema.

As stated in question 1, when the left ventricle fails as a pump, fluid is backed up into the pulmonary vasculature. When the pressure in the pulmonary vasculature exceeds 25 mm Hg or colloidal osmotic pressure, fluid begins to leak from the capillary bed into the interstitial spaces. When the buildup of pressure within the pulmonary bed is gradual, the lymphatic system is able to sequester the fluid away from the pulmonary bed (Goldman & Braunwald, 1998). However, when the increase in pressure is more acute, the fluid begins to leak into the alveoli. Classic signs and symptoms of pulmonary edema are extreme shortness of breath and respiratory distress, crackles, and pink frothy sputum. These signs and symptoms develop as the fluid begins to fill the alveoli and inhibit gas exchange, making the patient hypoxic. Also, as the fluid crosses into the alveoli, capillaries rupture, making the sputum pink tinged. When arterial blood gas levels are measured, the patient's arterial oxygen pressure (Pao_2) will be usually less than 60 mm Hg.

9. List the pharmacologic agents used in Mr. Arnold's care and explain their importance to his treatment.

The cornerstone of drug therapy for CHF is a diuretic plus an ACE inhibitor, with digoxin being added for patients who remain symptomatic (Massie & Amidon, 1998; Michael & Parnell, 1998). In patients such as Mr. Arnold who have a rapid onset of CHF and the development of pulmonary edema, vasopressors such as dobutamine and dopamine may be added in addition to nitroprusside. Other medications that may be added to the protocol include nitroglycerin and morphine sulfate.

Mr. Arnold's specific medication regimen included the following drugs.

Captopril (Capoten)

Captopril is an ACE inhibitor that is recommended for the treatment of CHF because it produces vasodilation and it blocks the RAS (Massie & Amidon, 1998; Michael & Parnell, 1998). By blocking the RAS and inhibiting angiotensin II, captopril promotes vasodilation. Also by blocking the RAS, aldosterone and subsequently ADH are inhibited and less fluid is retained. As the result of these actions, captopril reduces the preload and left ventricular filling pressures and moderately increases the CO. Long-term studies have indicated that captopril lessens symptoms and improves exercise tolerance (Massie & Amidon, 1998; Michael & Parnell, 1998). Caution should be used when captopril is started because it may cause significant hypotension. A starting dosage for captopril is 12.5 mg every 8 hours, and it can be increased to 25 to 100 mg three times daily (Massie & Amidon, 1998). In addition, because of the potential effects that ACE inhibitors have on renal function, the creatinine and potassium levels must be monitored closely.

Digitalis (Digoxin)

Digitalis is a cardiac glycoside that works by inhibiting the sodium-potassium pump. As a result, increased intracellular sodium is exchanged for extracellular calcium. The higher levels of intracellular calcium assist in increasing the force of the heart's contraction. Digitalis also inhibits atrioventricular conduction and is often used to decrease ventricular response to atrial fibrillation. Digoxin may be administered either orally or IV, but as in Mr. Arnold's case, when a rapid effect is desired to control atrial fibrillation, IV administration is preferred. Intravenously, the onset of digoxin's effect is 15 to 30 minutes, with a peak effect in 1½ to 3 hours. The initial dose of digoxin is 0.5 mg given over 20 minutes, with subsequent doses of 0.25 or 0.125 mg given after 3 hours (Massie & Amidon, 1998). When digoxin is given, it is important that digoxin toxicity be avoided. Studies have indicated that serum digoxin levels of 0.3 to 0.13 ng/ml are just as effective as levels in the range of 0.15 to 2.2 ng/ml (Michael & Parnell, 1998).

Dobutamine (Dobutrex)

Dobutamine is a sympathomimetic that stimulates both β- and α-adrenergic receptors. However, dobutamine is more specific to β_1-adrenergic receptors (myocardium) than to β_2-adrenergic receptors (peripheral vessels and bronchioles). At a dosage of 2.5 to 10 μg/kg/min, dobutamine increases contractility, stroke volume, and CO (Kotecki, 1999). At dosages greater than 10 μg/kg/min, β_2-adrenergic receptors are stimulated but not to the degree that β_1-adrenergic receptors are stimulated. Hence dobutamine was added to Mr. Arnold's regimen to improve contractility and decrease afterload by producing some vasodilation.

Dopamine (Intropin)

Although dopamine was not used in Mr. Arnold's case, it is important to discuss its use and dose-related effects. At a low dosage of 0.5 to 2 µg/kg/min, this inotropic agent increases renal perfusion, which aids in fluid elimination and preload reduction. At a dosage of 2 to 10 µg/kg/min, β-adrenergic receptors are stimulated, increasing contractility, stroke volume, and heart rate. Dosages greater than 10 µg/kg/min produce α-adrenergic effects that result in vasoconstriction, which increases blood pressure. At high dosage levels, however, this vasoconstriction leads to decreased renal perfusion (Kotecki, 1999). If dopamine had been added to Mr. Arnold's regimen, it would have been started at a low dosage to improve renal perfusion and hence increase the glomerular filtration rate and reduce fluid retention. Dopamine can also be used at moderate dosages to improve the force of contraction but at the expense of an increase in myocardial oxygen consumption. Consequently, dopamine is often not the drug of choice for improving the CO.

Furosemide (Lasix)

As stated previously, one of the cardinal features of CHF is retention of fluid. According to Massie and Amidon (1998), diuretics are the most effective means for treating the symptoms of CHF. Furosemide is a loop diuretic that has a rapid onset and is effective even in patients with severe renal insufficiency (Massie & Amidon, 1998). The dosage for furosemide can range from 20 to 320 mg/day in either single or divided doses. Because Mr. Arnold was developing pulmonary edema and he had evidence of the potential for poor gastric absorption, furosemide was administered IV. Complications that a clinician should be monitoring for are (1) volume depletion, (2) hypotension, (3) prerenal azotemia, and (4) hypokalemia, especially if digoxin is part of the medication therapy.

Nitroprusside (Nipride)

Nitroprusside is a potent venous as well as arterial dilator, and it reduces both preload and afterload and subsequently improves the CO. Nitroprusside is usually used only in the management of patients with acute decompensating CHF (Massie & Amidon, 1998). Because nitroprusside can produce profound hypotension, the dosage is usually titrated according to the patient's blood pressure, and it is often used in conjunction with dobutamine or dopamine to maintain vascular tone while improving the CO.

Nitroglycerin Ointment

Nitroglycerin is both a venous and arterial vasodilator, and consequently, it decreases both preload and afterload. According to Massie and Amidon (1998), nitroglycerin can be effective in relieving shortness of breath in patients with mild to moderate CHF. The standard dosage is 12.5 to 50 mg (1 to 4 inches) every 8 hours; however, to prevent the development of tolerance to nitrates, a 8- to 12-hour drug-free period should be used. When nitroglycerin is started, the dosage may need to be adjusted if hypotension or nitroglycerin-induced headaches develop.

10. Discuss long-term management of a patient with CHF.

Readmission rates to acute-care facilities of 25% to 47% have been reported (Dunbar, Jacobson, & Deaton, 1998). Although frequent readmissions and exacerbation of a patient's CHF result from a number of variables, insufficient patient and family education, inadequate self-monitoring and management, and noncompliance with dietary restrictions, medication regimens, and exercise recommendations have been cited as strong contributing factors (Dunbar et al, 1998). These factors emphasize the importance of patient and family teaching and counseling in helping the patient maintain the highest level of wellness possible and avoid rehospitalizations. Broad areas that need to be addressed include medications, diet, fluid restriction, activities of daily living, exercise, smoking cessation, and self-monitoring. In each of these categories, various teaching strategies, including verbal and written communication, tapes (audio and video), and Web sites (if appropriate), should be used. Because CHF is a chronic illness, these areas of content should be covered not only before discharge but also at each follow-up visit. Follow-up visits provide an excellent opportunity to reinforce appropriate behaviors and clarify misconceptions.

Specifically, the standard care for a patient with CHF includes moderate dietary sodium restriction and a graduated exercise program along with the medication regimen. Massie and Amidon (1998) recommend restriction of sodium to 2 g and a graduated exercise program to increase exercise capacity. As with any patient, it is important to obtain a complete history, including dietary habits, use of over-the-counter medications, and past exercise habits. By obtaining an accurate baseline, the clinician can individualize the patient teaching to maximize compliance. When teaching patients about dietary restrictions, the clinician must explain what sodium is and how to determine how much sodium is present in the patient's food intake. This includes teaching patients not only to read labels but also to learn what types of foods to avoid, such as canned or processed foods. In patients with more advanced CHF, fluid restriction may be added. When fluid restriction is instituted, the patient and family must learn how to determine an accurate intake. The patient and family should also be cautioned that ice in drinks must be calculated into the patient's daily intake record.

As previously stated, thorough patient teaching about the medication regimen is also critical. Patients need to know not only what their medications are and when to take them but also the possible side effects. In Mr. Arnold's case, it is important that he and his family have a complete understanding of the purpose of his digoxin, how to take his pulse, and what signs and symptoms may indicate digoxin toxicity. Also, because Mr. Arnold's medication regimen includes an ACE inhibitor, furosemide, and digoxin, his potassium levels need to be monitored carefully. In addition, Mr. Arnold needs to understand the purpose of his potassium supplements. Given his drug therapy, it would be advisable to counsel Mr. Arnold not to use a potassium-based salt substitute. For his nitroglycerin, Mr. Arnold needs to understand the purpose of having a drug-free period, usually at night, and know that he must notify his health care provider if he experiences frequent headaches.

Self-management strategies should be taught to each patient. This includes the ability to assess changes in shortness of breath or dyspnea, to recognize paroxysmal nocturnal dyspnea (PND), new onset of orthopnea, changes in weight, pedal edema, abdominal distension (ascites), blood pressure changes, nausea, and fatigue. For elderly patients, family members may be encouraged to note changes in mental status as a possible sign of an exacerbation of CHF. Specifically, for weight changes, patients need to be taught to weigh themselves every day, on the same scales, and at approximately the same time to be able to evaluate their fluid status. Patients need to be taught that a 2.2-lb increase in weight represents retention of 1 L of fluid. If a patient experiences a 2-lb increase in weight or greater over a 1- to 2-day period, he or she should be taught how to adjust the medication regimen appropriately as well as how to modify diet and fluid intake. If patients and their families have doubts or if self-regulation fails, they need to know when and how to contact their clinician or practitioner.

When a nurse or practitioner sees a patient in the clinic for follow-up, the same guidelines apply. The clinician needs to monitor vital signs, weight, breath sounds, capillary refill, jugular venous distension, hepatomegaly, ascites, 12-lead ECG changes, digoxin level, and electrolyte levels (including K^+, Na^+, and creatinine). A focused history needs to be obtained to assess compliance with diet, medications, and exercise and any problems the patient may have developed. By working closely with the patient and family, the hope is that patients can achieve and maintain their desired quality of life and avoid rehospitalizations.

11. Discuss new drug therapies for CHF that are on the horizon.

Although the cornerstone of pharmacologic intervention for systolic dysfunction is a diuretic plus an ACE inhibitor and digoxin, a number of recent studies support other potential therapies. Based on the pathophysiology of CHF, new treatments are being explored to (1) reduce SNS stimulation and (2) reduce the release of angiotensin II and aldosterone. One such therapy is the addition of a β-blocker to reduce the chronic overstimulation of the SNS. Research has shown that chronic SNS stimulation leads to reduced responsiveness of the myocardium to norepinephrine (Bristow, Roden, Lowes, Gilbert, & Eichhorn, 1998; Michael & Parnell, 1998). In addition, prolonged SNS stimulation leads to cardiac hypertrophy and remodeling, arrhythmias, impaired contractility, and overstimulation of the RAS. Early studies in the 1990s focused on metoprolol, but more recent work has focused on the use of carvedilol, bisoprolol, and bucindolol (Michael & Parnell, 1998). Both carvedilol and bucindolol are nonselective β-blockers that cause peripheral vasodilation. Bisoprolol is a β_1-selective antagonist. Although more research is needed to determine which β-blocker is most beneficial, studies have supported the use of either a β_1 selective blocker or a β-blocker that has peripheral vasodilation properties (Bristow et al, 1998; Michael & Parnell, 1998). If a β-blocker is added to a patient's drug regimen, it is important to titrate the dosages slowly to determine the most optimal dose for each patient.

Another drug that may be added to a patient's regimen, particularly if diastolic dysfunction is present, is a calcium channel blocker. In the Prospective Randomization Amlodipine Survival Evaluation study and the Vasodilator Heart Failure Trial III, amlodipine and felodipine, respectively, were shown to be effective when used in combination with an ACE inhibitor in a selected group of patients (Coodley, 1999; Michael & Parnell, 1998). However, it is important to note that calcium channel blockers have been shown to be detrimental for patients who have a systolic dysfunction.

Focusing on reducing the RAS stimulation, investigators have studied both angiotensin II blockers and aldosterone inhibitors. Research on an angiotensin II inhibitor has focused on losartan. Losartan is a peripheral vasodilator, and it reduces SVR. It also decreases aldosterone secretion and release of norepinephrine. It has been demonstrated that losartan can improve left ventricular function in certain subgroups of patients with CHF (Coodley, 1999). The primary aldosterone inhibitor that has been studied is spironolactone. According to Michael and Parnell (1998), when spironolactone was used in combination with a loop diuretic and an ACE inhibitor, less fluid retention occurred.

Although these new approaches to therapy show promising results, it is important to note that many of the studies were done on small sample groups or on selected subgroups of patients with CHF. Hence these additional modalities should be used cautiously until larger, multicenter studies can be conducted, but they do show promise for future management of patients with CHF.

CONGESTIVE HEART FAILURE

References

Albert, N. (1998). Advanced systolic heart failure: Emerging pathophysiology and current management. *Progress in Cardiovascular Nursing, 13*(3), 14-30.

American College of Cardiology/American Heart Association Task Force. (1995). Guidelines for the evaluation and management of heart failure. *Journal of the American College of Cardiology, 26*(5), 1376-1398.

Beattie, S., & Pike, C. (1996). Left ventricular diastolic dysfunction: A case report. *Critical Care Nurse, 16*(2), 37-50.

Bristow, M. R., Roden, R. L., Lowes, B. D., Gilbert, E. M., & Eichhorn, E. J. (1998). The role of third-generation beta-blocker agents in chronic heart failure. *Clinical Cardiology, 21*(Suppl. 1), I3-I13.

Coodley, E. (1999). Newer drug therapy for congestive heart failure. *Archives of Internal Medicine, 159*, 1177-1183.

Dunbar, S. B., Jacobson, L. H., & Deaton, C. (1998). Heart failure: Strategies to enhance patient self-management. *AACN Clinical Issues, 9*(2), 244-256.

Goldman, L., & Braunwald, E. (1998). *Primary cardiology*. Philadelphia, Saunders.

Konstam, M., Dracup, K., & Baker, D. (1996). *Quick reference guide for clinicians: Heart failure management of patients with left-ventricular systolic dysfunction*. (Publication No. 94-0613). Washington, DC: U.S. Department of Health and Human Services.

Kotecki, C. (1999). Heart failure. In L. Bucher & S. Melander (Eds.), *Critical care nursing*. Philadelphia: Saunders.

Massie, B., & Amidon, T (1998). Heart. In L. Tierney, S. McPhee, & M. Papadakis (Eds.), *Current medical diagnosis and treatment*. Stamford, CT: Appleton & Lange.

Michael, K. A., & Parnell, K. J. (1998). Innovations in the pharmacological management of heart failure. *AACN Clinical Issues, 9*(2), 172-191.

Moser, D. (1998). Pathophysiology of heart failure update: The role of neurohumoral activation in the progression of heart failure. *AACN Clinical Issues, 9*(2), 157-171.

Morelli, P. (1999). Cardiovascular anatomy and physiology in failure. In L. Bucher & S. Melander(Eds.), *Critical care nursing*. Philadelphia: Saunders.

Shapiro, S., & Brundage, B. (2000). Cardiac problems in critical care. In F. Bongard, & D. Sue, *Current critical care and diagnosis and treatment*. Stamford, CT: Appleton & Lange.

CHAPTER 10

CAROTID ENDARTERECTOMY

Pam B. Koob, RN, PhD, CFNP

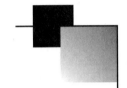

CASE PRESENTATION

Maxine Hamilton, age 62, has a history of coronary artery disease (CAD) and had four-vessel coronary artery bypass graft (CABG) surgery 4 years ago. Two years before her cardiac surgery, she had a silent inferior wall myocardial infarction (MI). This MI was not discovered until she was seen in her physician's office for her usual physical examination, which included an electrocardiogram (ECG) and cardiac enzyme determination. She did not remember having any unusual episodes of chest pain before the discovery of the MI, other than her usual "indigestion." She had been doing well since her CABG surgery, but during the past 6 months, Mrs. Hamilton has had at least three transient ischemic attacks (TIAs).

The first TIA involved numbness of her left arm and leg, dizziness, and a headache. The second TIA was identical. The third TIA did not include a headache, but she did again have numbness of her left arm and leg and dizziness. Each episode lasted approximately 15 minutes.

After the first TIA, Dr. Allen found bruits over the carotid arteries bilaterally and bright yellow plaques of cholesterol (Hollenhorst plaques) on retinal examination. After obtaining these findings, he performed a Doppler ultrasound of the carotid arteries and a computed tomography (CT) scan of the head to assist in determining the cause of the TIAs.

The results of the Doppler ultrasound and the CT scan indicated stenosis of both carotid arteries, which was more severe on the right side. After options were discussed with Mrs. Hamilton, a conservative medical approach was agreed on. Dr. Allen ordered aspirin (Bayer) 325 mg/day.

After the second TIA, Dr. Allen encouraged Mrs. Hamilton to consider surgery, but she declined. After the third TIA, Mrs. Hamilton agreed to have a cardiac catheterization and an arch angiography. Her precatheterization ECG revealed an old MI, with Q waves in leads II, III, and aV_F.

The cardiac catheterization revealed minimal (25%) occlusion of the right coronary artery. The remaining coronary vessels were 10% occluded. The two-vessel arteriogram report revealed bilateral carotid disease with 95% stenosis of the right internal carotid artery and 80% occlusion of the left internal carotid artery.

Intensive Care Unit Admission

After undergoing a right carotid endarterectomy, Mrs. Hamilton was admitted directly to the intensive care unit at 11:45 AM. Her initial postoperative vital signs and assessment revealed the following:

Height	162.5 (5 ft 5 in)	HR	80 bpm
Weight	63 kg (140 lb)	Respirations	24 breaths/min
BP	124/78 mm Hg	Temperature	36.8° C (98.2° F) (oral)

A clean dry dressing was placed over the right carotid area with a Jackson-Pratt drain in place. Her right neck area was slightly swollen.

The physician's orders were as follows:

- Cardiac monitor
- Continuous pulse oximetry
- Arterial line (A-line) for direct blood pressure (BP) measurement
- Oxygen at 2 L/min by nasal cannula
- 5% dextrose in 25% normal saline solution with 20 mEq KCl at 75 ml/hr
- Nitroprusside (Nipride) to keep BP below 140 (currently 10 ml/hr [33 µg/min] mixed as nitroprusside 50 mg in 250 ml of 5% dextrose in water).
- Complete blood count, blood urea nitrogen and K^+ levels, ECG, and chest x-ray film in the morning
- Meperidine hydrochloride (Demerol) 25 mg intramuscularly q3-4hr prn
- Head of bed elevated 30 degrees
- Neurologic checks every 15 minutes for 2 hours, every hour for 4 hours, every 2 hours for 6 hours, and then every 4 hours

At noon, 15 minutes after the initial assessment, the following data were obtained:

BP	172/92 mm Hg (cuff);	HR	98 bpm
	180/98 mm Hg (arterial line)	Respirations	26 breaths/min
		Temperature	37.2° C (98.9° F) (oral)

Breath sounds were clear, with a pulse oximetry reading of 96%. The trachea was midline with airflow auscultated over it. The ECG monitor revealed normal sinus rhythm at 98 bpm. The patient was easily aroused and oriented to person, place, and time. Handgrips were strong bilaterally with equal strength. Plantar flexion and dorsiflexion were intact. Mrs. Hamilton's speech was clear. Pupils were equal, round, and reacted to light. Cranial nerves were intact.

Other tests revealed the following:

Glucose	80 mg/dl	Na^+	139 mmol/L	Hgb	12.3 g/dl
BUN	11 mg/dl	K^+	3.9 mmol/L	Hct	39.3 %
Creatinine	0.9 mg/dl	Cl^-	106 mmol/L		

Nitroprusside (Nipride) was infused at 15 ml/hr (50 µg/min).

CAROTID ENDARTERECTOMY

Questions

1. How is carotid artery disease diagnosed? What is the best "medical" therapy?
2. Briefly describe the anatomy of the cerebral circulation and the pathophysiology of the carotid circulation that can require surgical intervention.
3. Define *carotid endarterectomy.*
4. Discuss the purpose and goal of carotid endarterectomy? Why was this procedure the best option for Mrs. Hamilton?
5. What is a stroke? What factors cause strokes?
6. What are the warning signs and symptoms of a stroke?
7. Mrs. Hamilton underwent the two most common diagnostic studies to determine blood flow and specific occlusion. Describe these studies and their typical findings. What are the risks and benefits of these studies?
8. Which study demonstrates when carotid endarterectomy should be selected over medical treatment? What criterion is used?
9. What are the clinical manifestations of atherosclerotic carotid artery disease? What are the three categories of patients with the disease?
10. Which patients are at greatest risk from carotid endarterectomy?
11. Define *TIA, amaurosis fugax,* and *reversible ischemic neurologic deficit (RIND).* What signs and symptoms did Mrs. Hamilton exhibit?
12. Describe the effect Mrs. Hamilton's hypertension could have postoperatively. What goals and treatment modalities would be expected?
13. Why do some patients develop postoperative hypotension? What are the nurse's responsibilities?
14. What should be included in Mrs. Hamilton's neurologic assessment?
15. Discuss how carotid endarterectomy can damage certain cranial nerves. What are the clinical manifestations of specific nerve damage? What precautions should be taken to prevent cranial nerve damage?
16. What are the signs of decreased cerebral functioning related to decreased cerebral blood flow that should be assessed in Mrs. Hamilton and immediately reported to the physician?
17. Twelve hours after surgery, the nurse notices a hematoma around Mrs. Hamilton's incision site. What causes a hematoma after a carotid endarterectomy? Discuss the danger posed by this finding.
18. What are other potential complications to keep in mind for Mrs. Hamilton?
19. What instructions should Mrs. Hamilton receive regarding restriction of neck movement immediately after surgery?
20. After surgery, Mrs. Hamilton made good progress and was discharged home the day after surgery. Discharge medications included nifedipine (Procardia) 20 mg orally every 8 hours and clopidogrel (Plavix) 75 mg daily. Describe the pharmacodynamics and clinical effects of these drugs. What instructions regarding her medications should be given to Mrs. Hamilton before her discharge?

CAROTID ENDARTERECTOMY

Questions and Answers

1. **How is carotid artery disease diagnosed? What is the best "medical" therapy?**

   Carotid artery disease is usually diagnosed in the office during a normal checkup by the primary health care provider. The primary care provider may include the following tests or examinations: history and physical examination, Doppler ultrasound imaging, oculoplethysmography, CT, arteriography and digital substraction angiography, and magnetic resonance angiography. Studies that can be done in the office are usually done first, and others are conducted from the least invasive to the most invasive in a stepwise fashion (Little & Meyer, 1997; Sacco, 1998).

   The best "medical" therapies for stroke prevention and the goals of treating carotid artery disease are smoking cessation, management of high blood pressure, blood glucose control for patients with diabetes, and antiplatelet medications such as aspirin, warfarin (Coumadin), or ticlopidine.

2. **Briefly describe the anatomy of the cerebral circulation and the pathophysiology of the carotid circulation that can require surgical intervention.**

   The brain receives 85% of its blood supply from the anterior circulation (bilateral carotid arteries) and 15% of its posterior blood supply from the posterior circulation (bilateral vertebral arteries). The common carotid arteries bifurcate extracranially into external and internal branches, with the external carotid artery carrying blood to the face and scalp and the internal carotid artery sending blood to the cerebral hemispheres. The internal carotid artery has four major intracranial branches: anterior cerebral artery, middle cerebral artery, ophthalmic artery, and posterior communicating artery (Clochesy, Breu, Cardin, Whittaker, & Rudy, 1996; Koob, 1999).

3. **Define *carotid endarterectomy*.**

   A carotid endarterectomy is the surgical removal of an atheroma (fatty plaque) at the carotid bifurcation in an attempt to prevent stroke (Ballotta, Da Giau, Saladini, & Abbruzzese, 1999; Loftus, 1997; Moore & Quinones-Baldrich, 1997; Mukherjee, 1998).

4. **Discuss the purpose and goal of carotid endarterectomy? Why was this procedure the best option for Mrs. Hamilton?**

   Carotid endarterectomy is the therapy of choice in symptomatic patients with high-grade internal carotid artery stenosis (Mayberg, 1997; Mukherjee, 1998; Rothwell, Slattery, & Warlow, 1997). The goal is removal of the atherosclerotic plaque formation in an effort to prevent stroke. Because of Mrs. Hamilton's high-grade stenosis and history of TIAs, the surgical procedure is indicated as the best option for preventing stroke or cerebrovascular accident (CVA) (Sacco, 1998).

5. **What is a stroke? What factors cause strokes?**

A stroke results from death of brain cells due to decreased blood flow to the brain. Sometimes, small pieces of plaque can break loose and obstruct an artery in the brain. A narrow opening in the carotid artery(ies) can be a source of blood clots that can easily travel to the brain, trap other blood clots, or cause total occlusion (Koob, 1999).

Patients with carotid artery stenosis who require a carotid endarterectomy have developed an obstruction of the blood flow to the brain. The obstruction usually occurs at the bifurcation of the common carotid artery and typically is a result of atherosclerosis. When fatty deposits are coated by fibrous tissue, a plaque develops, leading to stenosis. As this plaque increases in size, cerebral blood flow decreases. When the intimal lining of the artery is no longer intact, the plaque may become ulcerated and expose the roughened area. This, in turn, attracts more debris and can eventually lead to embolization. Cerebral blood flow decreases because of the narrowed vessel and release of microemboli from the atheroma occurs. If the emboli are of platelet origin, vasospasm and additional obstruction can occur as a result of the release of vasoactive substances such as thromboxane A_2 and create even further vasoconstriction. This further compromise to cerebral tissue leads to cerebral ischemia and infarction (Clochesy et al, 1996; Moore & Quinones-Baldrich, 1997; Sacco, 1998). Causative factors include atherosclerosis, fibromuscular dysplasia, aneurysms, trauma, Takayasu's arteritis, and spontaneous dissection.

6. **What are the warning signs and symptoms of a stroke?**

Signs and symptoms can include weakness/numbness of the face, arm, or leg; loss of vision or dimness, usually in one eye; difficulty speaking or understanding speech; severe headache; and dizziness, unsteadiness, or falls. Signs may last a few minutes and go away. If they last less than 24 hours, they are called transient ischemic attacks (TIAs) (Little & Meyer, 1997; Sacco, 1998).

7. **Mrs. Hamilton underwent the two most common diagnostic studies to determine blood flow and specific occlusion. Describe these studies and their typical findings. What are the risks and benefits of these studies?**

The most common studies include Doppler ultrasound of the carotid arteries and cerebral angiography. The Doppler ultrasound assesses peripheral arterial or cerebrovascular blood flow and velocity by picking up sound generated by blood moving through the underlying vessels. Vessels that are totally occluded do not transmit sound. No particular risk is associated with this study.

Cerebral angiography is performed by injecting a contrast material into one or more arteries to obtain radiographic visualization of the targeted circulation. Preprocedure care involves premedication and signing of an informed consent. Postprocedure care involves checking the site for bleeding or hematoma formation. A major complication of this procedure can be a stroke caused by accidental dislodging of an atherosclerotic plaque from the artery wall or a clot that formed at the end of the catheter or needle (Alspach, 1998; Little & Meyer, 1997).

8. Which study demonstrates when carotid endarterectomy should be selected over medical treatment? What criterion is used?

The North American Symptomatic Carotid Endarterectomy Trial (NASCET) has demonstrated that in patients with more than 70% occlusion of the internal carotid artery and a less than 6% surgical risk, carotid endarterectomy offers a clear benefit to the patient. The American Heart Association agrees and includes those who have had a mild stroke within the previous 6 months (Bahle, 1998; Gorelick et al, 1999; Kappelle, Eliasziw, Fox, Sharpe, & Barnett, 1999; Nemoto, 1999).

9. What are the clinical manifestations of atherosclerotic carotid artery disease? What are the three categories of patients with the disease?

Patients with atherosclerotic carotid artery disease may be seen with stroke or TIA or be asymptomatic. Three categories of patients have been identified by Moore and Quinones-Baldrich (1997): (1) patients with no symptoms but with a documented significant lesion or nonocclusive ulceration and no permanent neurologic deficits; (2) patients with TIAs, the most common sign of carotid artery disease; and (3) patients with completed cerebral infarction (Koob, 1999; Sacco, 1998).

10. Which patients are at greatest risk from carotid endarterectomy?

According to Rothwell et al. (1997), there is a 5% risk of stroke or death from the operative procedure, making the risk-versus-benefit balance somewhat delicate. These authors conducted a meta-analysis of all the published and unpublished literature from 1980 that was available to them and found that the following five clinical characteristics significantly increased a patient's risk with carotid endarterectomy: (1) surgery for CVA or TIA versus ocular ischemia by itself (amaurosis fugax or retinal artery occlusion), (2) female sex, (3) age older than 75 years, (4) systolic BP greater than 180 mm Hg, and (5) a history of peripheral vascular disease. They found no statistical evidence of linkage of diabetes mellitus, angina, recent MI, or current smoking to a higher surgical risk.

Three angiographic characteristics were found to be related to a higher risk of CVA or death. These were contralateral occlusion, stenosis of the intracranial section of the ipsilateral internal carotid, and stenosis of the ipsilateral external carotid artery.

11. Define *TIA, amaurosis fugax,* and *reversible ischemic neurologic deficit (RIND).* What signs and symptoms did Mrs. Hamilton exhibit?

A TIA is a temporary focal episode of neurologic dysfunction of vascular origin that may last from a few minutes up to 24 hours (Koob, 1999). By definition, neurologic examination must be normal or baseline within 24 hours. Typically, the neurologic deficit lasts 10 to 20 minutes and consists of hemiparesis with or without dysarthria, hemisensory loss, hemianopia, dysphasia, or monocular visual loss (Koob, 1999). Permanent damage is rarely associated with a TIA. When the symptoms are the same for each attack, the cause is usually the extracranial circulation. Patients with cardiac emboli tend to have variable symptoms. The most common symptoms are contralateral hemiparesis and/or hemiparesthesia, visual changes, receptive and/or expressive aphasia, vertigo, syncope, headaches, and ataxia. A classic symptom of carotid TIAs is transient spells of ipsilateral monocular blurring or blindness called *amaurosis fugax*. Amaurosis fugax is commonly referred to as a *retinal TIA* (Koob, 1999). A minor stroke lasts more than 24 hours but usually resolves.

A reversible ischemic neurologic deficit is neurologic dysfunction that lasts more than 24 hours but eventually resolves (Koob, 1999).

Symptoms accompanying Mrs. Hamilton's TIAs included dizziness, numbness of her left arm and leg, and a headache.

12. Describe the effect Mrs. Hamilton's hypertension could have postoperatively. What goals and treatment modalities would be expected?

Frequent changes in BP often occur during the immediate postoperative period. Baroreceptors located in the carotid sinus may have been disturbed during the surgical procedure, resulting in hypertension (Clochesy et al, 1996). Significant postoperative hypertension has been reported in the literature. Research indicates that hypertension usually occurs during the early postoperative period and generally lasts an average of 5 to 6 hours after surgery (Moore & Quinones-Baldrich, 1997; Sole, Hartshorn, & Lamborn, 1997).

One danger of hypertension includes rupture of the operative vessels. In addition, sustained hypertension puts the patient at risk for an intracerebral hemorrhage, edema, and stroke. Sodium nitroprusside and nitroglycerin are vasodilators commonly used to maintain the patient's BP within a range of 1 to 20 mm Hg of the patient's preoperative baseline (Blohme, Sandstrom, Hellstrom, Swedenborg, & Takolander, 1999; Katsung, 1998; Nemoto, 1999).

13. Why do some patients develop postoperative hypotension? What are the nurse's responsibilities?

Patients with chronic hypertension may develop reflex hypotension and bradycardia, which could require vigorous treatment with vasopressors. If hypotension occurs, the nurse must realize that this places the patient at risk for decreased cerebral blood flow and perfusion and can cause changes in mentation and increase the chances for neurologic deficits. The nurse must carefully titrate vasoactive drugs such as nitroprusside (Nipride) or nitroglycerin to avoid hypotension (Clochesy et al, 1996; Sole et al, 1997). If hypotension does occur and reducing the rate of the vasodilating drug being used is not effective, vasoactive drugs such as dobutamine or dopamine may be required (Nemoto, 1999).

14. What should be included in Mrs. Hamilton's neurologic assessment?

1. Level of consciousness and orientation
2. Ability to follow commands
3. Speech
4. Extremity movement and strength

5. Pupil size and reaction to light; visual field acuity
6. Cranial nerves
   - Ability to position the tongue midline (hypoglossal)
   - Ability to smile (facial)
   - Ability to speak (vagus)
   - Ability to raise arms and sustain for 3 seconds (spinal accessory) (Koob, 1999; Nemoto, 1999)

15. Discuss how carotid endarterectomy can damage certain cranial nerves. What are the clinical manifestations of specific nerve damage? What precautions should be taken to prevent cranial nerve damage?

Injuries to cranial nerves can occur from intraoperative trauma (e.g., inadvertent transection, retractor injuries) and edema, resulting in nerve compression. Cranial nerve damage occurs in 16% of patients undergoing carotid endarterectomy. These injuries usually resolve; however, 1% to 4% do not resolve (Nemoto, 1999; Pritz, 1998; Rothwell et al, 1997). The following cranial nerve injuries may occur:

- XII, hypoglossal (located under the carotid artery): inability to position the tongue midline
- X, vagus (laryngeal branch): hoarseness, loss of cough mechanism
- VII, facial (marginal mandibular branch): drooping of the lip ipsilateral to the surgery site
- XI, spinal accessory: inability to shrug shoulders

The presence of cranial nerve deficits should be determined before the patient is given any ice chips, water, or food. Once the gag reflex has returned, the patient should be given liquids only initially and cautiously when awake. The head of the bed should be elevated at all times. Suctioning equipment should be available and ready for use. In addition, the patient should be observed closely for respiratory difficulties or other signs of hypoxemia (Koob, 1999).

16. What are the signs of decreased cerebral functioning related to decreased cerebral blood flow that should be assessed in Mrs. Hamilton and immediately reported to the physician?

- Ipsilateral vascular-type headaches
- Decreased level of consciousness
- Unequal, dilated, or sluggish pupils
- Motor weakness or hemiplegia
- Visual disturbances
- Respiratory or breathing pattern changes
- Dysphasia
- Seizures
- Widening pulse pressure (late and ominous sign) (Clochesy et al, 1996; Nemoto, 1999; Sole et al, 1997)

17. Twelve hours after surgery, the nurse notices a hematoma around Mrs. Hamilton's incision site. What causes a hematoma after a carotid endarterectomy? Discuss the danger posed by this finding.

Development of a hematoma is a serious, potentially life-threatening complication. A hematoma in the neck area can contribute to airway occlusion, tracheal deviation, or rupture of the operative vessel. The patient should be monitored for bleeding and the following reported to the physician: edema, bright red drainage from the incision site, decreased hematocrit, and hypotension. In some cases, the patient may need additional surgery for reexploration and evacuation of the hematoma (Clochesy et al, 1996; Nemoto, 1999; Ouriel, Shortell, Illig, Greenberg, & Green, 1999; Pritz, 1999; Sole et al, 1997).

18. What are other potential complications to keep in mind for Mrs. Hamilton?

Stroke caused by embolization, thrombosis, or hemorrhage can occur. Also, post-operative MI is a major complication of carotid endarterectomy. Mrs. Hamilton is a potential candidate for an MI because of her history of preexisting cardiovascular disease. MI occurs infrequently but is the most common cause of death after carotid endarterectomy (0.8% to 3%); the risk of MI is increased in patients with a history of angina (13%) (Rothwell et al, 1997; Riggs & DeWeese, 1998).

19. What instructions should Mrs. Hamilton receive regarding restriction of neck movement immediately after surgery?

The patient should avoid any sharp turns of the neck. Nothing should be placed on the site that might cause injury or damage. The head should be supported at all times (Pritz, 1998; Riggs & DeWeese, 1998; Sole et al, 1997).

20. After surgery, Mrs. Hamilton made good progress and was discharged home the day after surgery. Discharge medications included nifedipine (Procardia) 20 mg orally every 8 hours and clopidogrel (Plavix) 75 mg daily. Describe the pharmacodynamics and clinical effects of these drugs. What instructions regarding her medications should be given to Mrs. Hamilton before her discharge?

According to Katsung (1998), calcium channel blockers, such as nifedipine, relax vascular smooth muscle, specifically arterioles and veins, without causing orthostatic hypotension and thus reduced BP. Peripheral vascular resistance is reduced, especially with nifedipine. Calcium channel blockers also reduce cardiac contractility and cardiac output in a dose-dependent fashion. Some research has indicated that calcium channel blockers may interfere with the development of atheromatous lesions. The most important adverse side effect is cardiac depression, including cardiac arrest, bradycardia, atrioventricular block, and congestive heart failure. Minor toxic effects caused by calcium channel blockers include flushing, edema, dizziness, nausea, and constipation. Mrs. Hamilton should be taught how to take her pulse before taking this drug and to report a pulse of less than 50 bpm to her physician, as well as the side effects just addressed (Mukherjee, 1998).

Clopidogrel (Plavix) blocks the binding of adenosine diphosphate to platelets, preventing arterial and venous thrombosis. It was approved for use by the U.S. Food and Drug Administration on November 17, 1997. Large clinical trials have shown a statistically significant reduction of death caused by stroke compared with aspirin.

Indigestion, nausea, vomiting, rash, and diarrhea are the most common adverse reactions (Katsung, 1998). Mrs. Hamilton should be instructed to report persistent symptoms to her doctor.

CAROTID ENDARTERECTOMY

References

Alspach, J. G. (Ed.). (1998). *American Association of Critical-Care Nurses: Core curriculum for critical care nursing* (5th ed.). Philadelphia: Saunders.

Bahle, J. (1998). Stroke prevention screening program. *Journal of Vascular Nursing, 16*(2), 35-37.

Ballotta, E., Da Giau, G., Saladini, M., Abbruzzese, E. (1999). Carotid endarterectomy in symptomatic and asymptomatic patients aged 75 years or more: Perioperative mortality and stroke risk rates. *American Vascular Journal, 13*(2), 158-163.

Blohme, L., Sandstrom, V., Hellstrom, G., Swedenborg, J., & Takolander, R. (1999). Complications in carotid endarterectomy are predicted by qualifying symptoms and preoperative CT findings. *European Journal of Vascular and Endovascular Surgery, 17*(3), 213-218.

Clochesy, J. M., Breu, C., Cardin, S., Whittaker, J., & Rudy, E. B. (Eds.). (1996). *Critical care nursing* (2nd ed.). Philadelphia: Saunders.

Gorelick, P. B., Sacco, R. L., Smith, D. B., Alberts, M., Mustone-Alexander, L., Rader, D., Ross, J. I., Raps, E., Ozer, M. N., Brass, L. M., Malone, M. E., Goldberg, S., Booss, J., Hanley, D. F., Toole, J. F., Greengold, N. L., & Rhew, D. C. (1999). Prevention of a first stroke: A review of guidelines and multidisciplinary consensus statement from the National Stroke Association. *Journal of the American Medical Association, 281*(12), 1112-1118.

Katsung, B. G. (Ed.). (1998). *Basic and clinical pharmacology.* Norwalk, CT: Appleton & Lange.

Kappelle, L. J., Eliasziw, M., Fox, A. J., Sharpe, B. L., & Barnett, H. J. (1999). Importance of intracranial atherosclerotic disease in patients with symptomatic stenosis of the internal carotid artery. The North American Symptomatic Carotid Endarterectomy Trial. *Stroke, 30*(2), 282-286.

Koob, P. B. (1999). The Neurological System. In C. J. Reeves, G. Roux, & R. Lockhart, R. (Eds.), *Medical-surgical nursing.* New York: McGraw-Hill.

Little, N. S., & Meyer, F. B. (1997). Indications for carotid endarterectomy. *Clinical Neurosurgery, 44,* 91-105.

Loftus, C. M. (1997). Carotid endarterectomy: How the operation is done. *Clinical Neurosurgery, 44,* 243-265.

Mayberg, M. R. (1997). Analysis of outcome in carotid endarterectomy trials. *Clinical Neurosurgery, 44,* 423-437.

Moore, W., & Quinones-Baldrich, W. (1997). Extracranial cerebrovascular disease: The carotid artery. In W. Moore & L. Bralow (Ed.), *Vascular surgery: A comprehensive review.* Philadelphia: Saunders.

Mukherjee, D. (1998). Carotid endarterectomy: Changing practice patterns. *Journal of Cardiovascular Surgery, 39*(6), 703-707.

Nemoto, E.M. (1999). No absolutes in neuromonitoring for carotid endarterectomy. *Stroke, 30*(4), 895, 896-897.

Ouriel, K., Shortell, C. K., Illig, K. A., Greenberg, R. K., & Green, R. M. (1999). Intracerebral hemorrhage after carotid endarterectomy: Incidence, contribution to neurologic morbidity, and predictive factors. *Journal of Vascular Surgery, 29*(1), 82-87, 87-89.

Pritz, M. B. (1998). Carotid endarterectomy. *Seminars in Neurology, 18*(4), 493-500.

Riggs, P. N., & DeWeese, J. A. (1998). Carotid endarterectomy. *Surgical Clinics of North America, 78*(5), 881-900.

Rothwell, P., Slattery, J., & Warlow, C. (1997). Clinical and angiographic predictors of stroke and death from carotid endarterectomy: A systematic review. *British Medical Journal, 315,* 1571-1577.

Sacco, R. L. (1998). Identifying patient populations at high risk for stroke. *Neurology, 51*(3, Suppl 3), 527-530.

Sole, M. L., Hartshorn, J., & Lamborn, M. (1997). *Introduction to critical care nursing.* Philadelphia: Saunders.

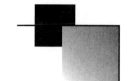

CHAPTER *11*

ACUTE RENAL FAILURE

Amy Reese Ramirez, RN, BSN, MSW, MSN, FNP •
Sheila Drake Melander, RN, DSN, ACNP-C, FCCM

CASE PRESENTATION

Sarah Banks, age 68, initially was admitted to the hospital for elective surgical repair of an abdominal aortic aneurysm. Her surgery was documented as uneventful. However, complications developed during her fifth postoperative day as a result of a small bowel perforation.

Postoperative Day 5

Vital signs and laboratory results were as follows:

BP	170/94 mm Hg	Hgb	10.1 g/dl
HR	110 bpm	Hct	30%
Respirations	30 breaths/min	RBCs	$3.5 \times 10^6/mm^3$
Temperature	38.6° C (101.4° F) (rectal)	WBCs	20,000/mm^3

Urine tests showed the following:

Creatinine	0.6 g/24 hr	Na$^+$	45 mmol/L
Osmolarity	460 mOsm/kg	K$^+$	15 mmol/L
Specific gravity	1.01	Cl$^-$	48 mmol/L
pH	9.0		

Results of serum measurements were the following:

Na$^+$	135 mmol/L	Creatinine	1.4 mg/dl
K$^+$	4.8 mmol/L	Uric acid	9 mg/dl
Cl$^-$	88 mmol/L	Phosphorus	5.2 mg/dl
Ca^{++}	6 mg/dl	Alkaline phosphatase	14.8 King-Armstrong units/dl
BUN	27 mg/dl		

Laboratory results and vital signs were telephoned to her physician. Her physician's orders included the following:

- Hydralazine (Apresoline) at 10 mg qid
- Gentamicin sulfate (Garamycin) IV at 5 mg/kg tid in divided doses
- Piperacillin sodium (Pipracil) 3 g q12h

Gastrointestinal Fistula Repair

As a result of an abnormal abdominal x-ray film, Mrs. Banks was returned to surgery for repair of a small bowel perforation. Four days after Mrs. Banks' bowel surgery, she developed a gastrointestinal fistula. She was again taken to surgery for repair of the fistula. Postoperatively, her blood pressure dropped to 80/52 mm Hg and her urine output was 20 ml/hr, requiring invasive monitoring. Mrs. Banks' oxygen saturations and arterial blood gas values dropped significantly. She required intubation and was transferred to the intensive care unit (ICU).

Intensive Care Unit Admission

After Mrs. Banks' admission to the ICU, the staff took a complete history that revealed her congestive heart failure. Mrs. Banks weighed 76.5 kg (170 lb) (preoperative weight was 71 kg [158 lb]) and had 2+ pitting edema in her lower extremities. Her skin was pale, shiny, and dry. She complained of nausea and stated that she "felt as if she had no energy left." Fluid intake for the past 24 hours was 1400 ml, and her output was 510 ml. Jugular vein distension was noted, and crackles were auscultated bilaterally in the lung bases. The initial cardiac rhythm was tachycardia with a rate of 110 bpm, a PR interval of 0.18 second, QRS complex of 0.14 second, and peaked T waves.

A fluid challenge was administered unsuccessfully. Despite volume replacement and diuretics, Mrs. Banks' renal status deteriorated further, and acute renal failure (ARF) was diagnosed. Dopamine (Intropin) was started at 2 µg/kg/min and dobutamine (Dobutrex) at 3 µg/kg/min, and continuous arteriovenous hemofiltration dialysis (CAVHD) was begun. Diagnostic data at this time were the following:

Weight	82 kg (182 lb)	Cl^-	98 mmol/L
BP	90-110 mm Hg (systolic)	Ca^{++}	7 mg/dl
HR	124 bpm	BUN	36 mg/dl
Urine output	15 ml/hr	Creatinine	3.9 mg/dl
Na^+	146 mmol/L	PAP	36/16 mm Hg
K^+	5.8 mmol/L	PAWP	15 mm Hg

After 4 days of CAVHD, blood urea nitrogen (BUN) and creatinine levels began falling, and blood pressure stabilized with a decrease in weight and edema. Electrolyte and laboratory values returned to normal limits. Total parenteral nutrition (TPN) was begun, and renal function continued to improve until CAVHD was discontinued 5 days later.

ACUTE RENAL FAILURE

Questions

1. Discuss the pathophysiology involved in ARF.
2. Describe the four phases in the clinical course of ARF.
3. Compare and contrast oliguric and nonoliguric renal failure.
4. What clinical assessment data support the diagnosis of ARF for Mrs. Banks? What other information may be useful in the diagnosis of ARF?

5.   What is the significance of the use of gentamicin sulfate (Garamycin) and piperacillin sodium (Pipracil) in Mrs. Banks' treatment regimen?
6.   Discuss the major nephrotoxic drug classifications, including risk factors and prevention of nephrotoxicity.
7.   What is the rationale for including dopamine (Intropin) in Mrs. Banks' treatment plan?
8.   Identify other pharmacologic agents used in the treatment of ARF and the rationale for their use.
9.   Discuss the dietary management of the patient in ARF.
10. Discuss the three different forms of dialysis used in the treatment of ARF, including the indications and contraindications for each. Why was CAVHD indicated for Mrs. Banks?
11. List nursing diagnoses appropriate for care of the patient with ARF.
12. What are the nursing responsibilities and potential complications related to CRRT?

ACUTE RENAL FAILURE

Questions and Answers

1.   Discuss the pathophysiology involved in ARF.

Definition

Bucher and Melander (1999) defined ARF as "the sudden deterioration in renal function usually associated with the loss of the kidney's ability to concentrate urine, as well as the retention and accumulation of nitrogen wastes." ARF accounts for 7% of the intensive care unit admissions and affects 20% of all critically ill patients (Stark, 1998, p. 545). The onset of ARF generally is sudden and is characterized by either anuria (<100 ml/24 hr), oliguria (100 to 400 ml/24 hr), or polyuria (>400 ml/24 hr). Oliguria is associated with 50% mortality in critically ill patients and 50% to 70% mortality after trauma or surgery. Nonoliguria with ARF presents a better prognosis and a lower mortality of 26% (Alspach, 1998). Because a successful treatment plan has not been established, the prevention of ARF remains the best approach (Stark, 1998).

Etiology

ARF can be classified as prerenal, postrenal, or intrarenal (Rakel, 1999). Prerenal failure results from decreased renal perfusion caused by hemorrhage, dehydration, decreased cardiac output, or fluid shifts. Postrenal failure is caused by an obstruction in the flow of urine from conditions such as benign prostatic hypertrophy, tumor, and bladder, renal, or ureteral calculi. Intrarenal failure is accompanied by tubular, interstitial, glomerular, or vascular renal tissue damage, such as that occurring in acute tubular necrosis (ATN), glomerulonephritis, renal vascular disease and interstitial nephritis.

According to Rakel (1999), the most common form of ARF in hospitalized patients is ATN resulting from ischemic or toxic damage to the nephrons. Patients at risk for developing ATN include those who have suffered a decrease in blood flow to peripheral organs, usually accompanied by hypotension and shock. Other risk factors include exposure to hemoglobin from mismatched blood transfusions, nephrotoxic drugs, radiographic contrast agents, poisons, heavy metals, and organic solvents (Lesko & Johnston, 1997).

Pathophysiology

The pathophysiology of ATN involves changes in renal hemodynamics, cellular metabolism, and nephron structure and function. A decrease in the mean arterial pressure (MAP) leads to decreased renal blood flow and perfusion pressure. As stated by McCance and Huether (1998), the kidney receives approximately 25% of the cardiac output, or 1200 ml/min. As a result of a decreased blood flow, ischemia may lead to a release of renin, activating the renin-angiotensin-aldosterone system. Once activated, this system causes the renal afferent arterioles to constrict and the glomerular blood flow, hydrostatic pressure, and filtration rate to decrease, which leads to tubular dysfunction and oliguria.

The amount of renal cell damage depends on the ischemic time period (Lesko & Johnston, 1997). Ischemia and hypoperfusion injury alter renal tubular cells, damaging the basement membrane. Cellular injury involves the depletion of adenosine triphosphate (ATP), oxygen free radical formation, loss of epithelial cell polarity, and increased calcium levels (Alspach, 1998). The depletion of ATP occurs within 30 seconds after ischemia, causing the loss of ionic composition, membrane integrity, and preservation of cellular volume (Alspach, 1998). The oxygen-free radicals are left unopposed during ischemic events, causing further disruption of cellular functioning. The passage of water, electrolytes, and other charged elements through the injured epithelial wall leads to a concentration defect. Increased calcium levels cause further renal vasoconstriction and a decrease in glomerular filtration rate (GFR) (Alspach, 1998).

In toxic ATN, toxins cause initial injury to the tubular cells. After this initial injury, the pathophysiologic characteristics of toxic and ischemic ATN are similar. However, the tubular basement membrane may not be damaged in toxic ATN, resulting in a faster healing process and regeneration (Alspach, 1998).

2. Describe the four phases in the clinical course of ARF.

The four phases of ARF include the (1) onset phase, (2) oliguric-anuric phase, (3) diuretic phase, and (4) convalescent or recovery phase.

Onset Phase

The onset phase can last from hours to days and is characterized by renal blood flow and oxygen consumption at 25% of normal, urine output at 30 ml or less per hour, and urinary sodium excretion greater than 40 mEq/L (Bucher & Melander, 1999). The most important factor affecting this phase is the alteration in systemic hemodynamics as evidenced by decreased cardiac output (Alspach, 1998).

Oliguric-Anuric Phase

The oliguric-anuric phase lasts about 8 to 14 days and is characterized by a further decrease in urine volume to 5% of normal. The oliguric phase occurs as a result of obstruction of the tubules, total reabsorption of urine filtration, tubular cell damage, and renal vasoconstriction (Alspach, 1998). The longer the patient remains in this phase, the poorer the prognosis. As reported by Alspach (1998), the nonoliguric phase is reflective of decreased tubular damage. Duration of this phase is generally short, with the patient reaching the recovery phase in 5 to 8 days.

Diuretic Phase

The diuretic phase appears when the sources of obstruction have passed, and a patent but nonfunctioning tubular epithelium and basement membrane remains (Stark, 1998). The urine is able to flow through the tubular space, but the cells cannot concentrate the urine. The high glomerular flow rate can contribute to a passive loss of electrolytes. Intravenous (IV) administration of crystalloids is necessary to maintain hydration during this phase (Bucher & Melander, 1999).

Convalescent or Recovery Phase

The convalescent or recovery phase begins with stabilization of laboratory values and can range from several months to 1 year (Bucher & Melander, 1999). During this phase, the edema is diminishing and the tubular cells begin to slowly resume functioning. Kidney functioning must be closely monitored to determine the final level of returning renal function (Stark, 1998).

3. Compare and contrast oliguric and nonoliguric renal failure.

Oliguric ATN

Oliguric ATN involves tubular damage, resulting in a tubular backleak of filtrate and tubular obstruction. During oliguria, the kidney is unable to concentrate urine, resulting in excretion of urine that is rich in sodium but lacking in excess volume, electrolytes, and waste (Stark, 1998). The patient exhibits fluid, electrolyte, and acid-base imbalances and requires frequent dialysis, resulting in a poorer prognosis.

Nonoliguric ATN

In contrast, tubular damage in the nonoliguric kidney is less severe. The presence of nonoliguria signals only epithelial damage to the tubules. There is no basement membrane damage, no cracks in the tubular wall, and no sloughing of cells obstructing the tubular space. The urine can pass freely in large volumes but cannot be concentrated. This explains the low specific gravity of 1.010 and the high level of urinary sodium (>40 mEq/L) (Stark, 1998). Therefore, when prevention of ATN in the critically ill patient is not possible, creation of a nonoliguric ATN by improving renal blood flow may help decrease the amount of tubular damage. Protective agents that can accomplish this include volume expanders, such as furosemide (Lasix), and dopamine (Intropin) (Stark, 1998).

4. What clinical assessment data support the diagnosis of ARF for Mrs. Banks? What other information may be useful in the diagnosis of ARF?

Assessment Data

Mrs. Banks' assessment information included jugular vein distension, pulmonary congestion, tachypnea, tachycardia, and intake and output imbalances. The cardiac monitor revealed peaked T waves and widened QRS complexes. Mrs. Banks also complained of lethargy and nausea and vomiting. Mrs. Banks' assessment data support the diagnosis of ARF (Bucher & Melander, 1999).

Patient History

Aspects of the patient's history that are important in diagnosing ARF include renal symptoms, systemic diseases, laboratory results, and medication history. Mrs. Banks had a history of cardiovascular disease and had experienced a hypotensive episode postoperatively along with sepsis. These findings in addition to the presence of other systemic diseases, such as hematopoietic or immunologic diseases, have a direct impact on the renal system. Also, Mrs. Banks was being treated with two nephrotoxic agents: gentamicin sulfate (Garamycin) and piperacillin sodium (Pipracil) (Alspach, 1998).

Laboratory Data

Laboratory studies for the evaluation of ARF include blood chemistry, complete blood count and smear, blood gas levels, urinalysis, and urine electrolyte levels (Rakel, 1999). Mrs. Banks' creatinine and BUN levels were both elevated. BUN levels are the least helpful of the two measures because the BUN concentration is often influenced by gastrointestinal bleeding, a high-protein diet, volume depletion, and catabolism (Rakel, 1999). Mrs. Banks was in an oliguric state; however, urine volume is not always a good measure of renal function because some patients may exhibit oliguric or polyuric renal failure. Patterns of urine output must be monitored to identify renal perfusion status. Mrs. Banks had elevations in sodium, potassium, chloride, phosphorus, uric acid, and alkaline phosphatase levels that support the diagnosis of ARF. A decreased calcium level and a high-normal magnesium level may also be evident in ARF (Rakel, 1999)

Urine laboratory values supporting ARF include the following:

- Decreased creatinine level and osmolality
- Increased sodium, potassium, and chloride levels
- Increased pH
- Fixed specific gravity and normal glucose and protein levels

It should be noted, however, that urinary laboratory values vary depending on the pathophysiologic changes involved. For example, with ATN, the urinary sodium level is usually elevated (Lesko & Johnston, 1997; Rakel, 1999).

Diagnostic Information

Noninvasive diagnostic procedures that should be performed for Mrs. Banks and other patients with ARF include fluid intake and output, daily weighing, and the kidney, ureters, and bladder x-ray examination. Invasive procedures that may be used include IV pyelography, computed tomography, renal angiography, renal scan, nephrosonography, and renal biopsy (Rakel, 1999).

5. **What is the significance of the use of gentamicin sulfate (Garamycin) and piperacillin sodium (Pipracil) in Mrs. Banks' treatment regimen?**

Gentamicin sulfate (Garamycin) and piperacillin sodium (Pipracil) are both nephrotoxic agents (Alspach, 1998). Piperacillin sodium, a penicillin, may lead to interstitial nephritis with ARF owing to a hypersensitive reaction. Gentamicin sulfate, an aminoglycoside, may lead to renal dysfunction with ATN. Aminoglycosides are major culprits in the development of nephrotoxic ATN. Aminoglycosides accumulate in the renal cortex and may not cause renal failure until after treatment is complete (McCance & Huether, 1998).

6. **Discuss the major nephrotoxic drug classifications, including risk factors and prevention of nephrotoxicity.**

Nephrotoxic Drug Classifications

Drug-induced ATN is a primary cause of ARF. Major nephrotoxic drugs include antibiotics, nonsteroidal antiinflammatory drugs (NSAIDs), and radiographic contrast media (Frazee, Rutecki, & Whittier, 1997a). To reduce the risk of antibiotic-induced drug toxicity, the patient should be given the shortest course with once-daily dosing; in addition, serum concentrations must be monitored carefully. Antibiotics should not be used in patients with known risk factors. Radiocontrast media are most likely to cause ARF in patients with preexisting renal damage, especially those with diabetes mellitus (Frazee et al, 1997a). Patients with congestive heart failure or poor renal perfusion or those who have been hospitalized recently are at greater risk for NSAID-induced ARF (Frazee, Rutecki, & Whittier, 1997b). Angiotensin-converting enzyme (ACE) inhibitors are also commonly associated with ARF (Frazee et al, 1997b). Patients at risk for ACE inhibitor–induced ARF include those with congestive heart failure or compromised left ventricular function and those receiving diuretics. The ACE inhibitor should be discontinued for these patients, and therapy should be focused on correcting renal blood circulation (Frazee et al, 1997b). Drugs that are highly insoluble in acidic urine, such as antineoplastics, may precipitate postrenal ARF. Prevention of this type of ARF involves alkalization of urine and hydration (Frazee et al, 1997b).

Prevention of Nephrotoxicity

Nephrotoxicity may be prevented by identifying risk factors, providing correct drug dosages, and monitoring serum drug levels. Serum creatinine and creatinine clearance levels should be monitored while a patient receives nephrotoxic agents. Alternative diagnostic measures should be considered before a contrast medium is used in patients at risk for renal dysfunction. The simultaneous use of more than one nephrotoxic agent should be avoided (Frazee et al, 1997a, 1997b).

7. **What is the rationale for including dopamine (Intropin) in Mrs. Banks' treatment plan?**

Dopamine (Intropin) dilates renal arterioles and increases renal blood flow and GFR. Dopamine is suggested for both the prevention and treatment of ARF in critically ill patients. Proponents suggest that low dosages between 0.5 and 2.5 µg/kg/min are useful for oliguric ARF. Caution must be taken with the use of dopamine, which can cause tachyarrhythmias, pulmonary shunting, and gut or digital necrosis (Thadhani, Pascual, & Bonventre, 1996).

8. **Identify other pharmacologic agents used in the treatment of ARF and the rationale for their use.**

Pharmacologic Management

In addition to dopamine (Intropin), loop diuretics such as furosemide (Lasix) and osmotic diuretics such as mannitol are used in the treatment of ARF when fluid overload is present (Rakel, 1999). Diuretics are used in ARF to increase urinary flow with the intent of flushing out the cellular debris causing tubular obstruction and possibly creating a nonoliguric ATN. Osmotic diuretics and loop diuretics have been found to dilate renal arteries by increasing the synthesis of prostaglandins, resulting in restoration of renal blood flow (Thadhani et al, 1996). Because the impact of a decrease in renal perfusion is greatest in the initial stages of

ARF, it is crucial to use diuretics as an early intervention. If administered early in the course of the ARF, both mannitol and furosemide can convert an oliguric state to a nonoliguric state. Patients with a response to these diuretics may have less severe renal damage than those with no response (Thadhani et al, 1996). Caution must be taken with the administration of dopamine. Even low-dose dopamine may cause severe complications, such as tachyarrhythmias and myocardial and peripheral ischemia (Rakel, 1999).

9. Discuss the dietary management of the patient with ARF.

According to Stark (1998), nutritional support is critical in the patient with ARF. Reasons include increased energy expenditure, extensive catabolic state, and the negative nitrogen balance. Tissue catabolism commonly develops in patients with ARF, which leads to increases in BUN levels, metabolic acidosis, and hyperkalemia. The patient requires a high-calorie, low-protein diet. The recommendation is 30 to 35 kcal/kg/day of carbohydrates and lipid supplementation. To diminish protein catabolism and reduce urea formation, 1.5 to 1.7 g of essential and nonessential amino acids should be administered (Stark, 1998). Salt and fluid restrictions are usually needed to match fluid input and output (Rakel, 1999). Continuous renal replacement dialysis therapy can assist in the management of large amounts of parental fluid infusions.

10. Discuss the three different forms of dialysis used in the treatment of ARF, including the indications and contraindications for each. Why was CAVHD indicated for Mrs. Banks?

The three dialysis options in the critically ill patient are hemodialysis, peritoneal dialysis, and continuous renal replacement therapy (CRRT).

Hemodialysis
Hemodialysis provides ultrafiltration for rapid water removal and diffusion for solute removal. It is indicated for uremia, electrolyte imbalances, fluid overload, and severe metabolic acidosis. Contraindications include hemodynamic instability, lack of access, and decreased clotting ability. Potential complications include fluid, electrolyte, and osmolar shifts and rebound hyperkalemia (Giuliano & Pysznik, 1998).

Peritoneal Dialysis
Peritoneal dialysis is a slow, efficient form of dialysis that involves an exchange of fluid and solutes between the peritoneal cavity and peritoneal capillaries. Peritoneal dialysis is indicated for uremia, fluid and electrolyte imbalances, and hemodynamic instability (Giuliano & Pysznik, 1998). It is not used in emergency situations unless all other forms of dialysis are unavailable or contraindicated. The disadvantages and complications of peritoneal dialysis are problems with access, less predictable removal of fluid, peritoneal drainage failure, slower removal of fluid than with other modes, and hyperglycemia caused by the hypertonic glucose in the dialysate. An advantage of peritoneal dialysis is that it requires less technical support and equipment than other renal replacement therapies (Giuliano & Pysznik, 1998).

Continuous Renal Replacement Therapy

Three forms of CRRT include slow continuous ultrafiltration, continuous arteriovenous hemofiltration, continuous venovenous hemofiltration, continuous venovenous hemodialysis (CVVHD), and continuous arteriovenous hemofiltration dialysis (CAVHD) (Alspach, 1998). CRRT is an ongoing therapy that may be used for days or months by allowing slow volume removal while maintaining hemodynamic stability. The hemofiltration options are designed primarily to remove water and some solutes, whereas the primary goal of the dialysis options is removal of solutes with the concomitant removal of water (Giuliano & Pysznik, 1998). CRRT is indicated for hypervolemic patients unresponsive to diuretics, patients who cannot tolerate rapid fluid shifts, and hemodynamically unstable patients with azotemia and/or uremia (Giuliano & Pysznik, 1998).

There are both advantages and disadvantages for using either CAVHD or CVVHD. CAVHD is slightly easier to execute than CVVHD because no pump is required. In CAVHD, a blood pump is not necessary because a pressure gradient is formed with blood flow from an artery to a vein. Hydrostatic pressure is exerted by the MAP, and negative pressure is created by the level of the drainage bag (Giuliano & Pysznik, 1998). The disadvantage of CAVHD is the need for a MAP of at least 60 mm Hg and the need for the placement of both an arterial and a venous catheter. With CAVHD, the patient's ultrafiltration rate depends on the MAP and the height of the collection device, making the management of the patient's intake and output of fluid difficult to balance (Giuliano & Pysznik, 1998).

CVVHD is powered by a pump rather than the MAP of the patient. The rate of ultrafiltration is more predictable because it depends on the set rate of the pump.

CRRT rather than traditional hemodialysis was an appropriate dialysis option for Mrs. Banks because of her hemodynamically unstable condition. Mrs. Banks also had a large daily fluid requirement that included TPN. Mrs. Banks' unresponsiveness to diuretic therapy also supported the need for CRRT.

11. List nursing diagnoses appropriate for care of the patient with ARF.

As cited by Bucher and Melander (1999), the following nursing diagnoses should be considered in the care of the patients with ARF:

- Alteration in urinary elimination
- Fluid volume deficit
- Fluid volume excess
- Altered nutrition: less than body requirements
- Risk for impaired skin integrity
- Knowledge deficit
- Decreased cardiac output
- Anxiety or fear
- Activity intolerance
- Body image disturbance
- Altered thought processes
- Risk for infection ineffective patient or family coping

12. What are the nursing responsibilities and potential complications related to CRRT?

Nursing Responsibilities

Before CRRT is begun, patient and family teaching concerning the procedure should be completed. Once the therapy has started, it is crucial to monitor the patient's hemodynamic status frequently to observe the patient's response to fluid removal. Any changes in heart rate, blood pressure, central venous pressure, and pulmonary capillary wedge pressure may indicate hypovolemia, requiring the need for a crystalloid infusion and adjustment of the ultrafiltration rate (McAlpine, 1998). Hemodynamic parameters should be measured every 15 minutes during the first hour of therapy and then every hour thereafter (McAlpine, 1998). The nurse should also monitor the partial thromboplastin times and observe the patient for any signs of bleeding. Electrolyte loss with ultrafiltration can be significant, indicating the need for close monitoring of electrolyte imbalances. Patients receiving CRRT therapy are at risk for hyponatremia, hypokalemia, hypocalcemia, and hypochloremia (McAlpine, 1998). The patient should also be monitored for acid-base imbalances. Drug levels must be monitored closely because CRRT may remove many of the drugs that are typically given to critically ill patients (Headrick, 1998).

The position and patency of the hemofilter and arteriovenous system must be checked frequently (Headrick, 1998). When a femoral catheter is used, the patient's legs must be positioned straight to avoid kinking of the catheter. Access sites must be inspected frequently for signs of infection or bleeding. A transparent permeable dressing should be applied and changed every 2 days or in accordance with the intravenous care and maintenance procedure (McAlpine, 1998). Fluid balance and electrolyte profiles should be calculated every 4 to 6 hours (McAlpine, 1998).

Prevention of Complications

Prevention of complications related to CRRT requires early intervention by the nursing staff. Restrictions on patient activity may lead to complications related to skin integrity, requiring a turning schedule via "log rolling." Dislodgment of the arterial catheter may lead to hemorrhage. Therefore patients receiving CRRT therapy may require restraints or sedation (Headrick, 1998). Sutures around the catheter and connection ports must be inspected frequently for patency (McAlpine, 1998). Thrombosis is another potential complication that requires close monitoring of distal extremity pulses and perfusion. Infection may be prevented by changing the occlusive dressing at the catheter site every 5 days, or according to hospital protocol. The site should be observed for signs of infection, and any lines and solutions should be changed according to hospital policy (McAlpine, 1998).

ACUTE RENAL FAILURE

References

Alspach, J. G. (1998). *American Association of Critical-Care Nurses: Core curriculum for critical care nursing* (5th ed.). Philadelphia: Saunders.

Bucher, L., & Melander, S. (Eds.). (1999). *Critical care nursing*. Philadelphia: WB Saunders.

Frazee, L. A., Rutecki, G. W., & Whittier, F. C. (1997a). Drug-induced acute renal failure: Keys to recognizing and treating intrarenal toxicity. *Consultant, 37*, 1592-1599.

Frazee, L. A., Rutecki, G. W., & Whittier, F. C. (1997b). Drug-induced acute renal failure: Recognizing and treating prerenal, postrenal, and pseudorenal injury. *Consultant, 37*, 1265-1268.

Giuliano, K. K., & Pysznik, E. (1998). Renal replacement therapy in critical care: Implementation of a unit-based continuous venovenous hemofiltration program. *Critical Care Nurse, 18*, 40-51.

Headrick, C. L. (1998). Adult/pediatric CVVH: The pump, the patient, the circuit. *Critical Care Nursing Clinics of North America, 10*, 197-207.

Lesko, J., & Johnston, J. R. (1997). Oliguria. *AACN Clinical Issues, 8*, 459-468.

McAlpine, L. (1998). CAVH: Principles and practical applications. *Critical Care Nursing Clinics of North America, 10*, 179-189.

McCance, K. L., & Huether, S. E. (1998). *Pathophysiology: The biological basis for disease in adults and children*. St Louis: Mosby.

Rakel, R. E. (Ed.). (1999). *Conn's current therapy*. Philadelphia: WB Saunders.

Stark, J. (1998). Acute renal failure: Focus on advances in acute tubular necrosis. *Critical Care Nursing Clinics of North America, 10*, 159-170.

Thadhani, R., Pascual, J., & Bonventre, J. V. (1996). Medical progress: Acute renal failure. *The New England Journal of Medicine, 334*, 1448-1460.

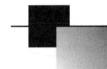

CHAPTER *12*
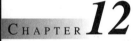

CHRONIC RENAL FAILURE
AND RENAL TRANSPLANTATION

Phyllis Ann Egbert, MSN, RNC, ACNP, CNN

CASE PRESENTATION

Richard Morgan, age 67, has end-stage renal disease (ESRD) caused by chronic pyelonephritis. He received hemodialysis at an outpatient clinic three times per week. He traveled with his wife approximately 75 miles to reach the clinic. A short experience with home dialysis was unsuccessful, and Mr. Morgan had begun to miss one and sometimes two clinic appointments each week. Mr. Morgan had no active malignancy or infectious process. He had a strong support system with siblings willing to donate a living donor kidney. He was financially secure through income and health insurance coverage.

Mr. Morgan arrived at the emergency department with a 2-day history of not feeling well, accompanied by nausea and vomiting. He was agitated and slightly confused. He was complaining of moderate to severe chest pain diffused over the precordium. Initial assessment revealed jugular vein distension, scattered crackles bilaterally throughout the lung bases, and pitting peripheral edema bilaterally in the lower extremities. Cardiac monitoring demonstrated sinus tachycardia with a rate of 116 bpm. A pericardial friction rub and an S_3 gallop were auscultated. His wife informed the nurse that Mr. Morgan missed his previous appointment for dialysis and was 8 kg (18 lb) heavier than his dry weight of 74 kg (164 lb). Current vital signs and laboratory results were as follows:

BP	180/110 mm Hg	K^+	7.3 mmol/L
HR	116 bpm	Cl^-	110 mmol/L
Respirations	36 breaths/min	CO_2	10 mmol/L
Temperature	38.7° C (101.6° F) (rectal)	Mg^{++}	1.3 mEq/L
Height	175 cm (5 ft 10 in)	PO_4^-	12 mg/dl
Weight	82 kg (182 lb)	Creatinine	26.9 mg/dl
RBCs	$3.1 \times 10^6/mm^3$	BUN	27 mg/dl
WBCs	$13,500/mm^3$	Glucose	95 mg/dl
Platelets	$226,000/mm^3$	pH	7.2
Hgb	8.5 g/dl	$Paco_2$	53 mm Hg
Hct	26%	Sao_2	85%
Na^+	136 mmol/L	HCO_3^-	10 mmol/L

Note: These values were in room air (21% oxygen).

The physician ordered admission to the medical intensive care unit for immediate hemodialysis. Oxygen was administered by a 40% face mask, and hemodialysis was initiated via a permanent arteriovenous (AV) fistula in the right forearm. An initial 4-hour dialysis treatment reduced Mr. Morgan's body weight to 76.5 kg (170 lb). After dialysis, Mr. Morgan was alert and oriented to place and person. Postdialysis assessment revealed the following: blood pressure 160/90 mm Hg, heart rate 94 bpm, and respirations 26 breaths/min. Mr. Morgan was given a diet restricted to 20 g of proteins and 1000 ml of fluids per day. His medication orders included the following:

- Aluminum carbonate (Basaljel) two tablets orally (PO) tid
- Ferrous sulfate (Iberet) 500 mg PO every morning
- Calcium carbonate (Os-Cal) two 250-mg tablets PO tid with meals

Hemodialysis was continued on a daily schedule of 4-hour sessions, and Mr. Morgan was transferred to the step-down unit. Mr. Morgan's condition progressively improved, and he was scheduled for discharge. Discharge assessment revealed the following:

BP	160/95 mm Hg	CO_2	15 mmol/L
HR	92 bpm	Ca^{++}	8.4 mg/dl
Respirations	20 breaths/min	Mg^{++}	2.3 mEq/L
Temperature	36.8° C (98.2° F)	PO_4^-	3.2 mg/dl
Weight	76.5 kg (170 lb)	Creatinine	12.6 mg/dl
RBCs	$4.1 \times 10^6/mm^3$	BUN	120 mg/dl
WBCs	$12,000/mm^3$	Glucose	125 mg/dl
Platelets	$226,000/mm^3$	pH	7.48
Hgb	9.1 g/dl	HCO_3^-	25 mmol/L
Hct	28.1%	Sao_2	95%
Na^+	136 mmol/L	$Paco_2$	30 mm Hg
K^+	5.8 mmol/L	Pao_2	135 mm Hg
Cl^-	98 mmol/L		

Note: These values were in room air (21% oxygen).

Mr. Morgan told his physician that he was unwilling to accept the limitations and restrictions in his life imposed by this illness and requested to have a kidney transplant. He informed the physician that he had discussed this at length with his three brothers and three sisters, and each is prepared to undergo testing to determine whether a transplant match is possible.

Six Months Later

The donor testing of Mr. Morgan's siblings resulted in a suitable kidney donor for his transplant. Six months after discharge, Mr. Morgan was readmitted to the transplant unit. Clinical and laboratory assessment revealed the following data:

BP	160/95 mm Hg	Cl^-	98 mmol/L
HR	92 bpm	CO_2	15 mmol/L
Respirations	20 breaths/min	Ca^{++}	8.4 mg/dl
Temperature	36.8° C (98.2° F)	Mg^{++}	2.3 mEq/L
RBCs	$4.1 \times 10^6/mm^3$	PO_4^-	3.2 mg/dl
WBCs	$12,000/mm^3$	Platelets	$226,000/mm^3$

Hgb	10.4 g/dl	Glucose	125 mg/dl
Hct	31.2%	HCO_3^-	25 mmol/L
Na^+	136 mmol/L	pH	7.48
K^+	5.8 mmol/L	Sao_2	95%
Creatinine	10.1 mg/dl	$Paco_2$	30 mm Hg
BUN	90 mg/dl	Pao_2	135 mm Hg

Note: These values were in room air (21% oxygen).

Preoperatively, Mr. Morgan was given methylprednisolone (Solu-Medrol), lymphocyte immune globulin (ATG), and azathioprine (Imuran). A right kidney was transplanted during an uneventful operation. Estimated blood loss was 200 ml. During the procedure, Mr. Morgan received 1400 ml of crystalloid intravenous solution and 3 U of packed red blood cells. He was transferred from the postanesthesia recovery room to the surgical intensive care. He received oxygen via a 40% face mask and dopamine at 2 μg/kg/min for renal perfusion. He had a Jackson-Pratt drain in the right flank and a Foley catheter to straight drainage. The initial postoperative assessment revealed the following clinical data:

BP	138/92 mm Hg	K^+	4.8 mmol/L
HR	92 bpm	Cl^-	92 mmol/L
Respirations	22 breaths/min	CO_2	18 mmol/L
Temperature	36.9° C (98.4° F)	PO_4^-	3.3 mg/dl
CVP	5 mm Hg	Creatinine	10.1 mg/dl
RBCs	$4.6 \times 10^6/mm^3$	BUN	90 mg/dl
WBCs	$12,500/mm^3$	pH	7.36
Platelets	$235,000/mm^3$	HCO_3^-	25 mmol/L
Hgb	11.1 g/dl	Sao_2	99%
Hct	33.5%	$Paco_2$	35 mm Hg
Na^+	131 mmol/L	Pao_2	138 mm Hg

Over the next 7 postoperative days, Mr. Morgan continued to improve. Blood urea nitrogen (BUN) and creatinine levels continued to drop, urine output averaged more than 100 ml/hr, and his condition was hemodynamically stable. Immunosuppression therapy included decreasing dosages of methylprednisolone, azathioprine 200 mg every day, and ATG 50 mg every 12 hours. On the seventh postoperative day, the relevant laboratory data were the following:

BP	138/92 mm Hg	Ca	8.5 mg/dl
HR	92 bpm	PO_4^-	3.3 mg/dl
Respirations	22 breaths/min	Creatinine	1.9 mg/dl
Temperature	36.9° C (98.4° F)	BUN	32 mg/dl
CVP	6 mm Hg	Intake	2250 ml
RBCs	$4.6 \times 10^6/mm^3$	Output (urine)	1050 ml
WBCs	$13,800/mm^3$	Output (Jackson-Pratt drain)	5 ml
Platelets	$296,000/mm^3$	Weight	76.5 kg (170 lb)
Hgb	12.9 g/dl	pH	7.36
Hct	36.7%	HCO_3^-	25 mmol/L
Na^+	135 mmol/L	Sao_2	99%
K^+	4.4 mmol/L	$Paco_2$	35 mm Hg
Cl^-	92 mmol/L	Pao_2	138 mm Hg
CO_2	22 mmol/L		

The Jackson-Pratt drain was removed. On the eighth postoperative day, Mr. Morgan began to complain of not feeling well; he had minimal abdominal tenderness on palpation and complained of nausea. His temperature fluctuated between 38.4° and 38.8° C (101.2° and 101.8° F). Urinary output dropped to an average of 55 ml/hr. Furosemide (Lasix) boluses did not improve his urinary output. On the 11th postoperative day, laboratory data revealed that his central venous pressure (CVP) was slightly elevated to 10.5 mm Hg and his weight was up to 82 kg (182 lb). His creatinine level was 7.1 mg/dl, and his BUN was 120 mg/dl. Muromonab-CD3 (Orthoclone OKT3) was started, and hemodialysis was initiated to support renal function for several days. Mr. Morgan's renal function showed progressive improvement. Cyclosporine was added to his immunosuppression therapy regimen. Mr. Morgan's laboratory data were as follows:

BP	138/92 mm Hg	Ca^{++}	8.5 mg/dl
HR	92 bpm	CO_2	22 mmol/L
Respirations	22 breaths/min	PO_4^-	3.3 mg/dl
Temperature	36.9° C (98.4° F)	Creatinine	1.9 mg/dl
CVP	6 mm Hg	BUN	31 mg/dl
RBCs	$4.6 \times 10^6/mm^3$	Intake	2250 ml
WBCs	$13,800/mm^3$	Output (urine)	1050 ml
Platelets	$296,000/mm^3$	Weight	76.5 kg (170 lb)
Hgb	9.5 g/dl	pH	7.36
Hct	28.7%	HCO_3^-	25 mmol/L
Na^+	135 mmol/L	Sao_2	99%
K^+	4.4 mmol/L	$Paco_2$	35 mm Hg
Cl^-	92 mmol/L	Pao_2	138 mm Hg

On the 28th postoperative day, Mr. Morgan was discharged home with the following regimen:

- Cyclosporine 100 mg/ml, 2.5 ml bid
- Ranitidine (Zantac) 150 mg hs
- Metoclopramide 10 mg hs
- Azathioprine (Imuran) 150 mg/day
- Nystatin 100,000 U/ml, 5-ml swish and swallow qid

CHRONIC RENAL FAILURE AND RENAL TRANSPLANTATION

Questions

1. Discuss the pathophysiology involved in chronic renal failure.
2. Discuss the typical laboratory findings seen with chronic renal failure.
3. Describe the symptoms of uremia that might be manifested by Mr. Morgan.
4. Describe how the relationship between calcium and phosphorus is altered in chronic renal failure.
5. Discuss the pathophysiology of aluminum toxicity in chronic renal failure.
6. Discuss the pathophysiology of pericarditis in chronic renal failure. Why was Mr. Morgan particularly prone to this complication?
7. Discuss the different forms of dialysis used in the treatment of renal failure,

including the indications and contraindications for each. Support the decision to use hemodialysis in treating Mr. Morgan.

8. Identify pharmacologic agents used to treat chronic renal failure and the rationale for their use.

9. Discuss the dietary management of the patient with chronic renal failure.

10. Identify clinical complications arising from noncompliance that were manifested by Mr. Morgan.

11. List nursing diagnoses appropriate for the care of the patient with chronic renal failure. Include nursing diagnoses appropriate for the care of the patient with a permanent AV fistula for dialysis access.

12. List the components of the teaching plan for the patient with chronic renal failure.

13. List the criteria used in the selection of patients for kidney transplantation.

14. Discuss hemodialysis and renal transplantation as alternative treatment modalities for Mr. Morgan. Support Mr. Morgan's decision to select renal transplantation rather than hemodialysis.

15. List the advantages and disadvantages of a living donor versus a cadaver donor. Why was it imperative that Mr. Morgan receive a living donor kidney?

16. Describe the cadaver kidney preservation process.

17. Briefly describe the surgical process of renal transplantation.

18. Discuss possible postoperative complications of renal transplantation.

19. List the nursing diagnoses appropriate for the care of the patient undergoing renal transplantation during the recovery period.

20. Discuss the pathophysiology of acute rejection. Describe the clinical manifestations of acute rejection in Mr. Morgan.

21. Discuss the immunosuppressive pharmacologic agents methylprednisolone, muromonab-CD3 (Orthoclone OKT3), and cyclosporine. Why did the physician add muromonab-CD3 and wait several days to begin cyclosporine?

22. List the components of the teaching plan for Mr. Morgan.

CHRONIC RENAL FAILURE AND RENAL TRANSPLANTATION

Questions and Answers

1. Discuss the pathophysiology involved in chronic renal failure.

The kidneys are paired organs located in the dorsal abdominal cavity in the retroperitoneal space in front of and on both sides of the spinal column between the 12th thoracic and third lumbar vertebrae. The right kidney is slightly lower than the left because the liver lies above it. The main function of the kidneys is to maintain proper fluid and electrolyte balance and remove metabolic wastes from the body. Fluid balance is achieved by the kidney's ability to concentrate or dilute urine. Electrolyte balance is achieved by the appropriate absorption and secretion of electrolytes within the tubular system of the nephron. Chronic renal failure may develop slowly over months or years or rapidly over many weeks. Irreversible kidney damage occurs when 85% to 90% of renal function is lost. The hallmark of renal failure is an increase in urea and other nonprotein nitrogens, which is termed *uremia* or *azotemia* (McCance & Huether, 1998). All body systems are affected by metabolic waste accumulation, fluid overload, and electrolyte imbalances. Initially, as the glomerular filtration rate (GFR) begins to fall, medication, diet, and fluid restrictions are used to maintain and support system function. However, with the loss of 90% of nephrons, GFR will decrease to 5 ml/min (normal is 125 ml/min), and symptoms of uremia (anorexia, nausea, vomiting, angina, dyspnea, insomnia, and loss of libido) will be seen. At this point, hemodialysis, peritoneal dialysis, or kidney transplantation are necessary to maintain the integrity of the body's internal environment (Bullock, 1996; Lakkis & Martinez-Maldonado, 1995).

2. Discuss the typical laboratory findings seen with chronic renal failure.

Normal values are the following:

Hct	40%-54% men; 37%-47% women	K^+	3.5-5.0 mEq/L
BUN	10-26 mg/dl	Cl^-	96-106 mEq/L
Creatinine	0.6-1.2 mg/dl	CO_2 (HCO_3^-)	24-30 mEq/L
Na$^+$	136-148 mEq/L	Ca^{++}	8.4-10.2 mg/dl
		Phosphate	2.7-4.5 mg/dl

Pertinent laboratory tests include a blood chemistry analysis, with particular attention to the complete blood count (CBC) and electrolyte, serum creatinine, BUN, calcium, and phosphorus levels to establish baseline data. Anemia is common with chronic renal failure because of the decrease in production of erythropoietin (a protein hormone produced by the kidneys to stimulate the bone marrow to produce red blood cells). It is not unusual to find hematocrit values of 20% to 25%. In addition, it is common to find serum potassium and phosphorus levels elevated and serum sodium and calcium levels decreased. BUN and serum creatinine levels are significantly elevated in patients with chronic renal failure. These patients demonstrate some degree of metabolic acidosis and decreased carbon dioxide (HCO_3^-) levels, because nonfunctioning kidneys can no longer produce new bicarbonate (Parker, 1998; Suki & Eknoyan, 1995).

3. Describe the symptoms of uremia that might be manifested by Mr. Morgan.

Uremia refers to the constellation of signs and symptoms associated with the deterioration of biochemical and physiologic functions that occur with renal failure. It results from the retention of substances that are ordinarily removed by healthy kidneys (urea, creatinine, and other organic and inorganic compounds) and derangements of hormonal and enzymatic homeostasis. Body systems affected by renal failure and possible clinical manifestations are as follows (Dubrow & Levin, 1995; Suki & Eknoyan, 1995; Vanholder, 1998):

- Genitourinary system: decreased urine volume, increased serum urea nitrogen level, and increased serum creatinine level
- Cardiovascular system: volume overload, pulmonary edema, hypertension, pericarditis, cardiomyopathy
- Neurologic system: encephalopathy, convulsions, altered mental state, memory loss, decreased muscle strength, psychosis, insomnia, neuropathy

- Hematologic system: anemia, thrombocytopenia
- Gastrointestinal system: anorexia, nausea, vomiting, gastritis, ulcers, uremic fetor (urine breath), constipation
- Integumentary system: yellow, gray-tinged skin, dryness, itching
- Skeletal system: bone demineralization, osteodystrophy, metastatic calcification

4. Describe how the relationship between calcium and phosphorus is altered in chronic renal failure.

Normal values are the following:

Serum phosphorus	2.7-2.4 mg/dl
Serum calcium	8.4-10.2 mg/dl
Calcium-phosphorus product	30-40 mg/dl

Approximately 98% of the total body calcium can be found within the bone, with the remaining 2% found in the plasma. It is the ionized plasma calcium level that controls the absorption of calcium from the gastrointestinal tract. Vitamin D must be metabolized by the kidney into its active form, 1,25-dihydroxycholecalciferol, to facilitate calcium absorption from the gastrointestinal tract. Plasma calcium and phosphorus exist in a reciprocal relationship so that when the phosphorus level decreases, the calcium level increases. The amount of phosphorus excreted by the kidney is directly proportional to the level of phosphorus in the plasma. Thus, if the serum phosphorus level is elevated, the kidneys increase the excretion of phosphorus to maintain the plasma level between 2.7 and 4.5 mg/dl. The parathyroid hormone plays a significant role in maintaining the calcium-phosphorus balance. When the serum calcium level decreases, parathyroid hormone is released by the parathyroid gland, which causes calcium to be released by the bone and phosphorus to be excreted by the kidney. With irreversible damage to the kidney, the complex relationship between calcium and phosphorus is severely altered. The kidney can no longer excrete the majority of phosphorus necessary to maintain balance; thus an elevated plasma phosphorus level occurs. The reciprocal relationship results in a decrease in plasma calcium. The state of hypocalcemia worsens because the kidney cannot metabolize the active form of vitamin D, which reduces calcium absorption from the gastrointestinal tract and impairs calcium mobilization from the bone. The parathyroid glands respond to the decreased plasma calcium levels and release parathyroid hormone to stimulate the reabsorption of calcium by the bone, which in turn increases the plasma calcium level. With both the serum calcium and phosphorus levels elevated, the calcium-phosphorus level is significantly elevated. If the calcium-phosphorus product exceeds 70 mg/dl, calcium phosphate crystals may precipitate in the brain, eyes, myocardium, lungs, skin, and bone. The increased production of parathormone may lead to further bone demineralization (McCarthy & Kumar, 1995; Parker, 1998).

5. Discuss the pathophysiology of aluminum toxicity in chronic renal failure.

Aluminum is a cation found in certain medications, such as aluminum-based phosphate binders (e.g., Amphojel, AlternaGEL, Basaljel), untreated tap water, fruits and vegetables grown in soil with high aluminum levels, food cooked in aluminum vessels, and unprocessed water used to prepare hemodialysis solution. Aluminum is absorbed from the gastrointestinal tract and partially excreted by the kidneys. About 80% of aluminum is protein bound, so it does not readily diffuse across the glomerular membrane for renal excretion. Patients undergoing dialysis are particularly prone to developing toxicity that results in bone disease, myopathy, encephalopathy, seizures, microcytic anemia, and myocardiomyopathy (Delmez, 1998; McCarthy & Kumar, 1995).

6. Discuss the pathophysiology of pericarditis in chronic renal failure. Why was Mr. Morgan particularly prone to this complication?

Pericarditis is inflammation of the visceral and parietal pericardial layers of the pericardium that develops as a result of toxic metabolic wastes found with renal failure. Toxins inflame and irritate the layers of the pericardium, causing a "rub" instead of gliding smoothly across each other during systole and diastole. Uremic pericarditis is commonly seen in patients who have not yet started dialysis. It is also seen during the first few months of dialysis therapy and in those whose dialysis is inadequate. The classic triad of symptoms for pericarditis is chest pain, fever, and pericardial friction rub. The chest pain is usually sharp and typically radiates over the left shoulder, neck, and left arm. The pain increases when the patient is supine, intensifies with deep breathing, and is relieved by sitting forward. The pericardial friction rub can be heard upon auscultation by placing the stethoscope's diaphragm over the left midsternal to lower sternal border; the amplitude may increase or decrease with inspiration or expiration. The most life-threatening complication of pericarditis is cardiac tamponade (Lancaster, 1995).

7. Discuss the different forms of dialysis used in the treatment of renal failure, including the indications and contraindications for each. Support the decision to use hemodialysis in treating Mr. Morgan.

Two major forms of dialysis are available for treatment of chronic renal failure: peritoneal dialysis and hemodialysis. Both techniques use diffusion, osmosis, and filtration via a semipermeable membrane to remove excess metabolic waste and excess fluid and electrolytes. Peritoneal dialysis uses the body's own peritoneal membrane in the abdominal cavity and requires placement of a catheter into the peritoneal cavity. The principle of osmosis is used to promote fluid shifts from the peritoneal vasculature into the dialysis solution. The osmotic gradient is created by the concentration of glucose in the peritoneal dialysis solution.

Hemodialysis is a process using an extracorporeal circuit and an artificial membrane (dialyzer) to mimic the functions of the glomerulus of the human kidney. It requires access to the central circulation, dialysis solution, treated water, dialyzer, and a dialysis machine (Salai, 1998). Either modality can be used in the treatment of acute or chronic renal failure. The patient should be given the choice after the risks and benefits of both have been explained. Mr. Morgan already had an AV fistula in his right forearm, which was created as a permanent access to his central circulation for hemodialysis.

8. Identify pharmacologic agents used to treat chronic renal failure and the rationale for their use.

Antianemics are drugs used to treat the anemia associated with decreased erythropoietin production by renal tissue; decreased red blood cell survival; chronic blood loss through blood sampling, dialysis, or gastrointestinal losses; and iron and vitamin B_{12} and folate deficiencies. Common antianemics include the following:

- Epoetin alfa (Epogen): glycoprotein that is biologically and immunologically identical to endogenous erythropoietin and functions by acting on erythroid tissues within the bone marrow to stimulate the differentiation of erythroid progenitor and early precursor cells
- Iron preparations: ferrous sulfate (Iberet, Feosol); iron dextran (InFed) injection; sodium ferric gluconate complex in sucrose (Ferrlecit) injection; polysaccharide iron complex (Niferex)
- Folic acid (Folvite)
- Pyridoxine (Pyridoxine hydrochloride)

Phosphate binding agents are used to bind phosphates in the gastrointestinal tract to facilitate their excretion via feces. Phosphate binding agents used include the following:

- Calcium acetate (PhosLo)
- Calcium carbonate (Os-cal, Tums)
- Aluminum hydroxide (Amphojel, ALternaGEL, Alucaps)
- Sevelamer hydrochloride (Renagel): the first calcium-free, aluminum-free phosphate binder

Vitamins are also used as supplements because of dietary restrictions, dialysis therapy, and metabolic imbalances. Important vitamins to replace are the following:

- All B with C
- Vitamin B complex with C
- Nephrocaps
- Nephro-Vite

Vitamin D supplementation and analogs are used to help normalize serum calcium and alkaline phosphatase levels and may also lower elevated parathyroid hormone levels. Patients with chronic renal failure can no longer convert vitamin D into the active form, contributing to the development of hypocalcemia and secondary hyperparathyroidism. Medications used to maintain homeostasis are the following:

- Ergocalciferol (Calciferol), least active
- Dihydrotachysterol
- 1,25-Dihydroxycholecalciferol/calcitriol (Rocaltrol), most active
- Calcitriol (Calcijex) injection
- Paricalcitol (Zemplar) injection

9. Discuss the dietary management of the patient with chronic renal failure.

A diet controlled for protein, phosphorus, or both may retard the progression of renal insufficiency to chronic renal failure. Hostetter (1998) and Kimmel (1998) report that a low-protein diet reduces intraglomerular pressure and capillary blood flow and decreases urinary protein loss, thus slowing the progression to chronic renal failure. The current recommendation for protein intake in patients with GFRs between 25 and 60 ml/min is 0.6 g/kg/day with two thirds provided as high-biologic value protein to meet the essential amino acid requirements and the recommendation for calorie intake is 35 to 50 kcal/kg. Patients with renal insufficiency are monitored for volume depletion or fluid overload. A minimum urinary volume of approximately 600 ml is required for the excretion of the average load of solids. Peripheral edema, hypertension, and congestive heart failure are potential complications that must be watched for. The diet for dialysis compensates for lack of kidney function, dialysate losses, and current nutritional status. The recommendations for the patient with renal failure is sodium intake of 1000 to 3000 mg/day, potassium intake of 2000 to 3000 mg/day, fluid intake to limit weight gains between dialysis treatments to 0.5 to 1.0 kg/day, and phosphorus intake of 600 to 1200 mg/day (McCann, 1998). Calorie and protein intake for patients receiving dialysis needs to be higher because the process of dialysis is catabolic. During hemodialysis, amino acid losses may exceed 10 to 12 g per treatment; with peritoneal dialysis, 5 to 15 g of amino acids and albumin are lost daily and 50% to 80% is as albumin. Recommendations for protein intake in patients receiving hemodialysis is 1.2 to 1.4 g/kg of body weight and 1.2 to 1.5 g/kg of body weight for patients receiving peritoneal dialysis (Alvestrand, 1995).

10. Identify clinical complications arising from noncompliance that were manifested by Mr. Morgan.

Mr. Morgan had an accumulation of uremic toxins resulting from noncompliance with his medical regimen. Mr. Morgan experienced nausea and vomiting, agitation, and confusion. In addition, he had chest pain, described as moderate to severe in intensity and diffusely located over the precordium. Pulmonary overload was revealed through neck vein distension, crackles scattered bilaterally throughout the lung bases, and pitting peripheral edema bilaterally in the lower extremities. He had a weight gain of 8 kg (17.6 lb). Cardiac monitoring demonstrated sinus tachycardia with a rate of 116 bpm. A pericardial friction rub and an S_3 gallop were auscultated. These symptoms are consistent with pericarditis. Laboratory values revealed metabolic acidosis, hyperkalemia, hyponatremia, hyperphosphatemia, hypocalcemia, and anemia.

11. List nursing diagnoses appropriate for the care of the patient with chronic renal failure. Include nursing diagnoses appropriate for the care of the patient with a permanent AV fistula for dialysis access.

- Fluid volume excess related to noncompliance with prescribed medical regimen
- Noncompliance with medical regimen related to limitations of disease
- Alteration in self-image related to skin changes and changes in lifestyle
- Impaired gas exchange related to pulmonary edema
- Alteration in nutrition: less than body requirements related to nausea and vomiting
- High risk for infection related to impaired defense barriers
- Alteration in self-image related to skin changes

- High risk for alteration in cardiac output related to uremic pericarditis and patency of the access (Molzahan, 1998)

12. List the components of the teaching plan for the patient with chronic renal failure.

- Compliance with components of medical regimen such as dialysis schedule and diet and fluid restriction
- Prevention of infection
- Regular exercise
- Maintenance of dialysis access: teaching about how to check for patency of the access, and signs and symptoms of infection
- Prevention of complications (Bucher & Melander, 1999)

13. List the criteria used in the selection of patients for kidney transplantation.

Renal transplantation is considered a viable alternative for treatment of ESRD when the patient does not have other medical problems that could increase the risks associated with the procedure. The usual age range of candidates for renal transplantation is 4 to 60 years. Patients at either end of the transplantation age continuum have an increased risk for complications. A thorough body systems assessment is performed before the person is considered for organ transplantation (Mudge, Carlson, & Brennan, 1998; Wilkinson, 1996).

The number of patients awaiting organ transplantation has increased dramatically from 1995 to 2000 because of the advances made in transplantation procedures. As of September 1999, 65,686 patients were awaiting vital organs for transplantation in the United States, with 43,142 of those awaiting cadaver kidney transplantation (United Network for Organ Sharing [UNOS], 1999). All potential organ recipients are entered into the national computer system through the United Network for Organ Sharing (UNOS). A point system has been instituted to allow equitable distribution of this scarce resource. Blood type compatibility between donor and recipient is mandatory.

Specific criteria have been established for potential kidney recipients. First, priority is given to the potential recipient with the best antigen match. Second, priority is also given to potential recipients who have preformed antibodies to major histocompatibility complex antigens because the presence of these antibodies can limit the number of kidneys for which the potential recipient would be eligible. Priority is also given to potential recipients who are considered "medical emergencies." The most common circumstance that qualifies a patient as needing an emergency kidney transplantation is the inability to maintain AV access for hemodialysis. The final criterion has to do with logistic factors based on the ease and rapidity with which the transplantation can be performed (Alspach, 1998; Katznelson, Terasaki, & Danovitch, 1996).

Organs from living-related donors provide the highest rates of renal graft survival. General physical criteria for donors include the absence of systemic disease and infection, no history of cancer, absence of hypertension and renal disease, and adequate renal function as evidenced by diagnostic studies. In addition, living-related donors must express a clear understanding of the associated surgery and a willingness to donate a kidney. Some transplant centers also require a psychiatric evaluation to determine the motivation of the donor.

14. Discuss hemodialysis and renal transplantation as alternative treatment modalities for Mr. Morgan. Support Mr. Morgan's decision to select renal transplantation rather than hemodialysis.

Hemodialysis and renal transplantation are alternative treatment modalities for Mr. Morgan. It is most often the patient's preference that determines the type of therapy instituted. Patients should consider which modality would best be suited to his or her physical condition and lifestyle. Mr. Morgan has no active malignancy or infectious process. He has a strong support system, with siblings willing to donate a living donor kidney. He is financially secure through income and health insurance coverage. Although Mr. Morgan has had difficulty complying with the medical regimen of hemodialysis because of transportation difficulties and distance to the health care facility, he stated that he is now willing to comply with the medical regimen after transplantation because these transportation issues will be eliminated.

Conservative medical management of ESRD with dialysis is costly. Although transplantation procedures are expensive, current success rates have made transplantation a cost-effective treatment option compared with traditional medical management. For example, a patient undergoing hemodialysis costs the federal government, through Medicare, about $53,000 per year. The cost of a kidney transplant is approximately $43,000 for the first year and $18,000 yearly for follow-up care. If the transplant functions for 5 years, the cost is $90,000 as opposed to $260,000 for 5 years of hemodialysis (U.S. Renal Data System [USRDS], 1999). Because Mr. Morgan was employed full-time before beginning dialysis and plans to return to work after the transplantation, other financial considerations are his potential earning power and the discontinuation of any disability benefits previously required.

One of the major obstacles to a successful renal transplant is finding a suitable donor. Blood relatives make the most compatible donors and result in an approximate 90% success rate for the patient (Mudge et al, 1998). Mr. Morgan had three brothers and three sisters consenting to be a donor if a transplant match was possible. It is imperative that Mr. Morgan receive a living donor kidney because the more similar the tissue antigens of the donor are to those of the recipient, the more likely it is that the transplant will be successful and immunologic rejection will be avoided.

Renal transplantation could also eliminate the lifestyle restrictions for the patient. Mr. Morgan was required to report to a community-based hemodialysis clinic 75 miles from his home three times each week. Approximately 24 hours each week were required for travel and treatment time. By choosing renal transplantation, Mr. Morgan hoped to alleviate the inconvenience and discomfort of the frequent dialysis treatments.

15. List the advantages and disadvantages of a living donor versus a cadaver donor. Why was it imperative that Mr. Morgan receive a living donor kidney?

Cadaver organ donors are those from previously healthy individuals who have suffered irreversible brain injury of a known cause. The most common causes of injury are cerebral trauma from motor vehicle accidents, gunshot wounds, intracerebral or subarachnoid hemorrhage, primary brain tumor, and anoxic brain damage resulting from drug overdose or cardiac arrest. The brain-dead donor must have effective cardiovascular function and must be supported on a ventilator to preserve organ viability. The donor must be free of extracranial malignancies, sepsis, and communicable diseases, including hepatitis, syphilis, tuberculosis, and human immunodeficiency virus infection (Alspach, 1998; Bucher & Melander, 1999; Rosenthal & Danovitch, 1996;). The age range of most suitable donors is newborn to 65 years. Age is generally less important than the quality of organ functions (Alspach, 1998; First, 1995).

Cadaver Donor Kidney

1. Advantages
   - Success rate of transplantation has improved to 85% to 90%.
   - Cadaver kidneys can maintain viability for as long as 72 hours after removal from the donor.
   - The average cost of transplant is $43,000 (same as that for living donor transplants).
2. Disadvantages
   - The potential organ recipient is placed on a national registry (UNOS) to allow equitable distribution of scarce organ supply.
   - The organ recipient may die while waiting for a kidney because of limited supply and great demand.
   - Few kidneys are available for transplantation, and surgery must be done as kidneys become available.
   - Recipients' physical and psychologic health may not be optimal.

Living-Related Donor Kidney

1. Advantages
   - The recipient is not placed on the national registry to wait for a kidney.
   - A living-related donor provides the highest rate of renal graft survival (90%).
   - The average cost is $43,000, and it is more cost-effective over the long term than hemodialysis.
   - Current research favors donor-specific blood transfusion, in which blood from the kidney donor is transfused into the recipient. This has improved graft survival, especially of organs from living donors.
   - Surgery can be scheduled electively to optimize the patient's state of health. The organ suffers less ischemia because it is not transported.
2. Disadvantages
   - Kidney removal from a living donor requires greater surgical care and is a delicate procedure that lasts 3 to 4 hours.
   - Donors experience more pain than recipients.
   - There is a small risk of complications or death for the donor.
   - The donor must have annual physical examinations for life to assess the function of the remaining kidney.
   - There is a psychologic impact for both the donor and the recipient.

At 67 years of age, if Mr. Morgan were to receive a living donor kidney, it would enhance his chances for a successful transplantation. The procedure could be scheduled electively, which would allow for an optimal state of health at the time of surgery. The living donor transplantation also would allow decreased ischemic time for the kidney by eliminating transport time.

16. Describe the cadaver kidney preservation process.

The cadaver donor nephrectomy is conducted as a sterile autopsy in the operating room. All arterial and venous vessels are carefully preserved (Bucher & Melander, 1999). The aorta and vena cava are cannulated from below and ligated above the renal arteries and veins. The cadaver kidneys are flushed with cold Ringer's lactate solution containing heparin 10,000 U/L. Once the transplantable kidney has been surgically removed, it is preserved in a sterile, iced electrolyte solution and transported to a transplant center. Kidneys can maintain viability for as long as 72 hours before they must be transplanted (Bucher & Melander, 1999; Rosenthal & Danovitch, 1996).

Preservation by Perfusion
The kidneys are perfused with a cold (6° to 10° C) solution at low flow, low pressure to provide the kidney with nutrients and oxygen and to remove products of metabolism. The kidneys can be preserved in this process for up to 72 hours (Rosenthal & Danovitch, 1996).

Preservation by Cold Storage
A high-potassium, low-sodium solution that resembles the electrolyte balance inside kidney cells is used to flush the kidney, and then the kidneys are stored in this solution in sterile plastic bags at temperatures of 6° C or less. The kidneys can be preserved in this process for up to 30 hours (Rosenthal & Danovitch, 1996).

17. Briefly describe the surgical process of renal transplantation.

After induction of anesthesia, the genitalia and abdominal skin are prepared and a Foley catheter is placed in the urinary bladder. The bladder is rinsed with a broad-spectrum antibiotic solution and gravity filled to capacity, and the catheter is clamped until the urinary tract reconstruction portion of the operation begins. Usually, the kidney graft is placed in the extraperitoneal area in the contralateral iliac fossa through a Gibson incision on the same side from which it was removed from the donor. The renal artery is attached to the hypogastric or internal iliac artery, and the renal vein is anastomosed to the external iliac vein. Mannitol (0.5 to 1 g/kg) is infused during and immediately after renal revascularization to act as an osmotic diuretic. The urinary tract reconstruction is by transvesical or extravesical ureteroneocystostomy. The recipient's own nonfunctioning kidney is usually not removed unless it is infected, greatly enlarged, or causing medically uncontrollable hypertension (Rosenthal, 1996).

18. Discuss possible postoperative complications of renal transplantation.

Numerous potential complications are associated with renal transplantation. Vascular complications nearly always require surgical intervention. Stenosis of the renal artery may occur, which is evident by the presence of hypertension, auscultation of a bruit over the artery anastomoses site, and decreased renal function. To correct stenosis of the renal artery, the clinician must surgically resect the involved artery and anastomose the kidney to another artery. Other vascular problems include vascular leakage and thrombosis, both of which require an emergency nephrectomy.

Wound complications include hematomas, abscesses, and lymphoceles. Genito-urinary tract complications such as ureteral leakage, ureteral fistulas, ureteral obstruction, calculus formation, bladder neck contractures, scrotal swelling, and graft rupture may also necessitate surgical intervention (Mudge et al, 1998). The most common and most life-threatening complication of renal transplantation is rejection. In tissue rejection, a reaction occurs between the antigens in the transplanted kidney and the antibodies and cytotoxic T cells in the recipient's blood. These immunologic substances treat the transplanted kidney as a foreign invader and cause tissue destruction, thrombosis, and eventual necrosis of the tissue (Bucher & Melander, 1999; Mudge et al, 1998).

19. List the nursing diagnoses appropriate to the care of the patient undergoing renal transplantation during the recovery period.

- Altered tissue perfusion related to rejection or acute tubular necrosis
- Potential for fluid volume excess related to intraoperative and postoperative fluid administration and/or inadequate urinary elimination
- Potential for fluid volume deficit related to excessive output, diuretic therapy, inadequate fluid administration, vomiting/diarrhea, and/or bleeding
- Altered patterns of urinary elimination related to bladder spasms, anatomical size, or obstruction due to clots, bladder leak, infection, or diabetic neurogenic bladder
- Potential for electrolyte imbalance related to level of renal function after transplantation, intraoperative blood transfusions, metabolic disorders associated with acidosis and hyperglycemia, or side effects of medications (e.g., cyclosporine, steroids)
- Potential for infection related to alterations in the immune system secondary to immunosuppressive therapy, presence of invasive lines and Foley catheter
- Potential for constipation or gastroparesis related to anesthesia, immobility, pain medication, fear of straining on defecation, presence of Foley catheter, inadequate dietary intake
- Altered comfort related to incisional pain and bladder spasms
- Alteration in nutrition: less than body requirements related to nausea and vomiting and postoperative pain
- Alteration in body image related to medication side effects and transplantation
- Alteration in self-image related to changes in lifestyle
- Potential for knowledge deficit related to the short/long posttransplant course, unfamiliar tests and procedures, home management, medications, rejection, and risk of infection
- Noncompliance with medical regimen related to limitations of disease and physical changes secondary to medication

20. Discuss the pathophysiology of acute rejection. Describe the clinical manifestations of acute rejection in Mr. Morgan.

The types of rejection are hyperacute, acute, and chronic. Hyperacute rejection occurs within 48 hours after transplant surgery. No treatment exists for this type of rejection, and after recognition of the problem, the rejected kidney is removed quickly to prevent further complications. Clinical manifestations include elevated temperature, elevated blood pressure, and pain at the transplant site (Amend,

Vincenti, & Tomlanovich, 1996; Bucher & Melander, 1999). Acute rejection usually occurs between 7 and 14 days after surgery but may occur up to 2 years after transplantation. The most common manifestations of acute rejection include oliguria or anuria, temperature greater than 37.8° C (100° F), enlarged and tender kidney, fluid retention, increased blood pressure, chronic fatigue, and changes in urinalysis and blood chemistry laboratory values. Acute rejection can be halted with early recognition and immediate administration of increased dosages of immunosuppressive drugs.

Chronic rejection occurs gradually over months to years. The clinical manifestations include gradually decreasing BUN levels and changes in serum electrolyte levels. No treatment exists for chronic rejection, and the patient is conservatively managed until renal function deteriorates and dialysis is required (Bucher & Melander, 1999; Nast & Cohen, 1996).

On the eighth postoperative day, Mr. Morgan began to demonstrate signs and symptoms of acute rejection. He complained of not feeling well, of minimal abdominal tenderness on palpation, and of nausea. His temperature fluctuated between 38.4° and 38.8° C (101.2° and 101.8° F). Urinary output dropped to an average of 55 ml/hr and did not improve with furosemide (Lasix) boluses. On the 11th postoperative day, laboratory data revealed that his CVP was slightly elevated to 10.5 mm Hg and his weight had increased to 82 kg (182 lb). His creatinine level was 7.1 mg/dl, and his BUN level was 120 mg/dl.

21. **Discuss the immunosuppressive pharmacologic agents methylprednisolone, muromonab-CD3 (Orthoclone OKT3), and cyclosporine. Why did the physician add muromonab-CD3 and wait several days to begin cyclosporine?**

Methylprednisolone (Solu-Medrol)

Methylprednisolone, a corticosteroid, acts as an antiinflammatory agent to prevent movement of leukocytes into tissue during resection. In addition, methylprednisolone limits antibody production and blocks the antigen-antibody complex formation. Numerous side effects of corticosteroids include infections, gastrointestinal tract bleeding, ulcers, pancreatitis, delayed wound healing, diabetes mellitus, psychosis, cataracts, fluid and electrolyte imbalances, and hypertension (*Physicians Desk Reference,* 1999).

Muromonab-CD3 (Orthoclone OKT3)

Muromonab-CD3 is a monoclonal anti–T-cell antibody that reacts with and blocks the function of all T cells, thereby reversing acute renal allograft rejection. The usual dosage of muromonab-CD3 is 5 mg/day. The drug is administered by intravenous bolus only. Muromonab-CD3 may not be given with any other drug. Side effects include respiratory complications such as acute pulmonary edema. This drug requires meticulous nursing assessment because it is given intravenously and reactions frequently occur with the first administration. Clinical manifestations of a reaction include fever, chills, dyspnea, and chest pain (*Physicians Desk Reference,* 1999).

Cyclosporine

Cyclosporine is a newer drug used to prevent and treat rejection of renal transplants. Cyclosporine works by interfering with T-cell growth and can be given orally or intravenously. If administered orally, the drug may be diluted in various liquids but should be taken 1 to 2 hours after meals at the same time each day to maintain a consistent absorption rate and thereby maintain a consistent blood level. The usual dosage of cyclosporine is 6 mg/kg in divided doses every 12 hours. Cyclosporine increases the risk of renal failure and hepatotoxicity.

Nursing responsibilities require observing for nephrotoxicity, hepatotoxicity, and potential malignancy, especially lymphoma. The nurse should monitor blood levels of the drug to ensure they are therapeutic but not toxic. Therapeutic trough levels range between 250 and 350 mg/ml. Six to eight weeks after renal transplantation, the dosage is usually decreased to 4 to 5 mg/kg (*Physicians Desk Reference,* 1999).

Muromonab-CD3 was added to Mr. Morgan's medical regimen on the 11th postoperative day, when Mr. Morgan's laboratory values indicated worsening signs of acute rejection. Muromonab-CD3 drug therapy was added to block cytotoxic human T cells and the generation of other T-cell functions. The symptoms of renal allograft rejection, such as those noted in Mr. Morgan's condition, are subtle and difficult to differentiate from similar symptoms of drug-induced nephrotoxicity. Cyclosporine was not administered immediately to Mr. Morgan because of the impaired renal function. After several days of hemodialysis to support renal function, Mr. Morgan's creatinine level had dropped to 1.9 mg/dl and cyclosporine was added to the regimen. Cyclosporine may be added to the medical regimen of acute rejection when the creatinine level is 2.5 mg/dl or less.

22.   List the components of the teaching plan for Mr. Morgan.

- Teach the patient the routine after a kidney transplant (e.g., what the patient will feel and see when he or she awakes from surgery, how often vital signs will be needed, and what type of a hospital unit he or she will be in after surgery).
- Inform the patient of the importance of all medications prescribed after transplantation, including purpose, side effects, dosage schedule, and frequency.
- Educate the patient about the laboratory values that will be monitored (e.g., BUN, creatinine, electrolytes, drug levels, CBC, platelets, and liver function studies) and discuss their importance.
- Teach the patient and family members the signs and symptoms of rejection (decreased urine output, pain over the kidney, a general feeling of illness, and weight gain) and the appropriate actions to take if any of these are seen.
- Teach the patient and the family members the signs and symptoms of infection, the importance of monitoring clinical manifestations, and the appropriate action to take if infection is suspected.
- Inform the patient and family members about dietary and fluid changes and/or restrictions.
- Arrange a consultation for nutritional support when convenient for the patient and family members.
- Educate the patient about the importance of skin care, use of sunscreen, and acne prophylaxis to prevent complications.
- Provide information stressing the importance of routine dental care, brushing, flossing, and gum care.
- Educate the patient and family members about family planning, use of contraceptives, and risks of pregnancy.
- Inform the patient of the importance of exercise and encourage the patient to establish a regular exercise routine.

- Teach health maintenance skills needed for monitoring the patient's health status and have the patient validate learning through return demonstrations (e.g., temperature, weight, blood pressure, pulse, glucose monitoring, incision care).
- Reinforce the importance of keeping all follow-up appointments with the physician or for diagnostic procedures.
- Provide information about kidney transplantation and local organizations and support groups.
- Provide information regarding the financial, psychologic, and rehabilitative resources available.
- Emphasize to the patient the importance of carrying medical alert information at all times.

CHRONIC RENAL FAILURE AND RENAL TRANSPLANTATION

References

Alspach, J. G. (Ed.). (1998). *American Association of Critical-Care Nurses: Core curriculum for critical care nursing* (5th ed.). Philadelphia: WB Saunders.

Alvestrand, A. (1995). Nutritional requirements of dialysis patients. In H. Jacobson, G. Striker, & S. Klahr (Eds.), *The principles and practice of nephrology* (2nd ed., pp. 761-766). St Louis: Mosby.

Amend, J. C., Jr., Vincenti, F., & Tomlanovich, S. J. (1996). The first two post-transplant months. In G. Danovitch (Ed.), *Handbook of kidney transplantation* (2nd ed., pp. 138-153). Baltimore: Williams & Wilkins.

Bucher, L., & Melander, S. (Eds). (1999). *Critical care nursing*. Philadelphia: Saunders.

Bullock, B. (1996). *Pathophysiology: Adaptations and alterations in function* (4th ed.). Philadelphia: JB Lippincott.

Delmez, J. A. (1998). Renal osteodystrophy and other musculoskeletal complications of chronic renal failure. In A. Greenburg (Ed.), *Primer on kidney diseases* (2nd ed., pp.448-455). San Diego: Academic Press.

Dubrow, A., & Levin, N. W. (1995). Biochemical and hormonal alterations in chronic renal failure. In H. Jacobson, G. Striker, & S. Klahr (Eds.), *The principles and practice of nephrology* (2nd ed., pp. 596-603). St Louis: Mosby.

First, M. R. (1995). Pretransplantation evaluation and preparation of donors and recipients. In H. Jacobson, G. Striker, & S. Klahr (Eds.), *The principles and practice of nephrology* (2nd ed., pp. 805-810). St Louis: Mosby.

Hostetter, T. H. (1998). Progression of renal disease. In A. Greenburg (Ed.), *Primer on kidney diseases* (2nd ed., pp.429-432). San Diego: Academic Press.

Katznelson, S., Terasaki, P. I., & Danovitch, G. M. (1996). Histocompatibility testing, crossmatching, and allocation of cadaveric kidney transplants. In G. Danovitch (Ed.), *Handbook of kidney transplantation* (2nd ed., pp. 32-54). Baltimore: Williams & Wilkins.

Kimmel, P. L. (1998). Management of the patient with chronic renal disease. In A. Greenburg (Ed.), *Primer on kidney diseases* (2nd ed., pp.433-440). San Diego: Academic Press.

Lakkis, F. G., & Martinez-Maldonado, M. (1995). Conservative management of chronic renal failure and the uremic syndrome. Renal osteodystrophy. In H. Jacobson, G. Striker, & S. Klahr (Eds.), *The principles and practice of nephrology* (2nd ed., pp. 614-620). St Louis: Mosby.

Lancaster, L. E. (1995). Systemic manifestations of renal failure. In L. E. Lancaster (Ed.), *Core curriculum for nephrology nursing* (3rd ed., pp. 73-108). Pitman, NJ: Jannetti.

McCance, K. L., & Huether, S. E. (1998). *Pathophysiology: The biologic basis for disease in adults and children* (3rd ed.). St Louis: Mosby.

McCann, L. (1998). *Pocket guide to nutrition assessment of the renal patient* (2nd ed.). New York: National Kidney Foundation.

McCarthy, J. Y., & Kumar, R. (1995). Renal osteodystrophy. In H. Jacobson, G. Striker, & S. Klahr (Eds.), *The principles and practice of nephrology* (2nd ed., pp. 1032-1045). St Louis: Mosby.

Molzahn, A. C. (1998). Psychosocial impact of renal disease. In J. Parker (Ed.), *Contemporary nephrology nursing* (pp. 269-284). Pitman, NJ: Jannetti.

Mudge, C., Carlson, L., & Brennan, P. (1998). Transplantation. In J. Parker (Ed.), *Contemporary nephrology nursing* (pp. 693-778). Pitman, NJ: Jannetti.

Nast, C. C., & Cohen, A. H. (1996). Pathology of kidney transplantation. In G. Danovitch (Ed.), *Handbook of kidney transplantation* (2nd ed., pp. 232-253). Baltimore, Williams & Wilkins.

Parker, K. P. (1998). Acute and chronic renal failure. In J. Parker (Ed.), *Contemporary nephrology nursing* (pp. 199-265). Pitman, NJ: Jannetti.

Physicians desk reference. (1999). Montvale, NJ: Medical Economics Co.

Rosenthal, J. T. (1996). The transplant operation and its surgical complications. In G. Danovitch (Ed.), *Handbook of kidney transplantation* (2nd ed., pp. 123-137). Baltimore, Williams & Wilkins.

Rosenthal, J. T., & Danovitch, G. M. (1996). Live-related and cadaveric kidney donation. In G. Danovitch (Ed.), *Handbook of kidney transplantation* (2nd ed., pp. 95-108). Baltimore, Williams & Wilkins.

Salai, P. B. (1998). Hemodialysis. In J. Parker (Ed.), *Contemporary nephrology nursing* (pp. 527-576). Pitman, NJ: Jannetti.

Suki, W. N., & Eknoyan, G. (1995). Conservative management of chronic renal failure and the uremic syndrome. In H. Jacobson, G. Striker, & S. Klahr (Eds.), *The principles and practice of nephrology* (2nd ed., pp. 614-620). St Louis: Mosby.

United Network for Organ Sharing (UNOS). (1999). Update. [Homepage]. http://www.unos.org.

U.S. Renal Data System [USRDS]. (1999). The 1999 annual data report [WWW document]. http://www.usrds.org/.

Vanholder, R. (1998). The uremic syndrome. In A. Greenburg (Ed.), *Primer on kidney diseases* (2nd ed., pp.403-407). San Diego: Academic Press.

Wilkinson, A. H. (1996). Evaluation of the transplant recipient. In G. Danovitch (Ed.), *Handbook of kidney transplantation* (2nd ed., pp. 109-122). Baltimore, Williams & Wilkins.

CHAPTER 13

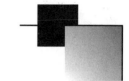

SUBARACHNOID HEMORRHAGE WITH ANEURYSM

Cinda Alexander, MSN, CCRN, CNRN, CNOR, CRNFA

CASE PRESENTATION

Connie, a 42-year-old white woman, was seen in the emergency department with complaints of severe left temporal headaches after collapsing at work. Initially, while at work, Connie was confused and incontinent of urine. After arrival in the emergency department, Connie was cooperative, her pupils were equal and reactive, and she was mildly disoriented. She stated that the headaches were "unlike any" she had experienced before. According to Connie's husband, Connie had experienced these headaches for about 3 to 4 weeks. Additional symptoms included nausea, photophobia, and a mildly stiff neck. A computed tomographic (CT) scan of the head without contrast material revealed a subarachnoid hemorrhage in the area of the internal carotid artery. Her serum Na^+ level was 130 mmol/L, K^+ level was 3.6 mmol/L, and Cl^- level was 106 mmol/L.

Initial assessment data after admission to the emergency department were as follows:

BP	152/78 mm Hg	Temperature	37.2° C (99° F)
HR	102 bpm	Sao_2	92% with room air
Respirations	22 breaths/min		

Neurologic signs were as follows:

- Lethargic, arouses to name
- Pupils equal and reactive
- Follows commands, moves all extremities equally
- Oriented to person only
- Glasgow Coma Scale score of 14

After admission and evaluation in the emergency department, Connie's condition was stabilized and she was transferred to the critical care unit. She was scheduled for an arteriogram the next day. Treatment with aminocaproic acid (Amicar) and nimodipine (Nimotop) was begun. Connie continued to complain of a generalized headache and neck stiffness. Assessment data were as follows:

BP   142/80 mm Hg   Temperature   37.2° C (99° F)
HR   84 bpm   Sao$_2$ 98% with room air
Respirations   24 breaths/min

Neurologic signs were as follows:

- Pupils equal and reactive
- Follows commands, moves all extremities equally, grasp equal
- Oriented to person and place
- Lethargic, arouses to name
- Glasgow Coma Scale score of 13

Connie's condition was stable throughout the night. Her arteriogram the next morning revealed a left vertebral posterior inferior cerebellar aneurysm. Connie and her family were present when the physician discussed the results of the arteriogram. Her treatment options were explored, and specific questions from the family were answered. Connie's neurologic status remained stable, and the decision to proceed with "early surgery" was made.

Surgery
At 10 AM the following morning, Connie underwent a craniotomy for a clip ligation of the left inferior cerebellar aneurysm.

Postoperative Course
Immediately after surgery, Connie's vital signs were stable. She recovered from the general anesthesia, responded to her name, and moved all extremities to command during the initial hour of recovery in the intensive care unit. Connie continued to show general recovery and recognized her family during the following hours. Several hours after surgery, she developed a sudden headache, confusion, and gross weakness in her right hand. Her vital signs were as follows:

BP   162/94 mm Hg   Respirations   32 breaths/min
HR   110 bpm   Temperature   38.3° C (101° F)

Neurologic signs included the following:

- Pupils equal and reactive
- Follows command and moves all extremities, right grasp weak
- Disoriented, speech inappropriate
- Glasgow Coma Scale score of 11

An emergency CT scan of the head demonstrated postoperative changes associated with the surgery, an aneurysm clip artifact, minimal air, and no obvious collection of blood. The transcranial Doppler study demonstrated an increased velocity in the left middle cerebral artery, greater than 120 cm/sec. With no obvious postoperative hematoma, a decision was made to repeat the arteriogram, which demonstrated apparent narrowing of the arteries. The clinician concluded that

Connie was experiencing a vasospasm. Her Na^+ level was 145 mmol/L, K^+ level was 3.9 mmol/L, and Cl^- level was 109 mmol/L.

After an arterial line and pulmonary artery (Swan-Ganz) catheter were inserted, hypervolemic/hyperfusion therapy was initiated and continued over the next 5 days. Connie's neurologic status stabilized and improved with this therapy. Connie was slowly weaned from this therapy, and her neurologic status remained stable for an additional 48 hours. Connie was then transferred to a neurosurgical step-down unit. Neurologically, she was alert and oriented, although easily confused if given multiple instructions. She moved all extremities to command; however, she has continued to demonstrate a mild weakness in her right hand and arm. She was discharged 8 days later to a rehabilitation unit with an anticipated discharge home after rehabilitation therapy.

SUBARACHNOID HEMORRHAGE WITH ANEURYSM

Questions

1. Discuss the clinical presentation of a subarachnoid hemorrhage.
2. Describe the incidence, risk factors, mortality, and morbidity associated with acute subarachnoid hemorrhage
3. Discuss how a subarachnoid hemorrhage is diagnosed.
4. Describe the pathophysiology involved and consequences of blood in the subarachnoid space.
5. Give the rationale for Connie's hyponatremia.
6. Describe how a subarachnoid hemorrhage is classified.
7. What therapeutic modalities should be anticipated for patients after subarachnoid hemorrhage? Give the rationale for each.
8. What parameters require close monitoring for patients after subarachnoid hemorrhage?
9. What are the general complications associated with aminocaproic acid (Amicar) and nimodipine?
10. What are the general "aneurysm precautions" observed for patients with a subarachnoid hemorrhage who may have a cerebral aneurysm?
11. Describe the pathophysiology of cerebral aneurysm.
12. Define the different types of aneurysms.
13. Discuss the secondary cerebral injuries associated with a ruptured aneurysm and subsequent subarachnoid hemorrhage.
14. Discuss the advantages and disadvantages of early versus late surgical intervention.
15. Discuss why nursing care is of particular importance after a craniotomy.
16. Describe the pathophysiology and incidence of rebleeding. When is rebleeding likely to occur?
17. Discuss clinical changes that should be anticipated if a patient is experiencing rebleeding.
18. Describe how rebleeding would be diagnosed.
19. Discuss the treatment for rebleeding. What is the duration of treatment?
20. Describe the pathophysiology and incidence of vasospasm. When is vasospasm likely to occur?

21. Discuss the causes of vasospasm.
22. Identify how cerebral vasospasm is diagnosed. Include clinical symptoms that should be anticipated.
23. Discuss the mortality and morbidity of vasospasm and rebleeding.
24. Discuss current treatment for vasospasm. What additional approaches are discussed in the literature?
25. How long should the treatment of vasospasm be continued, and how long will Connie remain at risk for vasospasm or rebleeding?
26. Discuss nonsurgical approaches available to patients unable to tolerate traditional surgical treatment.

SUBARACHNOID HEMORRHAGE WITH ANEURYSM

Questions and Answers

1. **Discuss the clinical presentation of a subarachnoid hemorrhage.**

Patients often report having sudden, severe, violent headaches, unlike any experienced before. Immediate loss of consciousness, nausea, vomiting, cranial nerve palsies, and focal neurologic deficits such as weakness of an extremity may also be present. Blood in the subarachnoid space produces signs and symptoms of meningeal irritation such as nuchal rigidity or stiff neck, photophobia, blurred vision, nausea and vomiting, headache, and fever. With the initial seepage of blood into the subarachnoid space, there may be a sudden onset of deep coma. As many as 40% of patients with subarachnoid hemorrhage have prodromal signs or warning symptoms, such as headache, that can indicate the occurrence of a small leakage of blood. However, these early symptoms are often ignored or attributed to other causes (Becker, 1998; Campbell & Edwards, 1997; Hickey, 1997).

2. **Describe the incidence, risk factors, mortality, and morbidity associated with acute subarachnoid hemorrhage.**

Subarachnoid hemorrhage occurs in 25,000 to 30,000 North Americans annually; of these, 50% to 60% die. One third of these deaths occur before the person enters the health care system. An additional 20% to 30% sustain permanent neurologic damage and disability. The average age of occurrence is 50 years, with patients ranging from 35 to 60 years (Becker, 1998; Campbell & Edwards, 1997; Hickey, 1997). Johnston, Selvin, and Gress (1998) reported that mortality decreased between 1997 to 1994 in the United States. Mortality is reported to be higher in women and African Americans. Risk factors include smoking, hypertension, and alcohol use (Becker, 1998). The major causes of death associated with aneurysmal subarachnoid hemorrhage are rebleeding and vasospasm (Lanzino & Kassell, 1998).

3. **Discuss how a subarachnoid hemorrhage is diagnosed.**

Diagnosis is based on history, clinical presentation, and a number of diagnostic procedures. Lumbar puncture may be used to confirm blood in the cerebrospinal fluid (CSF), which circulates in the subarachnoid space. The spinal fluid is bloody grossly and xanthochromic (a yellow discoloration of the CSF) after centrifugation. Lumbar puncture is avoided if intracranial hypertension is suspected because of the risk of brain herniation (Romeo, 1993; Wojner, 1999). A CT scan within 48 hours of the bleeding episode can demonstrate the blood in the subarachnoid space in 75% to 85% of all patients. Magnetic resonance imaging may be used to identify the subarachnoid blood and inner structures of the brain. Magnetic resonance angiography with intravenous gadolinium is a noninvasive approach to image cerebral vasculature and perhaps provide useful screening for suspected aneurysm or arteriovenous malformation. A four-vessel cerebral angiogram is the mainstay of diagnosis and usually is able to provide a definitive diagnosis of aneurysm or arteriovenous malformation. Cerebral angiography visualizes both intracranial and extracranial vessels. Contrast medium is injected, and a series of radiographic films is recorded (Baxter, Cohen, & Maravilla 1998; Hickey, 1997; Van Tatenhove & Kelley, 1999).

4. Describe the pathophysiology involved and consequences of blood in the subarachnoid space.

The pathophysiology of subarachnoid hemorrhage is complex and not well understood but includes a number of events. *Subarachnoid hemorrhage* is arterial blood that has extravasated into the subarachnoid space, which normally contains CSF. Subarachnoid hemorrhage as a result of a ruptured aneurysm usually occurs around the circle of Willis at a point of bifurcation of the arterial vessels (Rusy, 1996). The amount of bleeding may range from small amounts to large amounts that extend beyond the site of leakage, flooding into cisterns and the ventricular system. Blood is an irritant to brain tissues that initiates an inflammatory response and cerebral edema. Studies suggest there is a rapid rise in intracranial pressure as well as a reduction of cerebral blood flow after a subarachnoid hemorrhage. There is often an abnormality in the cerebral vasculature response to partial pressure of carbon dioxide ($Paco_2$), suggesting a disturbance in autoregulation. Patients with subarachnoid hemorrhage are often hypertensive after the initial bleeding episode, probably as a result of the release of catecholamines into the circulatory vasculature. This hypertension maintains or improves the cerebral perfusion pressure. Fibrin, platelets, and fluid around the point of arterial rupture, usually an aneurysm, seal off the tear (Hickey, 1997; Macdonald, 1996). After a subarachnoid hemorrhage, neurologic injury occurs immediately as a result of blood seeping into adjacent tissues or may be delayed as a result of a secondary event such as rebleeding or vasospasm. Estimates are that 45% of patients who survive the initial bleeding episode will have a transient loss of consciousness. This probably is caused by either intracranial hypertension and increased intracranial pressure or transient cardiac arrhythmias as a result of blood around the brainstem (Kirsch, Diringer, Borel, & Hanley, 1989; Macdonald, 1996; McKhann & LeRoux, 1998; Wojner, 1998).

5. Give the rationale for Connie's hyponatremia.

According to Segatore (1993), hyponatremia is the most common electrolyte imbalance found in patients with subarachnoid hemorrhage. Hyponatremia is associated with a high incidence of brain ischemia and infarction. The pathogenesis of hyponatremia after subarachnoid hemorrhage remains unclear; it is probably caused by cerebral salt wasting or the syndrome of inappropriate secretion of antidiuretic hormone (ADH) (Dorsch, 1996; McKhann & LeRoux, 1998; Segatore, 1993).

6. Define how a subarachnoid hemorrhage is classified.

The Hunt and Hess classification system is most commonly used to "grade" the severity of a subarachnoid bleeding episode in terms of clinical presentation and significance. The grades range from grade I (asymptomatic or minimal headache) to grade V (deep coma, extension abnormal, and moribund appearance). Timing of surgery may be judged by the presenting grade and clinical progression. The higher grades are associated with much higher mortality and morbidity (Campbell & Edwards, 1997; Hickey, 1997; Wojner, 1998, 1999).

7. What therapeutic modalities should be anticipated for patients after subarachnoid hemorrhage? Give the rationale for each.

After stabilization and control of systemic blood pressure, bed rest and aneurysm precautions are instituted. Elastic stockings or antithrombotic pumps may be used to counter the effects of bed rest and hemostasis. Normal hydration is supplemented with intravenous therapy. Drug therapy includes the following (Feigin, Rinkel, Algra, Vermeulen, & Van Gijn, 1998; Hickey, 1997; Kirsch et al, 1989; Sikes & Nolan, 1993):

- *Anticonvulsants:* used prophylactically to prevent seizures because blood in the subarachnoid space is an irritant to the surrounding tissues.
- *Steroids:* are controversial but may be used if the patient shows signs of increased intracranial pressure, focal neurologic deficits, or cerebral edema.
- *Calcium channel blocker:* used prophylactically to reduce or minimize the threat of vasospasm and subsequent secondary ischemia.
- *Antifibrinolytic therapy:* is controversial but used to prevent clot lysis at the point of rupture. Agents such as aminocaproic acid or tranexamic acid reduce the risk of rebleeding during the first 2 weeks after rupture. The clot reinforces the wall of the aneurysm. If this therapy is used, it is initiated immediately upon diagnosis of a subarachnoid hemorrhage. Antifibrinolytic agents are discontinued upon ligation of the aneurysm.
- *Analgesics:* used to control the headaches and pain associated with meningeal irritation.
- *Mild sedative:* possibly used if the patient is agitated and at risk for increased intracranial pressure because of combativeness.
- *Stool softener:* used to prevent straining for bowel movements and initiation of Valsalva's maneuver, which may trigger increased intracranial pressure.

8. What parameters require close monitoring for patients after subarachnoid hemorrhage?

Neurologic and vital signs are assessed for evidence of complications such as hydrocephalus, increased intracranial pressure, rebleeding, or vasospasm. The nurse also monitors for complications associated with prolonged bed rest. Detailed clinical assessment is paramount in the care of these patients to detect any early, subtle changes in neurologic status that may indicate secondary complications.

9. What are the general complications associated with aminocaproic acid (Amicar) and nimodipine?

Aminocaproic acid (Amicar) has been associated with an increase in hydrocephalus and vasospasm. Calcium channel blockers are associated with hypotension, which can induce cerebral ischemia in the patient after subarachnoid hemorrhage. Calcium antagonists significantly limit the effectiveness of vasopressor drugs used to maintain systemic blood pressure (Feigin et al, 1998; Kirsch et al, 1989, LeRoux & Winn, 1998).

10. What are the general "aneurysm precautions" for patients with a subarachnoid hemorrhage who may have a cerebral aneurysm?

Aneurysm precautions include the following (Hickey, 1997):

- Place the patient in a quiet room.
- Control the room lighting to prevent strong, direct light.
- Allow reading and TV watching if these activities do not overstimulate the patient.
- Maintain good oxygen and carbon dioxide exchange; supplemental oxygen is usually ordered.
- Maintain head of bed elevation, generally 20 to 30 degrees to augment cerebral venous drainage.
- Maintain bed rest, possibly with bathroom privileges (avoid straining for bowel movements).
- Restrict visitors and discuss with visitors the importance of a calming, supportive environment.
- Schedule nursing care and diagnostic tests to avoid overstimulating the patient.

11. Describe the pathophysiology of cerebral aneurysm.

Cerebral aneurysms are saccular outpouchings of the walls of a cerebral artery. The causes of cerebral aneurysms are unclear. However, at least three theories have been identified in the literature. The congenital theory suggests that a congenital weakness exists in the wall of the artery's medial layer allowing an outpouching. The degenerative theory suggests that a local weakness develops in the intima as a result of hemodynamically induced degenerative changes. In midlife, the vessel develops an outpouching of the intimal layer caused by hemodynamic stress on the weakened area (usually due to arteriosclerosis). Aneurysms often occur in the area of the circle of Willis at a point of bifurcation or a junction of the arteries. Rupture often occurs in association with physical activities or strain. Clinical studies suggest a seasonal variation for aneurysmal rupture in the spring and fall as well as a circadian cycle of increased episodes in the morning or evening. Also, there is a component of genetic predisposition (Becker, 1998; Campbell & Edwards, 1997; Connolly & Solomon, 1998; Dorsch, 1996; Hickey, 1997; Rusy, 1996; Walters & Lancton, 1999).

12. Define the different types of aneurysms.

Types of aneurysms are best classified by their shapes. Common classification by shape is as follows (Hickey, 1997; Rusy, 1996; Walters & Lancton, 1999 Wojner, 1998):

- *Berry:* most common, berry shaped with a neck or stem
- *Saccular:* saccular outpouching
- *Fusiform:* outpouching without a neck or stem
- *Traumatic:* associated with head trauma
- *Mycotic:* caused by septic emboli
- *Charcot-Bouchard:* microscopic, associated with hypertension, and often located in the brainstem and basal ganglia
- *Dissecting:* generally associated with atherosclerosis; blood is forced between the intimal layer and medial layer

13. Discuss the secondary cerebral injuries associated with a ruptured aneurysm and subsequent subarachnoid hemorrhage.

Rebleeding

Rebleeding occurs when an aneurysm releases additional blood into the subarachnoid space. With each additional rupture episode, patient mortality increases dramatically. Rarely do patients survive the third episode of a rupture and rebleeding (McKhann & LeRoux, 1998).

Hydrocephalus and Increased Intracranial Pressure

Subarachnoid hemorrhage and subsequent clot(s) in the subarachnoid space may interfere with the flow and reabsorption of CSF via the arachnoid villi. Large clots may mechanically interfere with the flow of blood through the ventricular system, resulting in hydrocephalus, increased intracranial pressure, and reduced cerebral blood flow. The clinical presentation is generally a decrease or change in the level of consciousness (Hickey, 1997; Kirsch et al., 1989; LeRoux & Winn, 1998; McKhann & LeRoux, 1998).

Seizures

Seizures after a subarachnoid hemorrhage are more common in younger adults with a ruptured aneurysm and may occur in up to 25% of patients. Seizures associated with subarachnoid hemorrhage are divided into initial, early, and late. Initial seizures occur at the time of the rupture. Early seizures occur within 2 weeks, and late seizures usually occur more than 2 weeks after the initial hemorrhage. In the acute setting, seizures are often followed by rebleeding, probably because of the increased cerebral blood flow and perfusion pressure. Prophylactic anticonvulsant therapy is generally advocated but remains controversial, and often phenytoin (Dilantin) is the drug of choice (Kirsch et al, 1989; LeRoux & Winn, 1998; McKhann & LeRoux, 1998).

Vasospasm

Vasospasm is a narrowing of the vessels in the area of the subarachnoid hemorrhage. Vasospasm can lead to cerebral ischemia and a cerebral infarct (Bell & Kongable, 1996; Kirsch et al, 1989, Mayberg, 1998; Rusy, 1996).

Hypothalamic Dysfunction

Hypothalamic dysfunction may be exhibited as hyponatremia resulting from a disturbance in the regulation of ADH. Referred to as the syndrome of inappropriate secretion of ADH, this condition exists when the neurons of the supraoptic hypothalamic secrete ADH unrelated to true serum osmolarity or intravascular volume. Water is retained by the kidneys, and hyponatremia or hypervolemia results. Electrocardiogram changes may occur as a result of an overstimulated sympathetic system (McKhann & LeRoux, 1998; Segatore, 1993).

14. Discuss the advantages and disadvantages of early versus late surgical intervention.

Traditionally, surgical repair of the aneurysm was delayed 7 to 14 days to allow cerebral edema to subside and to allow for medical stabilization of the patient. However, during the waiting period, the peak incidence of both rebleeding and vasospasm occurs. With improvements in microsurgical techniques and neuroanesthesia, the trend now is toward early surgery (i.e., within 1 to 3 days).

Early surgery enables the prevention of rebleeding and aggressive treatment with hypervolemia and hypertension for any vasospasm as necessary (Mendel & Carter, 1994). Early surgery consists of removal of the subarachnoid clot, which perhaps minimizes the vasospastic reaction to the clot (Hosoda, Fujita, Kawaguchi, Shose, Hamano, & Iwakura, 1999; Lanzino & Kassell, 1998). Early surgery is associated with a higher risk probably because of the technically difficult nature of surgery on an edematous brain. Miyaoka, Sato, and Ishii (1993) suggest in a retrospective analysis of 1622 cases that early surgery for patients with grade I and II aneurysms was not a major factor in predicting outcome. However, early surgery for patients with grade III and IV aneurysms does appear to provide additional benefits of preventing a rebleeding episode and allowing for aggressive treatment of vasospasm and clot removal at the time of surgery. The International Study on the Timing of Aneurysm Surgery (ISTAS) conducted during the 1980s indicated that good recovery was significantly higher in the early surgery group when the data collected by the North American Centers were analyzed separately. Early surgery allows for the concomitant removal of intraparenchymal hematoma. Delayed surgery may be considered based on the size and location of the aneurysm. Early surgery is not indicated for giant and technically difficult to approach aneurysms. Elderly patients and those with significant comorbidity may require a delayed approach (Lanzino & Kassell, 1998).

15. Discuss why nursing care is of particular importance after a craniotomy.

Overall and serial evaluation of neurologic status is critical to detect any changes associated with development of a postoperative intracranial blood clot. Airway maintenance is essential because these patients often have difficulty controlling their airway because of neurologic deficits. Evaluation of increased intracranial pressure related to cerebral edema is critical, particularly after suctioning or painful procedures. Electrolyte imbalances are also a concern postoperatively after a craniotomy because of the diuresis that occurs intraoperatively. As patients recover after a craniotomy, nutrition and complications of bed rest must be assessed carefully. Postoperative pain, particularly headache, requires attention with judicious use of pain medication (Romeo, 1993; Wojner, 1999).

16. **Describe the pathophysiology and incidence of rebleeding. When is rebleeding likely to occur?**

Rebleeding occurs when the fibrin-platelet clot is displaced by either hypertension or fibrinolysis. Women, patients in poor premorbid health, patients with elevated systolic blood pressures, and patients with a high clinical grade on the Hunt and Hess scale are more likely to have a rebleeding episode. Patients with aneurysms are at risk for rebleeding until the aneurysm is clipped or treated in some fashion. Peak incidence for rebleeding is 24 to 48 hours after the aneurysm (Hickey, 1997; Kirsch et al, 1989; LeRoux & Winn, 1998; McKhann & LeRoux, 1998; Rusy, 1996). Rebleeding occurs in as many as 30% of all patients with aneurysms, and the mortality is 45% (Lanzino & Kassell, 1998).

17. **Discuss clinical changes that should be anticipated if a patient is experiencing rebleeding.**

The clinical presentation of rebleeding is generally profound, with gradual or sudden deterioration in neurologic status. Patients may complain of increased pain associated with a headache. Often, there may be a sudden onset of nausea and vomiting and a rise in systolic blood pressure and intracranial pressure (Dorsch, 1996; McKhann & LeRoux, 1998).

18. **Describe how rebleeding is diagnosed.**

The definitive diagnosis of rebleeding is made by a second CT scan. The results of the second scan are compared with the initial CT scan. The second CT scan can also reveal evidence of increasing subarachnoid hemorrhage, which is indicative of a rebleeding episodes.

19. **Discuss the treatment for rebleeding. What is the duration of treatment?**

Ideally, treatment consists of prevention. The definitive prevention is surgical clip ligation of the aneurysm. The efficacy of prophylactic treatment while waiting for surgical intervention is controversial. Antifibrinolytic agents such as aminocaproic acid (Amicar) may be administered with the initial diagnosis of subarachnoid hemorrhage to prevent clot lysis. Aminocaproic acid is discontinued intraoperatively once the clip is in place. The placement of Guglielmi detachable coils provides some protection against rebleeding during the acute phase (Martin, 1998; McKhann & LeRoux 1998; Nelson, 1998).

20. **Describe the pathophysiology and incidence of vasospasm. When is vasospasm likely to occur?**

Vasospasm is a narrowing of the arteries in the area of the aneurysm and subarachnoid hemorrhage. The specific cause of vasospasm is debated in the literature. A correlation is suggested between the incidence of vasospasm and the amount of blood released into the subarachnoid space. The extent of the clot (when located in the basal cisterns and cerebral fissures) should be considered when evaluating the probability of spasm. Subarachnoid clots larger than 3 by 5 mm in the basal cisterns or layers of blood 1 mm or thicker in the area of the cisterns have a high correlation with spasm (Bell & Kongable, 1996; Hickey, 1997). The following have a high incidence of vasospasm: patients with a high clinical grade on the Hunt and Hess scale and patients with hyponatremia, hypovolemia, electroencephalogram abnormalities, increased cerebral blood flow velocity, decreased regional cerebral blood flow, or fibrinogen degradation products greater than 80 μg/ml in the CSF (Sikes & Nolan, 1993). Vasospasm is also associated with a loss of autoregulation, tissue ischemia, and ultimately, tissue infarction. The onset of vasospasm is usually 3 to 14 days after the initial subarachnoid hemorrhage, with a peak around day 7. The threat of vasospasm persists for up to 3 weeks (Bell & Kongable, 1996; Campbell & Edwards, 1997; Dorsch, 1996; Hickey, 1997; Kirsch et al, 1989; Rusy, 1996).

21. Discuss the causes of vasospasm.

The cause of vasospasm is still unknown; however, a dominant theory exists. Once the clot in the subarachnoid space begins to break down, spasmodic agents are released, resulting in vasospasm. Theories of etiology include the following:

- Biochemical process resulting in contraction of arterial muscle cells
- Release of spasmodic substances during the breakdown of erythrocytes and platelets in the subarachnoid blood
- Release of mitogenic substances from platelets, resulting in structural vessel changes
- An inflammatory process resulting in vasculopathy

There is also much interest in the role that oxygen-free radicals may play in the development of vasospasm (Campbell & Edwards, 1997; Mayberg, 1998).

22. Identify how cerebral vasospasm is diagnosed. Include clinical symptoms that should be anticipated.

Sequential neurologic assessment is crucial to identify the clinical symptoms of vasospasm. The clinician must carefully observe for lethargy, confusion, restlessness, disorientation, new headaches, hemiparesis, seizures, labile blood pressure, change in speech, elevated fever, or slight leukocytosis, all of which are indicative of the onset of vasospasm. The transcranial Doppler study may detect vessel narrowing with elevated velocities. The demonstrated increase in velocity may often precede clinical symptoms. With deterioration of neurologic function and no radiographic evidence of rebleeding, a second angiogram provides definitive diagnosis of vasospasm. Other causes of a change in condition (e.g., electrolyte imbalance, development of hydrocephalus) must be considered as well (Bell & Kongable, 1996; Campbell & Edwards, 1997; Manno, 1997; Mayberg, 1998).

23. Discuss the mortality and morbidity of vasospasm and rebleeding.

Mortality and morbidity related to vasospasm is high, approaching 50%. Among those who survive the initial subarachnoid hemorrhage, 40% will develop clinical symptoms of vasospasm, resulting in delayed cerebral ischemia. Morbidity is associated with the degree of cerebral ischemia, infarction, and permanent neurologic injury. Mortality associated with rebleeding is as high as 70% and increases with each episode of rebleeding. Patients rarely survive a third rebleeding event. Morbidity is associated with the location and degree of cerebral tissue injury with each event and can be quite severe (Campbell & Edwards, 1997; Hickey, 1997; Kirsch et al, 1989; McKhann & LeRoux, 1998; Rusy, 1996).

24. Discuss current treatment for vasospasm. What additional approaches to the treatment of vasospasm are discussed in the literature?

Current modalities of treatment are focused on increasing cerebral perfusion pressure using hypervolemic/hypertensive therapy and pharmacologic agents to dilate cerebral arteries, improve rheologic findings, and maximize cardiac performance (Campbell & Edwards, 1997; Hickey, 1997; Sikes & Nolan, 1993).

Hypervolemic/hypertensive therapy is also referred to as *hyperdynamic therapy* or *triple-H therapy.* This consists of induced hypervolemia, hemodilution, and hypertension. The goal is to increase cerebral blood flow, cerebral perfusion pressure, and cerebral microcirculation. Much of the improvement in mortality associated with subarachnoid hemorrhage has been attributed to aggressive treatment of vasospasm after the clip ligation of the aneurysm. Vasopressor agents such as dopamine or phenylephrine (Neo-Synephrine) may be useful to elevate systolic blood pressure. Hypervolemia is induced with combined use of colloids (albumin) or crystalloids (5% dextrose in lactated Ringer's solution [D5LR] or in normal saline). Intravenous solutions such as D5LR may be given at high rates (125 to 300 ml/hr). Triple-H therapy is not without risk and hazards. The patient must be monitored carefully for complications such as pulmonary edema, congestive heart failure, cerebral edema, increased intracranial pressure, myocardial infarction, intracerebral hemorrhage, and systemic complications of prolonged vasopressor administration. Guidelines for hypervolemic/hypertensive therapy are as follows (Campbell & Edwards, 1997; Hickey, 1997; Mayberg, 1998; Mendel & Carter, 1994; Rusy, 1996):

- Central venous pressure >10 mm Hg
- Pulmonary capillary wedge pressure 14 to 20 mm Hg
- Hematocrit 33% to 38%
- Heart rate >70 bpm
- 30% rise in mean arterial blood pressure (130 to 150 mm Hg)
- Systolic blood pressure 160 to 200 mm Hg

Despite the interest in a variety of drugs to prevent the narrowing of arteriole walls, the results have not been promising. The greatest interest is currently in the use of calcium antagonists. Of the calcium channel blockers available, nimodipine is currently the drug of choice. Nimodipine is more potent than nifedipine (Procardia), is lipid soluble, readily crosses the blood-brain barrier, and perhaps has fewer systemic effects from hypotension.

Nimodipine promotes collateral circulation, reduces platelet aggregation, and blocks calcium influx into single nerve cells, thus promoting an antispasmodic effect. Nimodipine enhances the cardiac function by reducing afterload. Treatment is continued for 21 days. The typical dosage is 60 mg every 4 hours orally. Although other calcium channel blockers (e.g., nicardipine, AT877) are available, the drug of choice remains nimodipine (Feigin et al, 1998).

Rheology is the study of blood's ability to flow. Patients with a subarachnoid hemorrhage often have increased blood volume within the brain tissue, suggesting microstagnation. Increased hematocrit, erythrocyte aggregation, platelet aggregation, plasma viscosity, and shear rate affect blood viscosity. The hematocrit is the easiest to manipulate and is done so by hemodilution. Crystalloids and colloids are used in conjunction to provide hemodilution and hypervolemic therapy to increase the cerebral perfusion to the tissues deprived by vasospasm. Plasma protein fraction (Plasmanate), 5% albumin, hetastarch (Hespan), or dextran may also be used (Sikes & Nolan, 1993).

Additional drugs may be used to maximize cardiac performance and promote supported hypervolemic/hypertensive therapy. The mean arterial blood pressure is elevated to the point at which the clinical condition of the patient improves and is then titrated down to the point at which neurologic status is maintained. Therapy can be much more aggressive in patients who have clipped or surgically secured aneurysms once the threat of rebleeding has been removed.

Inotropic and vasoconstrictive therapy may be necessary to support the desired elevation in blood pressure. Dopamine (Intropin) (3 to 10 µg/kg/min), dobutamine (Dobutrex) (2.5 to 10 µg/kg/min), and phenylephrine hydrochloride (Neo-Synephrine) (10 to 100 µg/min) are commonly used. Atropine sulfate may be necessary to block vagal bradycardia induced by hypervolemia. Vasopressin (Pitressin) may be used to keep urine output at less than 200 ml/hr and to prevent diuresis as a response to hypervolemia. Cardiac pharmacologic management such as digitalis (Digoxin) may be necessary for the patient at risk for pulmonary compromise and cardiac failure with the added stress of hypervolemia therapy (McKhann & LeRoux, 1998; Sikes & Nolan, 1993).

Cerebral angioplasty is indicated for patients who do not improve with conventional therapy. This investigative therapy involves temporary balloon dilation of the affected arterial segment(s). Arterial dilation is immediate and permanent. Complete recovery has been reported using this technique. Possible use of oxygen-free radical scavengers (lazaroids) is being considered to prevent cellular damage. Intracisternal injection of the drug recombinant tissue plasminogen activator is also under evaluation (Mendel & Carter, 1994; Sikes & Nolan, 1993). This may reduce vasospasm by improving the process of clot lysis and clearance, thus preventing prolonged exposure to perivascular blood and the release of oxyhemoglobin (Bell & Kongable, 1996; Mayberg, 1998; McKhann & LeRoux, 1998; Rusy, 1996).

25. How long should the treatment of vasospasm be continued, and how long will Connie remain at risk for vasospasm or rebleeding?

Hypervolemic therapy is maintained until stabilization of the patient's condition and resolution of the acute phase. Calcium antagonists are usually continued for 21 days.

The risk for rebleeding is present until the aneurysm is surgically treated by clip ligation or clamp of the main feeder artery. In patients with untreated aneurysms after the first year, the risk of rebleeding is cumulative at 3% for each year. The risk for vasospasm is present for approximately 21 days, then the incidence drops off dramatically (LeRoux & Winn, 1998).

26. Discuss nonsurgical approaches available to patients unable to tolerate traditional surgical treatment.

Endovascular occlusion is an option for patients unable to undergo traditional surgical treatment. Coil embolization has been advocated for poor-grade patients (Hunt and Hess scale), advanced age, medically instability, difficult location of the aneurysm, and so on. One approach is the placement of platinum Guglielmi detachable coils within the aneurysmal sac. Thrombosis around the coil promotes occlusion of the aneurysm. There are many questions regarding long-term stability and recurrence after coil treatment. Another option includes treatment with stereotactic radiosurgery (LeRoux & Winn, 1998; Martin, 1998; Nelson, 1998; Walters & Lancton, 1999).

SUBARACHNOID HEMORRHAGE WITH ANEURYSM

References

Baxter, A., Cohen, W. A., & Maravilla, R. (1998). Imaging of intracranial aneurysms and subarachnoid hemorrhage. *Neurosurgery Clinics of North America, 9*(3), 445-462.

Becker, K. J. (1998). Epidemiology and clinical presentation of aneurysmal subarachnoid hemorrhage. *Neurosurgery Clinics of North America, 9*(3), 435-444.

Bell, T., & Kongable, G. (1996). Innovations in aneurysmal subarachnoid hemorrhage: Intracisternal t-PA for the prevention of vasospasm. *Journal of Neuroscience Nursing, 25*(2), 107-214.

Campbell, P., & Edwards, S. (1997). Hyperdynamic therapy: The nurse's role in the treatment of cerebral vasospasm. *Journal of Neuroscience Nursing, 29*(5), 318-326.

Connolly, E., & Solomon, R. (1998). Management of symptomatic and unsymptomatic unruptured aneurysms. *Neurosurgery Clinics of North America, 9*(3), 509-524.

Dorsch, N. (1996). Special problems associated with subarachnoid hemorrhage. In J. R. Youmans (Ed.), *Neurological surgery* (pp. 1438-1448). Philadelphia: Saunders.

Feigin, V., Rinkel, G., Algra, A., Vermeulen, M., & Van Gijn, J. (1998). Calcium antagonist in patients with aneurysmal subarachnoid hemorrhage. *Neurology, 50*(4), 876-881.

Hickey, J. (1997). *Neurological and neurosurgical nursing.* Philadelphia: JB Lippincott.

Hosoda, K., Fujita, S., Kawaguchi, T., Shose, Y., Hamano, S., & Iwakura, T. (1999). Effects of clot removal and surgical manipulation on regional cerebral blood flow and delayed vasospasm in early aneurysm surgery for subarachnoid hemorrhage. *Surgical Neurology, 51*(1), 81-88.

Johnston, S., Selvin, S., & Gress, D. (1998) The burden, trends, and demographics of mortality from subarachnoid hemorrhage. *Neurology, 50*(5), 1413-1418.

Kirsch, J., Diringer, M., Borel, C., & Hanley, D. (1989). Cerebral aneurysms: Mechanisms of injury and critical care interventions. *Critical Care Clinics, 5*(4), 755-772.

Lanzino, G., & Kassell, N. (1998). Surgical treatment of the ruptured aneurysm. *Neurosurgery Clinics of North America, 9*(3), 541-547.

LeRoux, P. & Winn, H. (1998). Management of the ruptured aneurysm. *Neurosurgery Clinics of North America, 9*(3), 525-540.

Macdonald, R. (1996). Pathophysiology and clinical evaluation of subarachnoid hemorrhage. In J. R. Youmans (Ed.), *Neurological surgery* (pp. 1224-1242). Philadelphia: Saunders.

Manno, E. (1997). Transcranial Doppler ultrasonography in the neurocritical care unit. In M. N. Diringer (Ed.), *Critical care clinics* (pp. 79-104). Philadelphia: Saunders.

Martin, N. (1998). The combination of endovascular and surgical techniques for the treatment of intracranial aneurysms. *Neurosurgery Clinics of North America, 9*(4), 897-916.

Mayberg, M. (1998). Cerebral vasospasm. *Neurosurgery Clinics of North America, 9*(3), 615-628.

McKhann, G., & LeRoux, P. (1998). Perioperative and intensive care unit care of patients with aneurysmal subarachnoid hemorrhage. *Neurosurgery Clinics of North America, 9*(3), 595-610.

Mendel, R. & Carter, L. (1994). Evaluation and treatment of clinical vasospasm following subarachnoid hemorrhage. *Contemporary Neurosurgery, 16*(6), 1-6.

Miyaoka, M., Sato, K., & Ishii, S. (1993). A clinical study of the relationship of timing to outcome of surgery for ruptured cerebral aneurysms. *Journal of Neurosurgery, 79,* 373-378.

Nelson, P. (1998). Neurointerventional management of intracranial aneurysms. *Neurosurgery Clinics of North America, 9*(4), 879-896.

Romeo, J. (1993). Patients with craniotomies. In J. M. Clochesy, C. Breu, S. Cardin, E. B. Rudy, & A. A. Whittaker (Eds.), *Critical care nursing* (pp. 788-793). Philadelphia: Saunders.

Rusy, K. (1996). Rebleeding and vasospasm after subarachnoid hemorrhage: A critical care challenge. *Critical Care Nurse, 16*(1), 41-47.

Segatore, M. (1993). Hyponatremia after aneurysmal subarachnoid hemorrhage. *Journal of Neuroscience Nurses, 25*(2), 92-99.

Sikes, P., & Nolan, S. (1993). Pharmacologic management of cerebral vasospasm. *Critical Care Nurse Quarterly, 15*(4), 78-88.

Van Tatenhove, J., & Kelley, C. (1999). Neurodiagnostic tests. In L. Bucher & S. Melander (Eds.), *Critical care nursing* (pp.824-842). Philadelphia: Saunders.

Walters, K. & Lancton, M. (1999). Cerebral aneurysms and other cerebrovascular disorders. *Nursing Clinics of North America, 34*(3).

Wojner, A. (1998). Neurovascular disease. In M. R. Kinney, S. B. Dunbar, J. A. Brooks-Brunn, N. Molter, & J. M., Vitello-Cicciu (Eds.), *AACN's clinical reference for critical care nursing* (pp. 733-768). St Louis: Mosby.

Wojner, A. (1999). Neurovascular disorders. In L. Bucher & S. Melander (Eds.), *Critical care nursing* (pp. 913-939). Philadelphia: Saunders.

CHAPTER 14

HEAD TRAUMA AND SUBDURAL HEMATOMA

Cinda Alexander, MSN, CCRN, CNRN, CNOR, CRNFA

CASE PRESENTATION

Amy, a 27-year-old right-handed woman, was involved in a motor vehicle accident. Amy was an unrestrained passenger in a car that swerved off the road and struck a tree. Amy was ejected from the car and was found unconscious by the emergency medical service personnel.

After being placed on a spinal board and in a Philadelphia collar, Amy was transported by helicopter to the nearest emergency room trauma center. Amy was somewhat combative and unresponsive to commands at arrival. Her pupils were reactive bilaterally (left > right). Her respiratory rate was 40 breaths/min and labored. Subsequently, an endotracheal tube was placed, and mechanical ventilation was started. Additional treatment included placement of a subclavian intravenous (IV) line, arterial catheter, and Foley catheter. Initial evaluation of her cervical spine revealed no abnormal findings, and the long spine board and Philadelphia collar were removed. Amy's diagnostic data were as follows:

BP	90/40 mm Hg	Temperature	36.7° C (98° F)
HR	100 bpm	Pupils reactive	left > right
Respirations	40 breaths/min	Glasgow Coma Scale score	9

Amy's initial computed tomographic (CT) scan of the head revealed a left temporal cerebral contusion with a midline shift of brain structures. The CT scan also revealed a left temporal parietal subdural hematoma (SDH).

After surgical removal of the hematoma, Amy was transferred to the critical care unit. Intubation and mechanical ventilation were continued. An intracranial pressure (ICP) monitoring device was placed. The following were her diagnostic data after surgery:

ICP	25 mm Hg	pH	7.48
BP	130/88 mm Hg	P_{CO_2}	40 mm Hg
HR	100 bpm	P_{O_2}	434 mm Hg
Respirations	12 breaths/min	HCO_3^-	20.4 mmol/L
Temperature	37.8° C (100° F)		

Ventilator settings were as follows:

TV   700 ml
Rate   12/min
Fio_2 100 %

As Amy recovered from the general anesthesia, she opened her eyes to speech, verbalized incomprehensible sounds, and exhibited abnormal general flexion to obtain a Glasgow Coma Scale score of 8. Over the next 2 hours, Amy's body temperature increased to 38.3° C (101° F). Despite hyperventilation, Amy's ICP remained elevated. Her serum osmolality was 282 mOsm/L, K^+ level was 3.9 mmol/L, and Na^+ level was 139 mmol/L. Postoperative orders included the following:

- Fluid restriction to maintain patient's osmolality between 305 and 315 mOsm/L
- Furosemide (Lasix) 20 mg q6h, IV
- Mannitol (Osmitrol) 25 to 50 g periodic bolus
- Phenytoin (Dilantin) 100 mg IV q6h

Amy's ICP remained elevated for more than 72 hours; then gradually, her pressure stabilized. After 2 weeks in the intensive care unit, Amy was transferred to a neurologic step-down unit and then to a head injury rehabilitation unit.

HEAD TRAUMA AND SUBDURAL HEMATOMA

Questions

1. Where does head trauma rank as a cause of death in the United States? What are the statistics associated with head trauma? Include morbidity and mortality information.
2. Identify the leading causes of head injury.
3. What is the rationale for Amy being placed on a long spine board with a Philadelphia collar?
4. What is the Glasgow Coma Scale? How is this scale helpful?
5. Differentiate the types of skull fractures associated with head trauma. What clinical presentations and pathophysiology are pertinent in these types of trauma?
6. Identify special considerations that are necessary for patients with basilar skull fractures for placement of an endotracheal or nasogastric tube.
7. List and describe the focal injuries associated with traumatic head injury. Include the mechanism of injury and clinical presentation associated with each.
8. List and describe the diffuse injuries associated with traumatic head injury.
9. Discuss the significance of a midline shift.
10. Identify the types of SDHs. Include the pathology and clinical presentation of SDH.
11. What surgical intervention is indicated for patients with SDH?
12. Define ICP. What methods are available for monitoring ICP? Describe the potential complications of ICP monitoring.

13. What factors determine when an ICP monitoring device is placed?
14. List and describe possible secondary injuries with head injury.
15. Based on Amy's arterial blood gas results, what ventilator changes should be anticipated? What is the desirable arterial carbon dioxide pressure ($Paco_2$) range in the presence of increased ICP?
16. Discuss the effect hyperventilation has on cerebral blood flow and increased ICP.
17. Describe the pathophysiology of intracranial hypertension. What is the general cause of increased ICP in patients with acute head injury?
18. What is autoregulation and how does it impact cerebral blood flow and ICP?
19. Given an ICP of 25 mm Hg and blood pressure of 120/72 mm Hg, calculate Amy's cerebral perfusion pressure (CPP). Is the CPP an acceptable value? Discuss the drawbacks of using CPP values.
20. Discuss the medical management that should be anticipated for patients with head injuries. Include the rationale and identify at least one potential complication associated with each.
21. Define and discuss the clinical significance of posturing such as abnormal flexion and abnormal extension.
22. Describe the relevance of controlling hyperthermia in the management of patients with head injuries.
23. What nursing management actions are essential to prevent or minimize the effects of secondary injury in patients with head injuries?
24. What are the potential extracranial effects of increased ICP?
25. Which cranial nerves must be intact before the patient eats or drinks?

HEAD TRAUMA AND SUBDURAL HEMATOMA

Questions and Answers

1. Where does head trauma rank as a cause of death in the United States? What are the statistics associated with head trauma? Include morbidity and mortality information.

Head trauma is the third leading cause of death in the United States. It is estimated that more than 10 million head injuries occur each year. Approximately 750,000 hospitalizations and 100,000 to 150,000 deaths are associated with head injury. Of all trauma-related deaths, 70% involve a head injury. Mortality from head injury alone is estimated to be approximately 50%. Most of these deaths occur before the person enters the health care system. The incidence of head injury is three times greater in males than in females, and peak incidence is at age 15 to 24 years (Guidelines for the Management of Severe Head Injury, 1995; McNair, 1999; Sullivan, Schefft, Warm, & Dember, 1994; Walleck, 1993).

2. Identify the leading causes of head injury.

Motor vehicle accidents are the leading cause of head injury with alcohol or drug consumption often associated as a contributing factor. Other causes include shootings, falls, assaults, and sporting accidents (Mansfield, 1997; March, 1999).

3. **What is the rationale for Amy being placed on a long spine board with a Philadelphia collar?**

It is known that Amy was traveling in a vehicle and was not wearing a seat belt. It is also known that after the automobile she was riding in hit a tree, Amy was ejected from the vehicle. It is well documented that there is a strong correlation between spinal cord trauma and head trauma or general trauma. Therefore, if head or spinal trauma is suspected, it is always recommended that victims at the site of an accident be placed on a spinal board and in a Philadelphia collar to prevent any secondary trauma to either the spine or the head and neck area. Motor vehicle accidents account for 47.7% of all spinal cord injuries (Hickey, 1997). There is a higher incidence of spinal cord injury associated with victims who are ejected from the vehicle as in Amy's case.

4. **What is the Glasgow Coma Scale? How is this scale helpful?**

The Glasgow Coma Scale is a standardized scale used to evaluate neurologic response. The scale is divided into three sections designed to assess consciousness, verbal abilities, and motor response. The scores range from 3 to 15, with 15 representing normal function. It is generally accepted that a score of 8 or less constitutes coma. The scale is a useful tool to communicate the patient's neurologic condition after a rapid assessment (Hartshorn, Byers, & Goddard, 1993; March, 1999; McNair, 1999; Nikas, 1998).

5. **Differentiate the types of skull fractures associated with head trauma. What clinical presentations and pathophysiology are pertinent in these types of trauma?**

Skull fractures are categorized as linear, depressed, or basilar and may be simple, comminuted, or compound in nature. The presence of a skull fracture does not delineate the degree of injury to the brain structures within the skull (Davis & Briones, 1998).

Linear Skull Fracture
Linear skull fractures are nondisplaced fractures of the skull. Most linear skull fractures are not displaced and do not require intervention unless they extend into a major sinus or across a major vascular channel (March, 1999; Nikas, 1998). If there is a fracture across a major vascular channel, such as the middle meningeal artery in the temporal parietal area, the patient should be evaluated carefully for acute epidural bleeding.

Depressed Skull Fracture
A depressed skull fracture is characterized by an inward depression of the outer table of the skull. Patients will have an open laceration in the area of the depression and varying degrees of neurologic alterations based on the degree of brain tissue involvement. Surgical intervention may be necessary to remove bone fragment from the meninges or brain tissue. The area of tissue and compression by the bony fragments can become a source of irritability and seizure

focus (Hartshorn et al, 1993, March, 1999). If the fracture is severe, clinical presentation may extend to seepage of cerebrospinal fluid (CSF) and brain tissue from the fracture site.

Basilar Skull Fracture

A basilar skull fracture is located at the base of the skull. If the fracture is significant, the underlying dura may be torn, which allows direct communication with the subarachnoid space and brain tissue. Infection and meningitis are of major concern with this type of fracture. Clinical presentation may include the following (March, 1999; Walleck, 1993; Davis & Briones, 1998):

- Seepage of CSF from the nose (rhinorrhea)
- Bilateral periorbital ecchymosis (raccoon eyes) if the anterior fossa is involved
- Leakage of CSF from the ears (otorrhea) if the middle fossa is involved
- Ecchymosis of the mastoid sinus (battle sign) if the posterior fossa is involved

6.   Identify special considerations that are necessary for patients with basilar skull fractures for placement of an endotracheal or nasogastric tube.

The inherent risk associated with endotracheal intubation and passage of a nasogastric tube is penetration through the fracture site and passage into the brain itself. Precautions include the use of the oral route for intubation and nasogastric tubes to minimize this risk. In addition, the nose should never be suctioned for removal of drainage in patients with basilar skull fractures (Walleck, 1993).

7.   List and describe the focal injuries associated with traumatic head injury. Include the mechanism of injury and clinical presentation associated with each.

The most common focal injuries associated with head injury are laceration, contusion, and intracranial hematomas (Butterworth & DeWitt, 1989; Hickey, 1997; Mansfield, 1997; March, 1999).

Contusions and Lacerations

A *contusion* is bruising of the brain. Contusions can be mild, involving a small portion of the brain tissue with minimal clinical symptoms, or they can be large, usually in the case of impact injuries, where the size increases as a result of edema and may produce significant increases in ICP. Injury to the brain usually results from accelerations and decelerations of the brain within the cranial vault. Contusions and lacerations tend to occur in the frontal and temporal areas and are commonly associated with skull fractures. A laceration is the tearing of brain parenchyma and is often associated with a depressed skull fracture. The significance of contusions and lacerations and severity of the neurologic injury are related to the degree of secondary insults such as edema, hemorrhage, and ischemia (Butterworth & DeWitt, 1989; March,1999).

Hematomas

Intracranial hematomas are classified as extradural or intradural. Extradural hematomas are referred to as *epidural* and generally are arterial in nature, usually occurring from a laceration of the middle meningeal artery. The clot forms between the inner table of the skull and the outer dura. Clinical symptoms develop quickly and are manifested as a sudden deterioration of consciousness, a fixed and dilated ipsilateral pupil, and hemiplegia or paresis. SDHs *(intradural)* form when there is bleeding between the dura and arachnoid layers. SDHs are generally venous in nature and often result from tears of cortical bridging veins but can result from bruising of the cortical tissue as well. The bleeding creates direct pressure and irritation of the cortical tissue. Clinical presentation includes a significantly depressed level of consciousness, pupillary changes (unequal to dilated and fixed), headache, agitation, confusion, and motor deficits. The degree of symptoms usually depends on the location and size of the clot formation (March, 1999; Walleck, 1993).

8. List and describe the diffuse injuries associated with traumatic head injury.

Concussion

A *concussion* is a transient, temporary condition of the brain without any structural damage. The clinical symptoms usually include a brief (generally seconds) loss of consciousness, confusion, and some amnesia. However, concussion can be severe enough to induce brief respiratory arrest, pronounced confusion, and severe amnesia. Concussions can be graded I through IV, with IV being the most severe. Clinical presentation and the lack of adequate supervision at home may necessitate hospitalization (March, 1999).

Diffuse Axonal Injury

Diffuse axonal injury (DAI) is a shear injury to the white matter with stretching and tearing of the reticular activating fibers. Microscopic focal lesions in the white matter include axon contraction balls throughout white matter, gathering of microglial cells, followed by degradation of long tracts. Microhemorrhagic or necrotic lesions appear in the corpus callosum and in the dorsolateral part of the upper brainstem (Liau, Bergsneider, & Becker, 1996; McNair, 1999; Sahuquillo-Barris, Lamarca-Ciuro, Vilata-Castan, Rubio-Garcia, & Rodriguez-Pazos, 1988). Clinical presentation includes deep and profound coma, abnormal posturing, increased ICP, hypertension, and hyperthermia. The hallmark of DAI is immediate and prolonged coma without radiographic identification of a specific cause (Butterworth & DeWitt, 1989; Crow, 1991; Davis & Briones, 1998; Mansfield, 1997; March, 1999; Walleck, 1993).

9. Discuss the significance of a midline shift.

A midline shift on a CT or magnetic resonance imaging scan indicates that the delicate structures of the central portion of the brain, such as the ventricles and brain stem, have been displaced laterally. Brain tissue displacement is poorly tolerated and leads to areas of ischemia, diffuse edema, and shearing of structures (Liau et al, 1996; McNair, 1999; Walleck, 1993).

10. **Identify the types of SDHs. Include the pathology and clinical presentation of SDH.**

SDHs are classified as acute, subacute, and chronic, with mortality ranging from 52% to 90% (March, 1999; Walleck, 1993; Wilberger, Harris, & Diamond, 1991). Acute SDH generally occurs within 48 hours of the initial injury. Clinical presentation is usually progressive, with possible headache, symptoms of increased ICP, pupillary and motor changes, and marked coma.

Subacute SDH develops 2 to 24 days after the initial injury. SDHs are often difficult to diagnose and are strongly indicated by failure to regain consciousness after head trauma.

Chronic SDH can develop from minor head trauma. Often, chronic SDH is associated with the elderly population because of cerebral atrophy, which can result from a minor fall or bump of the head. In the chronic state, the blood clot becomes encased within a membrane. Clinical symptoms generally are subtle and vague, with progressive confusion, drowsiness, headache, seizures, and hemiparesis. Symptoms associated with chronic SDH may not become apparent until several weeks to months after the initial injury. Persons with alcoholism are prone to chronic SDH formation as a result of frequent falls and changes in clotting factors associated with alcoholism (Hickey, 1997; March, 1999; McNair, 1999; Walleck, 1993).

11. **What surgical intervention is indicated for patients with SDH?**

Small SDHs can be treated medically because they can be reabsorbed if there is no evidence of significant increased ICP or shifting of brain structures. Acute SDH is surgically treated by craniotomy and removal of the clot. The greater the thickness of the clot and the greater the midline shift, the higher the morbidity and mortality (Zumkeller, Behrmann, Heissler, & Dietz, 1996). Subacute SDH may require a craniotomy flap or may be treated by burr holes if the clot has degenerated into a thick viscous liquid. Chronic SDH is treated with burr holes and placement of a temporary drain. Persistent chronic SDH may require a craniotomy flap to remove the membrane flap (Walleck, 1993).

12. **Define ICP. What methods are available for monitoring ICP? Describe the potential complications of ICP monitoring.**

ICP is a dynamic state of equilibrium that exists among the three components within the cranial vault: blood, brain, and CSF. Any increase in one component necessitates a decrease in another component for the dynamic equilibrium to remain constant; otherwise, an increase in ICP occurs (Monro-Kellie doctrine).

Various methods are available to measure ICP, including catheters and transducer setups that measure pressure from the epidural area, subdural area, subarachnoid space, tissue, and intraventricular spaces. The major complication associated with ICP monitoring is infection. Generally, the more invasive the method, the greater the risk of serious consequences of infection. Other complications associated with ICP monitoring include hematoma and migration of the catheter or device (Davis & Briones, 1998; Nikas, 1998; Van Tatenhove & Kelley, 1999).

13. What factors determine when an ICP monitoring device is placed?

Indications for an ICP monitor are somewhat controversial. General guidelines for placement include the following (Andrews, 1998; Butterworth & DeWitt, 1989; Van Tatenhove & Kelley, 1999):

- A Glasgow Coma Scale score of ≤8
- Intradural hematomas or contusions
- Demonstrated cerebral edema on CT scan
- Midline shifts

The Guidelines for the Management of Severe Head Injury (1995) indicate that ICP monitoring is appropriate if the CT scan is abnormal. In addition, if the CT scan is normal, ICP monitoring is appropriate if two or more of the following are noted:

- Age older than 40
- Motor posturing
- Systolic blood pressure <90 mm Hg

14. List and describe possible secondary injuries with head injury.

Secondary insults precipitated by brain trauma may include hypoxia, hypercapnia, hypotension, and cerebral edema or intracranial hypertension. Secondary processes may be immediate or delayed and are mediated by biochemical and cellular responses to the initial insult (Davis & Briones, 1998; Mansfield, 1997; March, 1999; McNair, 1999; Wright, 1999).

Hypoxia
Brain injury often leads to irregular and inadequate respiratory efforts. Early management of the airway at the scene of injury and aggressive respiratory support is critical. Hypoxemia contributes to neurologic damage because the brain compensates for a deceased oxygen supply by increased cerebral blood flow. This offers a luxury perfusion to the uninjured tissue and contributes to increased cerebral blood volume, thus increasing ICP (March, 1999; McNair, 1999). The Guidelines for the Management of Severe Head Injury (1995) recommend that hypotension (systolic blood pressure <90 mm Hg) or hypoxia (arterial oxygen pressure [Pao_2] <60 mm Hg) must be avoided and corrected immediately.

Hypercapnia
Carbon dioxide is a potent cerebrovasodilator that will increase cerebral blood flow and contribute to increased intracranial hypertension.

Hypotension
Hypotension is often the result of multisystem injury and overall blood loss. The mean arterial pressure (MAP) must be sufficient to maintain cerebral perfusion. Systemic hypotension contributes to general cerebral hypoperfusion (March, 1999).

Intracranial Hypertension
Cerebral edema associated with head trauma may be local or diffuse. Cerebral edema exaggerates the amount and severity of neurologic injury and leads to increased ICP. Intracranial hypertension is a major complication and is the most common cause of death associated with brain injury. Most of the care of patients with head injuries is

focused on control of ICP (Andrews, 1998; Bouma, Muizelaar, Bandoh, & Marmarou, 1992; Hickey, 1997; Marion & Letarte, 1997). Wilberger et al. (1991) found that control of increased ICP after removal of an SDH was a variable more critical to the patient's outcome than timing of surgery for removal of the clot.

15. Based on Amy's arterial blood gas results, what ventilator changes should be anticipated? What is the desirable arterial carbon dioxide pressure ($Paco_2$) range in the presence of increased ICP?

Ventilator changes to reduce the $Paco_2$ include increasing the rate (frequency) or tidal volume. Decreasing the fraction of inspired oxygen (Fio_2) to minimize the effect of oxygen toxicity is also indicated.

16. Discuss the effect hyperventilation has on cerebral blood flow and increased ICP.

Hyperventilation, a cornerstone in the management of traumatic brain injury, assists with the reduction of carbon dioxide, a potent cerebrovasodilator. With a reduction of $Paco_2$, there is vasoconstriction of the cerebral blood vessels, decreased cerebral blood volume, and thus decreased ICP. Severely lowered $Paco_2$ levels have a potential for causing ischemia and infarction (Walleck, 1993). Because traumatic brain injury is associated with a reduction of cerebral blood flow in the initial 24 hours after injury, hyperventilation is not without risk. Chronic use of hyperventilation of less than $Paco_2$ of 25 mm Hg should be avoided because it may contribute to cerebral ischemia in an already compromised brain (Guidelines for the Management of Severe Head Injury, 1995; Mansfield, 1997; Walleck, 1993; Wright, 1999; Yundt & Diringer, 1997).

Guidelines for the Management of Severe Head Injury (1995) include the following:

- Chronic, prolonged hyperventilation ($Paco_2$ of =25 mm Hg) should be avoided
- Prophylactic hyperventilation ($Paco_2$ =35 mm Hg) should be avoided the first 24 hours after injury

17. Describe the pathophysiology of intracranial hypertension. What is the general cause of increased ICP in patients with acute head injury?

The Monro-Kellie hypothesis describes the skull encasing a closed system with three components: blood, CSF, and brain tissue. If the volume of any of these three components increases without a concurrent decrease in one of the other, increased ICP will result. Normal ICP is 0 to 15 mm Hg. Some variations may be associated with the type of monitoring device used. *Intracranial hypertension* is a sustained increase in ICP greater than 15 mm Hg caused by the following conditions:

- Conditions that increase brain volume such as hematomas or cerebral edema
- Conditions that increase cerebral blood flow, including hyperemia and hypercapnia

- Conditions that increase CSF volume such as increased production of CSF, decreased absorption, and obstruction hydrocephalus

Cerebral edema is a common complication of moderate to severe brain injury that can result in intracranial hypertension and reduction of cerebral blood flow. Eisenhart (1994) describes three major causes of cerebral edema: increased cerebral blood flow, biochemical changes at the cellular level, and brain ischemia.

Initially, after acute head injury, cerebral blood flow increases, with an associated increase in ICP or intracranial hypertension, because there is engorgement of the brain tissue. As the ICP elevates, there is an associated tissue ischemia. Cerebral edema is also triggered at the cellular level via chemical changes and the release of excitatory amino acids. The state of increased pressure is further complicated by hypotension, resulting in decreased oxygenation to the tissues, and hypercapnia, resulting in cerebrovasodilation (Hickey, 1997; Nikas, 1998). Treatment now focuses on management of brain tissue perfusion and promotion of cerebral perfusion (Davis & Briones, 1998; Mansfield, 1997; March, 1999; McNair, 1999). However, according to the Guidelines for the Management of Severe Head Injury (1995), ICP treatment should be initiated at an upper threshold of 20 to 25 mm Hg. In addition, interpretation and treatment of ICP should be correlated by frequent clinical review of the cerebral perfusion pressure (CPP) data. Cerebral blood flow must be maintained at a minimal level to ensure adequate tissue perfusion. Because cerebral blood flow is difficult to measure in the clinical setting, the CPP can be estimated and used as an index (see question 19).

18. What is autoregulation and how does it impact cerebral blood flow and ICP?

Autoregulation is the automatic change in cerebral blood vessels in response to varying systemic pressures to maintain a continuous perfusion pressure gradient to the tissues without wide fluctuation of flow. The reflex maintains constant perfusion despite wide variations in systemic MAP. When autoregulation is disrupted, as may be the case in traumatized brain tissue, that area of tissue is dependent on systemic pressure for perfusion (Hickey, 1997; March, 1999; McNair, 1999; Rosner, 1995; Walleck, 1993).

19. Given an ICP of 25 mm Hg and blood pressure of 120/72 mm Hg, calculate Amy's CPP. Is the CPP an acceptable value? What are the drawbacks of using CPP values?

To calculate MAP:

$$\frac{\text{Systolic} + (2 \times \text{Diastolic})}{3} = \text{MAP}$$

To calculate CPP: MAP − ICP = CPP

$$\frac{120 + (2 \times 72)}{3} = 88 \text{ mm Hg (MAP)} \qquad 88 - 25 = 63 \text{ mm Hg (CPP)}$$

The focus has shifted from the single measurement of ICP to management of cerebral perfusion. Controversy exists over the "minimal" acceptable CPP value.

Generally, 60 mm Hg is considered \ the lowest acceptable value. Once ICP rises and CPP begins to fall, cerebral tissue is deprived of sufficient blood flow, and ischemia and infarction occur. If the ICP rises too high, the brain tissue herniates, followed by ischemia and infarction. If the herniation process continues without intervention, death caused by brainstem compression is usually the result (Kirsch, Diringer, Borel, Hart, & Hanley, 1989; Liau et al, 1996; March, 1999; Walleck, 1993). The recommendation of the Guidelines for the Management of Severe Head Injury (1995) is to maintain a CPP of 70 mm Hg.

20. **Discuss the medical management that should be anticipated for patients with head injuries. Include the rationale and identify at least one potential complication associated with each.**

CSF Drainage

A ventriculostomy will allow the drainage of CSF as well as ICP monitoring. Generally, the drainage point, or the point at which the CSF should drain via the ventriculostomy, is set for 20 mm Hg. The drainage point may be lowered to 15 mm Hg to promote additional CSF drainage if there is an increase in ICP (Hickey, 1997; Marion & Letarte, 1997). A serious complication of a ventriculostomy is infection or ventriculitis. Generally, a ventriculostomy in place longer than 7 to 10 days is associated with a significantly higher incidence of infection. Care should be taken to not allow "overdrainage" of the CSF and subsequent collapse of the ventricles.

Hyperventilation

Hyperventilation is induced to decrease the $Paco_2$ and promote vasoconstriction of cerebrovasculature, thereby decreasing cerebral blood flow and ICP. However, severe reduction of $Paco_2$, below 20 mm Hg, can cause hypoxia and tissue ischemia or infarction (Nikas, 1998). Hyperventilation should be used judiciously only if uncontrolled ICP is present (Eisenhart, 1994; March, 1998).

Osmotic Diuretics

Osmotic diuretics decrease brain edema by creating a vascular gradient promoting movement of water from brain tissue into the vascular compartment. Hyperosmolarity and renal failure are potential complications of this treatment. Mannitol is the drug of choice because of its rapid onset of action (Guidelines for the Management of Severe Head Injury, 1995; Hickey, 1997; March, 1997; Marion & Letarte, 1997). Serum osmolarity should be maintained below 320 mOsm. The Guidelines for the Management of Severe Head Injury (1995) suggest that an intermittent bolus may be more effective than a continuous IV infusion.

Loop Diuretics

Loop diuretics, such as furosemide (Lasix), are often used in combination with osmotic diuretics. The benefits probably relate to the ability of loop diuretics to reduce total body fluid and shifting of extravascular space, preventing acute pulmonary edema and congestive heart failure that can be a complication of osmotic therapy (March, 1999). Amy's hydration status must be evaluated carefully because the overuse of loop diuretics can lead to severe dehydration.

Fluid Management

Fluid restriction remains controversial in the care of patients with head injuries. Too much fluid restriction may result in severe dehydration. The patient's osmolality is the best guide for fluid therapy with a goal of 305 to 315 mOsm/L (normal 280 to 300 mOsm/L) with the goal of euvolemia (Hickey, 1997).

Glucocorticosteroids

The Guidelines for the Management of Severe Head Injury (1995) state that use of glucocorticosteroids is not recommended for improving outcome or reducing ICP in patients with severe brain injury. Steroids are still widely used in the treatment of brain tumors. Side effects associated with large doses of steroids include decreased resistance to infection and gastrointestinal hemorrhage (Hickey, 1997; March, 1998).

Barbiturate Therapy

Barbiturate therapy for coma is still considered for patients with uncontrolled ICP associated with cerebral edema. Barbiturates lower ICP; however, the mechanism is not well understood. Barbiturates are associated with numerous complications, including hypotension and decreased cardiac output (Kelly, Nikas, & Becker, 1996; Kirsch et al, 1989; Walleck, 1993). An ICP monitoring device must be used during barbiturate therapy so that the nurse can evaluate the patient's neurologic status because the patient is in a drug-induced coma (Guidelines for the Management of Severe Head Injury, 1995; March, 1999).

Seizure Control

Posttraumatic epilepsy occurs in 5% to 20% of patients with head injuries. The more severe the injury, the greater the likelihood of seizure activity. Seizures may occur early, within the first 7 days, or late after brain injury. Late posttraumatic seizures should not be treated prophylactically with anticonvulsants (Guidelines for the Management of Severe Head Injury, 1995; March, 1999). Risk factors to assess include intracranial hematoma, focal neurologic deficits, posttraumatic amnesia lasting more than 24 hours, depressed skull fracture, and age younger than 5 years. The treatment of early posttraumatic seizures may reduce secondary injury and ischemia. Seizure activity in the presence of brain injury can lead to a severe elevation in ICP and place increased metabolic demands on a compromised brain. Phenytoin (Dilantin) is the drug of choice for seizure control. Potential adverse effects of IV phenytoin are hypotension and cardiac arrhythmias.

Sedation, Analgesics, and Neuromuscular Blockade

Benzodiazepines are the most commonly used sedatives. Propofol is the most popular. Because sedatives do not provide analgesia, consideration must be given for pain control. Parenteral narcotics, such as small doses of morphine or fentanyl, may be used. Short-acting neuromuscular blockade (e.g., with vecuronium) may be used to counteract the ICP response to stimulation associated with activities such as personal care or suctioning (Fowler, Hertzog, & Wagner, 1995; Hickey, 1997; March, 1998; Marion & Letarte, 1997). Potential complications of these agents include hypotension and respiratory depression.

Neuroprotectants

There is much interest in investigational drugs called *neuroprotectants*. These drugs are thought to treat or control the pathologic response to the secondary insult of ischemia (March, 1999). As ischemia occurs in an injured brain, it is believed that there are biochemical processes that trigger a "neurotoxic cascade" of reactions. These biochemical changes may include the release of excitatory amino acids as well as the generation of oxygen-free radicals. The eventual result is cellular damage and destruction, which may not be restricted to the initially injured cells. Pharmacologic agents such as oxygen-free radical scavengers, glutamate antagonists, calcium channel blockers, nonglucocorticosteroids, and excitatory amino acid antagonists are now being studied in various trial phases (Eisenhart, 1994; Guidelines for the Management of Severe Head Injury, 1995; March, 1999; McNair, 1999).

21. Define and discuss the clinical significance of posturing such as abnormal flexion and abnormal extension.

Noxious stimuli can initiate abnormal, stereotypical motor responses referred to as *posturing*. Posturing, such as abnormal extension and abnormal flexion, is often associated with abnormal brainstem function and damage to the cerebral hemisphere.

Decortication is the hyperflexion of the upper extremities and the hyperextension of the lower extremities. Decortication, also referred to as *flexion abnormal,* may indicate damage to the cerebral hemispheres and internal capsule. Decerebration is the hyperextension of both the upper and lower extremities and internal rotation of the upper extremities. Decerebration, also referred to as *extension abnormal,* can indicate brainstem dysfunction. The presence of abnormal posturing does not clearly predict the outcome after acute head injury. However, it emphasizes the need for close neurologic monitoring because the brain has been severely compromised (Hartshorn et al, 1993).

22. Describe the relevance of controlling hyperthermia in the management of patients with head injuries.

Hyperthermia increases metabolic activity in the brain tissue, resulting in a greater oxygen demand. This leads to an increase in cerebral blood flow and production of carbon dioxide in a brain already compromised by cerebral edema and increased ICP (March, 1999; Walleck, 1993).

23. What nursing management actions are essential to prevent or minimize the effects of secondary injury in patients with head injuries?

Walleck (1993) outlines the following guidelines for patient care:

- *Patient positioning:* Patient position should always promote venous drainage from the brain. The head, neck, and chest are maintained in alignment to prevent obstruction of the jugular veins and twisting of the neck. The head of the bed is usually elevated. According to Feldman et al. (1992), elevation of the head at 30 degrees significantly reduces ICP without compromising cerebral blood flow and CPP.
- *Ventilation:* Airway management and pulmonary toilet are important protocols to manage patients with head injuries and prevent pulmonary complications.
- *Hyperventilation and oxygenation:* Hyperventilation and oxygenation before and after pulmonary suctioning can minimize the negative effects of suctioning. Caution must be observed to prevent overhyperventilation, which may lead to $Paco_2$ values less than 25 mm Hg.

- *Maintenance of blood pressure:* Hemodynamic stability is critical in the patient with a head injury to prevent wide fluctuations in MAP. Appropriate treatment of hypotension with IV fluids and pharmacologic agents and ongoing assessment of the MAP are indicated.
- *Normothermia:* Monitoring and maintenance of normal body temperature are necessary to prevent the effects of a hypermetabolic state on ICP.
- *Neurologic assessment:* Ongoing assessment of the patient's neurologic function is paramount to detect subtle changes that may indicate deterioration of the patient's condition. Serial evaluation and collaboration among caregivers are critical to ensure that any changes in status are noted.
- *Physical care:* There has been much interest in the literature as to the effects of personal care such as bathing, oral hygiene, and range of motion on ICP. Individualization based on patient response is necessary to determine which activities are well tolerated and which should be avoided. Generally, it is accepted that physical activities should be spaced to allow the patient recovery time and to prevent compounded effects on the ICP.

24. What are the potential extracranial effects of increased ICP?

The following are major extracerebral effects of traumatic brain injury (March, 1999).

Pulmonary Effects

- *Hypoxia:* Hypoxia occurs as a result of ventilation-perfusion mismatch or pulmonary shunt.
- *Noncardiogenic pulmonary edema:* Cerebral ischemia triggers a response of sympathetic discharge that alters capillary permeability in the lungs and creates an increase in atrial pressure.
- *Acute respiratory distress syndrome (ARDS):* ARDS is a common complication of patients with head injuries, resulting in an increase in dead space, a decrease in pulmonary compliance, and formation of hyaline membrane.
- *Aspiration pneumonitis:* In patients with head injuries, the airway is often not guarded because of a depressed level of consciousness, leaving them at risk for aspiration.
- *Fat emboli:* Fat emboli are often associated with long bone fractures seen in patients with multiple trauma.
- *Pulmonary contusion:* Pulmonary contusion often accompanies head injury caused by multiple trauma.

Cardiovascular Effects

- *Hyperdynamic cardiovascular response:* Hyperdynamic cardiovascular response is a cardiovascular effect associated with head trauma, a state of elevated cardiac output, increased heart rate, and increased blood pressure.
- *Posttraumatic hypertension:* Posttraumatic hypertension is precipitated by increased sympathetic activity, resulting in increased systolic blood pressure associated with Cushing's phenomenon.

Gastrointestinal Effects

- *Pancreatitis:* Pancreatitis is a gastrointestinal effect caused by blunt trauma to the abdomen that may be difficult to diagnose because of the patient's decreased level of consciousness.
- *Stress ulceration:* Stress ulceration may be present as erosive gastritis or gastrointestinal bleeding resulting from increased acidity.

Electrolyte and Metabolic Derangements

- *Hyponatremia:* Hyponatremia is associated with diarrhea, vomiting, gastric suction, and syndrome of inappropriate secretion of antidiuretic hormone.
- *Hypernatremia:* Hypernatremia usually represents water loss and may also be the result of diabetes insipidus.
- *Potassium deficits:* Deficiencies may be related to inadequate potassium replacement, diuretics, or alkalemia.
- *Thyroid and adrenal malfunction:* Trauma to the hypothalamus and pituitary glands results in thyroid and adrenal malfunction.

Nutrition

- *Autocatabolic state:* Autocatabolic state is an effect of increased ICP caused by stress-related hypermetabolism and gluconeogenesis.
- *Coagulation abnormalities:* Disseminated intravascular coagulation (DIC) is the most common coagulopathy associated with severe head trauma, especially with acute SDH and contusions. The cause of DIC is high thromboplastic activity of brain tissue.

25. Which cranial nerves must be intact before the patient eats or drinks?

It is essential that the nurse evaluate the following cranial nerves before the patient eats or drinks:

- Cranial nerve V (trigeminal): chewing
- Cranial nerve VII (facial): facial muscles
- Cranial nerves IX and X (glossopharyngeal and vagus): gag and swallowing
- Cranial nerve XII (hypoglossal): tongue

Only if these cranial nerves are intact bilaterally can the patient take nourishment by mouth (Walleck, 1993).

HEAD TRAUMA AND SUBDURAL HEMATOMA

References

Andrews, B. T. (1998). Intensive care for the neurosurgical patient. *Contemporary Neurosurgery, 20*(3), 1-6.

Bouma, G. J., Muizelaar, J. P., Bandoh, K., & Marmarou, A. (1992). Blood pressure and intracranial pressure-volume dynamics in severe head injury: Relationship with cerebral blood flow. *Journal of Neurosurgery, 77,* 15-19.

Butterworth, J. F., & DeWitt, D. S. (1989). Severe head trauma: Pathophysiology and management. *Critical Care Clinics, 5*(4), 807-819.

Crow, W. (1991). Aspects of neuroradiology of head injury. *Neurosurgery Clinics of North America, 2*(2), 321-340.

Davis, A. E. & Briones, T. L. (1998). Intracranial disorders. In M. R. Kinney, S. B. Dunbar, J. A. Brooks-Brunn, N. Molter, & J. M. Vitello-Cicciu (Eds.), *AACN's clinical reference for critical care nursing* (pp. 685-710). St Louis: Mosby.

Eisenhart, K. (1994). New perspectives in the management of adults with severe head injury. *Critical Care Nurse Quarterly, 17*(2), 1-12.

Feldman, Z., Kanter, M., Robertson, C. S., Contant, C. F., Hayes, C., Sheinberg, M. A., Villareal, C. A., Narayan, R. K., & Grossman, R. G. (1992). Effect of head elevation on intracranial pressure, cerebral perfusion pressure, and cerebral blood flow in head-injured patients. *Journal of Neurosurgery, 76,* 207-211.

Fowler, S. B., Hertzog, J., & Wagner, B. (1995). Pharmacological interventions for agitation in head-injured patients in the acute care setting. *Journal of Neuroscience Nursing, 27*(2), 119-123.

Guidelines for the Management of Severe Head Injury: A joint initiative of: The Brain Trauma Foundation, The American Association of Neurological Surgeons, The Joint Section on Neurotrauma and Critical Care. (1995). URL http://www.braintrauma.org/guidelines.nsf.

Hartshorn, J. C., Byers, V. L., & Goddard, L. (1993). Nervous system injury. In J. Hartshorn, M. Lamborn, & M. I. Noll (Eds.), *Introduction to critical care nursing* (pp. 246-267). Philadelphia: Saunders.

Hickey, J. V. (1997). *Neurological and neurosurgical nursing.* Philadelphia: JB Lippincott.

Kelly, D. F., Nikas, D. L., & Becker, D. P. (1996). Diagnosis and treatment of moderate and severe head injuries in adults. In J. R. Youmans (Ed.), *Neurological surgery* (pp. 1618-1718). Philadelphia: Saunders.

Kirsch, J. R., Diringer, M. N., Borel, C. O., Hart, G. K., & Hanley, D. F. (1989). Medical management and innovations. In K. A. Gould (Ed.), *Critical care nursing clinics of North America* (pp. 143-151). Philadelphia: Saunders.

Liau, L. M., Bergsneider, M., & Becker, D. P. (1996). Pathology and pathophysiology of head injury. In J. R. Youmans (Ed.), *Neurological surgery* (pp. 1549-1594). Philadelphia: Saunders.

Mansfield, R. T.(1997). Head injuries in children and adults. In M. M. Parker (Ed.), *Critical care clinics* (pp.611-625). Philadelphia: Saunders.

March, K. (1999). Acute head injury. In L. Bucher & S. Melander (Eds.), *Critical care nursing* (pp.843-868). Philadelphia: Saunders.

Marion, D. W. & Letarte, P. B. (1997). Management of intracranial hypertension. *Contemporary Neurosurgery, 19*(3), 1-6.

McNair, N. D. (1999). Traumatic brain injury. *Nursing Clinics of North America, 34*(3), 637-659.

Nikas, D. L. (1998).The neurologic system. In J. G. Alspach (Ed.), *American Association of Critical-Care Nurses: Core curriculum for critical care nursing* (pp.339-463). Philadelphia: Saunders.

Rosner, M. J. (1995). Introduction to cerebral perfusion pressure management. *Neurosurgery Clinics of North America, 6*(4), 761-774.

Sahuquillo-Barris, J., Lamarca-Ciuro, J., Vilata-Castan, J., Rubio-Garcia, E., & Rodriguez-Pazos, M. (1988). Acute subdural hematoma and diffuse axonal injury after severe head trauma. *Journal of Neurosurgery, 68,* 894-900.

Sullivan, T. E., Schefft, B. K., Warm, J. S., & Dember, W. N. (1994). Closed head injury assessment and research methodology. *Journal of Neuroscience Nursing, 26*(1), 27-29.

Van Tatenhove, J. C., & Kelley, C. B. (1999). Neurodiagnostic tests. In L. Bucher & S. Melander (Eds.), *Critical care nursing* (pp.824-842). Philadelphia: Saunders.

Walleck, C. A. (1993). *Patients with head injury and brain dysfunction* (pp. 677-706). Philadelphia: Saunders.

Wilberger, J. E., Harris, M., & Diamond, D. L. (1991). Acute subdural hematoma: Morbidity, mortality, and operative timing. *Journal of Neurosurgery, 74,* 212-218.

Wright, M. M. (1999). Resuscitation of the multitrauma patient with head injury. *AACN Clinical Issues, 10*(1), 32-43.

Yundt, K. D., & Diringer, M. N. (1997). The use of hyperventilation and its impact on cerebral ischemia in the treatment of traumatic brain injury. In M. N. Diringer (Ed.), *Critical care clinics* (pp.163-184). Philadelphia: Saunders.

Zumkeller, M., Behrmann, R., Heissler, H. E., & Dietz, H. (1996). Computed tomographic criteria and survival rate for patients with acute subdural hematoma. *Neurosurgery, 39*(4), 708-712.

CHAPTER 15

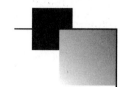

EPIDURAL HEMATOMA

Cinda Alexander, MSN, CCRN, CNRN, CNOR, CRNFA

CASE PRESENTATION

David, age 24 years, was driving home from a party late at night when he lost control of his car and hit a tree. On impact, his head hit the windshield. A witness to the accident stated that David was unconscious for at least 5 minutes but was awake when the paramedics arrived on the scene at 3 AM.

On arrival at the emergency department (ED), David was awake and restless with little memory of the accident. He was slightly combative with the ED staff, and his breath was reported to smell of alcohol. A small laceration was observed on his left temple. Skull x-ray films identified a left-sided temporal fracture. Vital signs were as follows:

BP	128/80 mm Hg	Respirations	22 breaths/min
HR	88 bpm	Temperature	36.6° C (97.8° F)

David was admitted to the neurologic critical care unit for observation. He remained alert and oriented throughout the night, with no changes noted in his neurologic status. However, at 9 AM, the assessment revealed that David was very irritable and did not know the date or time. He became drowsy and was mumbling incoherently. The physician on call was notified, and an immediate computed tomographic (CT) scan was ordered, which revealed a left-sided epidural hematoma (EDH).

Emergency Surgery

David was immediately taken to the operating room, where a craniotomy was performed to remove the clot. He tolerated the procedure well and was returned to the neurologic critical care unit after surgery.

Postoperative Course

After surgery, David was drowsy but arousable to voice. His pupils were equal and reactive. A large head dressing was in place with no signs of drainage noted. An arterial line was placed, and a peripheral intravenous line of 5% dextrose in lactated

Ringer's solution was infusing at 100 ml/hr. David was also receiving oxygen at 3 L/min via nasal cannula. Diagnostic data were as follows:

BP	90/60 mm Hg (arterial line)	pH	7.35
HR	92 bpm	Pao_2	82 mm Hg
Respirations	24 breaths/min	$Paco_2$	35 mm Hg
Temperature	37.7° C (99.7° F)	Sao_2	95%
HCO_3^-	28 mmol/L		

Two days later, David was awake and alert with no neurologic deficits noted. Vital signs remained stable. The arterial line was discontinued, and he was tolerating a regular diet. He was transferred to the neurologic unit and discharged 1 day later.

EPIDURAL HEMATOMA

Questions

1. Describe the pathophysiology of EDH.
2. What is the classic clinical picture of EDH?
3. What diagnostic modalities are used to identify an EDH?
4. Discuss the options for surgical intervention in patients with EDH.
5. Discuss the incidence of and mortality associated with EDH. What prognostic indicators may be assessed to predict outcome?
6. Discuss the nursing responsibilities for monitoring and assessment of the patient with EDH.

EPIDURAL HEMATOMA

Questions and Answers

1. Describe the pathophysiology of EDH.

EDH is a collection of blood between the inner periosteum of the skull and the dura mater. Most EDHs result from arterial bleeding; however, venous bleeding from damage to the meningeal vein or dura sinus is also a potential source. The most common location for an EDH is the temporal fossa. Other sites may include the subfrontal region or occipital-suboccipital area. A temporal fracture may lead to a laceration of the meningeal artery because the temporal region is the thinnest portion of the skull. An epidural hemorrhage occurs as a result of the bleeding meningeal artery. An EDH may lead to cerebral displacement and uncal herniation rather than direct brain injury. The hematoma can push the temporal lobe medially, causing herniation of the uncus and hippocampal gyrus over and through the tentorial notch. The result is a compromised blood supply that suppresses brainstem functions (Hickey, 1997; March, 1999; McNair, 1999; Nikas, 1998).

2. What is the classic clinical picture of EDH?

The classic picture of EDH consists of a brief loss of consciousness as a direct result of the injury, followed by a lucid interval. An estimated 30% to 50% of patients will experience the lucid period (Nikas, 1998). The lucid interval can last anywhere from a few minutes to hours and is followed by a depression in the level of consciousness. Additional symptoms may include ipsilateral pupillary changes progressing to fixed and dilated pupils with simultaneous contralateral motor weakness or paresis. As the mass effect continues, the patient's level of consciousness will rapidly deteriorate (Hickey, 1997; March, 1999; McNair, 1999).

3. What diagnostic modalities are used to identify an EDH?

In the patient with EDH, a CT scan will reveal an area of density that indicates the location and extent of the hematoma. As the clot expansion strips the dura away from the inner table of the skull, it takes on a biconvexity appearance with sharp margins on CT imaging (Crow, 1991). The CT scan allows rapid identification of the hematoma, so treatment can be initiated quickly with a resulting reduction in mortality and morbidity for these patients. After the initial evaluation, there is a need for clinical vigilance and subsequent examinations, even though the initial CT scan may be normal, because the EDH may not have yet developed in the patient. Because most patients with EDH have a skull fracture, typically in the thin squamous portion of the temporal area, an x-ray film of the head and neck is diagnostically beneficial (Hickey, 1997, March, 1999; McNair, 1999).

4. Discuss the options for surgical intervention in patients with EDH.

According to Lee, Hung, Wang, Chung, and Chen (1998), a delay in evacuation of a hematoma increases the morbidity and mortality of patients with EDH after clinical symptoms of herniation develop. Surgical removal of the clot is necessary to minimize any neurologic deficit by preventing herniation or a shift in brain tissue. A craniotomy consists of incising through the scalp and muscle and creating a bone flap to expose the dura mater. At this time, the clot can be removed and the damaged vessel repaired. A small, thin EDH may not require surgical intervention and can be treated with observation (Hickey, 1997; McNair, 1999).

5. Discuss the incidence of and mortality associated with EDH? What prognostic indicators may be assessed to predict outcome?

The overall mortality for EDH is reported to be between 9.4% and 33%. With increased access to CT imaging, mortality of less than 10% can be expected. Traumatic EDH accounts for 0.2% to 6% of all head injuries. Lee et al. (1998) identified the following prognostic indicators for unfavorable functional outcome:

- A longer period of herniation until operative decompression
- Associated brain injury such as diffuse axonal injury
- Greater clot density (>50 ml) and degree of midline shift (>10 mm)

- Total obliteration of the basal cisterns
- Reoperative motor response of abnormal posturing

6. Discuss nursing responsibilities for monitoring and assessment of the patient with EDH.

It is beneficial to obtain a thorough patient history, including the type of injury involved, level of consciousness at time of injury, baseline vital signs, behavior, and motor function, to identify any significant changes in assessment from the baseline. The most reliable indicator of neurologic function is level of consciousness. The Glasgow Coma Scale is the most reliable scale for assessing the level of consciousness by assessing the patient's best eye opening and verbal and motor responses. Scale scores range from 3 to 15. The lower the score, the more severe the head injury. Pupil size and reaction to light should be assessed frequently for changes. Ipsilateral pupil dilation is an indication of herniation from a hematoma, lesion, or edema and is often a late sign.

Blood pressure and heart rate must be assessed frequently to ensure that brain tissues are adequately perfused. Bradycardia, systolic hypertension, and bradypnea are the set of clinical manifestations known as *Cushing's triad;* however, these are late signs of increased ICP. Bradycardia, junctional escape rhythms, and idioventricular rhythms can occur in patients with cerebral hemorrhage and increased ICP. Therefore continuous cardiac monitoring is required. Respiratory patterns must be assessed frequently to identify possible herniation.

Urine output, serum sodium, and osmolarity levels must be monitored to rule out the syndrome of inappropriate secretion of antidiuretic hormone, which may be a secondary effect of head injury (Hickey, 1997; March, 1999; McNair, 1999; Nikas, 1998).

Patients may sustain traumatic brain injury at the time of the initial trauma. Additional treatment may be required for head trauma. The reader is referred to Chapter 14 for information regarding traumatic brain injury.

EPIDURAL HEMATOMA

References

Crow, W. (1991). Aspects of neuroradiology of head injury. *Neurosurgery Clinics of North America, 2*(2), 321-340.

Hickey, J. V. (1997). *Neurological and neurosurgical nursing.* Philadelphia: JB Lippincott.

Lee, E., Hung, Y., Wang, L., Chung, K., & Chen, H. (1998). Factors influencing the functional outcome of patients with acute epidural hematomas: Analysis of 200 patients undergoing surgery. *The Journal of Trauma: Injury, Infection, and Critical Care, 45*(5), 946-952.

March, K. (1999). Acute head injury. In L. Bucher & S. Melander (Eds.), *Critical care nursing* (pp.843-868). Philadelphia: Saunders.

McNair, N. D. (1999). Traumatic brain injury. *Nursing Clinics of North America, 34*(3).

Nikas, D. L. (1998).The neurologic system. In J. G. Alspach (Ed.), *American Association of Critical-Care Nurses: Core curriculum for critical care nursing* (5th ed., pp. 339-463). Philadelphia: Saunders.

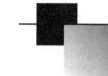

CHAPTER *16*

GASTROINTESTINAL TRACT BLEEDING

Cynthia S. Goodwin, RN, MSN

CASE PRESENTATION

James Jones, age 44 years, was transferred from the emergency department (ED) to the intensive care unit (ICU) with a diagnosis of probable gastrointestinal (GI) tract bleeding. The ED history states that he had been seen as an outpatient 1 week ago because of epigastric pain after heavy alcohol consumption at a New Year's party. He stated he had been "hung over and nauseated" for 48 hours and has had severe epigastric pain since the party. Gastritis was diagnosed, and he was sent home with antiemetic and antacid medications and advised to stop smoking. Although he returned to his job as a commodities trader, he has not felt well since the party. He has been taking two buffered aspirin two to three times daily for epigastric pain in addition to his prescribed medications. He returned to the ED because of nausea, two episodes of vomiting large amounts of "dark brown" liquid, and complaints of extreme weakness. He also experienced dizziness when he stood or sat up abruptly.

Vital signs at admission and laboratory data at 6 PM were as follows:

BP	96/60 mm Hg lying; 84/50 mm Hg standing	Temperature tympanic	37.9° C (100.2° F)
HR	102 bpm	Hgb	12.5 g/dl
Respirations	20 breaths/min	Hct	40%
		WBCs	1200/mm^3

Emergency Department Record

A 14-gauge nasogastric tube (NGT) was placed, and 350 ml of dark-brown guaiac-positive "coffee grounds" liquid returned. His stomach was lavaged with 500 ml of normal saline (NS), and the drainage subsequently became clear.

Mr. Jones' ICU admission orders were as follows:

1. Monitor electrocardiogram, vital signs, and intake and output every hour.
2. Maintain bed rest.

Time	HR (bpm)	Respirations (breaths/min)	BP (mm Hg)	Other Client Data
		TABLE 16-1 Vital Signs and Flow Sheet Data		
7 PM	112	16	104/64	
8 PM	115	18	100/60	Temperature 37.9° C (100.2° F)
9 PM	120	20	98/60	
10 PM	120	20	100/60	Hgb 12.3 g/dl
				Hct 36%
11 PM	120	20	96/54	Sleeping
Midnight	112	20	92/50	Temperature 36.7° C (98° F) (tympanic)
				Voided 120 ml amber urine

3. Suction NGT at low intermittent setting; for active bleeding, notify physician and irrigate with 30 ml of NS q2h. and prn until drainage becomes clear.
4. Give nothing by mouth (NPO) except for sips with oral medications.
5. Give medications orally (PO); clamp NGT for 30 minutes after administration of medication.
6. Give magnesium hydroxide (Mylanta) 30 ml q4h PO.
7. Give cimetidine (Tagamet) 300 mg q6h PO.
8. Give promethazine (Phenergan) 25 mg IV q6h prn for nausea.
9. Start intravenous (IV) infusion of 5% dextrose in lactated Ringer's solution (D5LR) at 100 ml/hr.
10. Schedule for esophagogastroduodenoscopy (EGD) at 7 AM in GI laboratory.
11. Measure hemoglobin (Hgb) and hematocrit (Hct) at 9 PM.
12. Perform complete blood count and platelet count, prothrombin time, partial thromboplastin time, chemistry 12, electrolytes, and urinalysis in the morning.

Mr. Jones had an uneventful evening. His medical record reflected the data shown in Table 16-1.

At midnight, his NGT was clamped to administer medication. When the NGT was unclamped at 12:30 AM, 300 ml of bloody drainage returned. He became restless and anxious. His skin was pale and moist. Oxygen was started by nasal cannula at 4 L/min. Vital signs at 12:30 AM were as follows:

BP	84/50 mm Hg lying
HR	126 bpm
Respirations	28 breaths/min

The physician was called, and the following orders were received:

1. Lavage the NGT with saline until clear.
2. Immediately measure Hgb and Hct and call results.
3. Type and crossmatch for 2 units of packed red blood cells (PRBCs); type and screen for an additional 4 units of PRBCs.
4. Place a triple-lumen subclavian IV line.
5. Measure central venous pressure (CVP) hourly; if it is less than 10 mm Hg, give 500 ml of NS IV fluid challenge and repeat the fluid challenge once if needed.
6. Anchor a Foley catheter and measure urine amount hourly.
7. Notify the gastroenterologist and surgeon.

TABLE *16-2*	Vital Signs and Flow Sheet Data					
Time	HR (bpm)	Respirations (breaths/min)	BP (mm Hg)	CVP (mm Hg)	Urine Output	Other Client Data
2 AM	120	26	84/50	10	30	
3 AM	116	24	90/58	12	75	
4 AM	112	20	94/62	12	90	
5 AM	110	18	96/64	12	94	
6 AM	110	18	98/62	13	80	
7 AM	104	18	98/64	12	68	Hgb 10.1 g/dl Hct 28%

The interventions were carried out. No urine was obtained from the catheter. Assessment and laboratory data at 1 AM were as follows:

CVP   8 mm Hg
Hgb   9.8 g/dl
Hcy   24%

At 1:30 AM after two 500-ml fluid challenges, Mr. Jones' CVP was 12 mm Hg and he had urine output of 30 ml/hr. D5LR was infusing at 50 ml/hr in a peripheral line and NS at 150 ml/hr in a central line. The physician ordered 2 units of PRBCs, which Mr. Jones received at 2 AM. His chart reflected the data shown in Table 16-2.

At 7:10 AM, Mr. Jones was transported to the GI laboratory for the EGD. The gastroenterologist found diffuse gastritis with a 2-cm duodenal ulcer. No clots were visible, and the ulcer was not actively bleeding. A biopsy specimen taken from the gastric wall tested positive for *Helicobacter pylori,* and a culture and sensitivity test were then performed.

Pharmacologic treatment for *H. pylori* was instituted, along with histamine-receptor antagonists and supplemental antacids. Mr. Jones' physicians chose to treat him conservatively with medication, and Mr. Jones progressed well. He was released from the ICU to the step-down unit in 24 hours and discharged home after 3 days.

GASTROINTESTINAL TRACT BLEEDING

Questions

1. What is the incidence of and mortality associated with acute GI tract bleeding?
2. Identify common causes of GI tract bleeding and list predisposing factors specific to Mr. Jones.
3. Discriminate between the characteristics of upper and lower GI tract bleeding.
4. What complication did Mr. Jones experience?
5. Which factors determine whether blood products will be administered to a patient with GI tract bleeding?

6. Mr. Jones' Hgb and Hct values dropped dramatically from admission to 7 AM. Discuss the drop in Hgb and Hct values in relation to Mr. Jones' blood loss.

7. If a patient continues to have active bleeding from the GI tract despite conservative management, what other medical procedures might be implemented?

8. Identify pharmacologic therapy commonly used in the treatment of GI tract bleeding.

9. What are the indications and types of surgical procedures for upper GI tract bleeding?

10. Identify six nursing diagnoses appropriate for Mr. Jones.

11. What is the incidence of *H. pylori* infection in gastritis and duodenal ulcers?

12. What is the treatment of choice for *H. pylori* infection?

GASTROINTESTINAL TRACT BLEEDING

Questions and Answers

1. What is the incidence of and mortality associated with acute GI tract bleeding?

More than 300,000 Americans with acute GI tract bleeding are admitted to hospitals each year, with an overall mortality of 10% (Savides & Jensen, 2000). Half the episodes are caused by peptic ulcers, and esophageal varices are the second leading cause. Mortality from bleeding esophageal varices ranges from 40% to 70% (Thelan, Lough, Urden, & Stacy, 1998). For all causes of GI tract bleeding, mortality is greater in those who are either older than age 60, who are in shock upon admission, who have a rebleeding episode within 72 hours, or whose red nasogastric aspirate fails to clear (Zuckerman, 1999).

2. Identify common causes of GI tract bleeding and list predisposing factors specific to Mr. Jones.

Causes of acute upper GI tract bleeding include gastric and duodenal ulcers, esophageal varices, erosive gastritis or esophagitis, Mallory-Weiss tears, angiomas of the stomach or small bowel, and aortoenteric fistulas. Common causes of acute lower GI tract bleeding include colonic angiomas (angiodysplasia), diverticula, and internal hemorrhoids.

Less common causes of GI tract bleeding include gastrointestinal cancer, inflammatory bowel disease, bowel infarction with perforation, and stress ulcers. Contributing factors may include liver disease, bleeding disorders, a history of abdominal aortic aneurysm repair, and nonsteroidal antiinflammatory drug or anticoagulation therapy. Mr. Jones' predisposing factors included alcohol ingestion, smoking, aspirin intake, and a stressful job.

3. Discriminate between the characteristics of upper and lower GI tract bleeding.

Bleeding above the duodenojejunal junction is defined as upper GI bleeding. Upper GI tract bleeding is characterized by *hematemesis* (vomiting bright or dark red blood) or vomiting old digested blood, a dark material that looks like coffee grounds. Bleeding from the stomach and esophageal sources is common, and in 90% of bleeding duodenal ulcers, blood also refluxes into the stomach (Eastwood, 1998). Bleeding below the ligament of Treitz seldom results in vomiting of blood.

Lower GI bleeding from the colon, rectum, or anus is characterized by *hematochezia* (rectal passage of red blood or mahogany-colored stool) (Eastwood, 1998). *Melena*, the passage of black or tarry stools, can result from either upper orlower GI tract bleeding (Gawlinski & Hamwi, 1999). In massive rapid upper GI tract bleeding, the patient may have both hematemesis and hematochezia.

4. What complication did Mr. Jones experience?

Mr. Jones experienced hypovolemia as a result of acute blood loss. His tachypnea, tachycardia, low CVP, orthostatic hypotension, low urine output, skin color changes, and restlessness indicated a class III hemorrhage, with a 30% to 40% loss of blood volume and moderately severe hemorrhagic shock (Gawlinski & Hamwi, 1999).

5. Which factors determine whether blood products will be administered to a patient with GI tract bleeding?

Blood administration is based on the level of shock, the response to IV fluid replacement, and changes in Hgb and Hct levels. Unstable vital signs after infusion of 2 L of crystalloid fluid replacement indicate the need for blood replacement. An Hgb value less than 10 mg/dl and a Hct less than 25% are also indicators for blood replacement. The amount of bloody drainage and the presence of active bleeding are also considered. PRBCs are commonly used because they decrease exposure to plasma antibodies and the risk of fluid volume overload (Bucher & Melander, 1999).

6. Mr. Jones' Hgb and Hct values dropped dramatically from admission to 7 AM. Discuss the drop in Hgb and Hct values in relation to Mr. Jones' blood loss.

Hgb and Hct values are poor indicators of the severity or rapidity of blood loss (Thelan et al, 1998, p. 940). Initial Hgb and Hct values will not match the degree of blood loss because it takes 48 to 72 hours for intravascular and extravascular equilibration to occur (Zuckerman, 1999). In Mr. Jones' case, the drop in Hgb and Hct values probably reflected some actual blood loss. However, part of the decrease, which occurred despite his receiving 2 units of PRBCs, was caused by hemodilution from fluid replacement therapy.

7. **If a patient continues to have active bleeding from the GI tract despite conservative medical management, what other medical procedures might be implemented?**

Therapies that may be used to treat acute GI bleeding include the following:

- Iced saline NGT lavage is sometimes used. However, evidence suggests that iced saline actually prolongs bleeding and increases clotting time compared with no lavage and that saline lavage resolves clots but does not halt bleeding (Zuckerman, 1999).
- Endoscopic hemostasis can be achieved via coagulation by cautery or injection of sclerosing agents. Electrocoagulation is achieved with heater probes, photocoagulation, or laser therapy, which is more expensive than traditional electrocoagulation. Sclerosing agents such as ethanolamine, sodium tetradecyl sulfate, or other solutions can also be injected into bleeding sites.
- Band ligation can be used during endoscopy to treat esophageal varices. This method is as effective as sclerotherapy in achieving initial hemostasis and reducing rebleeding rates. Small elastic "O" rings are placed around the varices, causing strangulation, sloughing, and fibrosis (Zuckerman, 1999).
- Vasopressin infusion acts to constrict arteries and contract the bowel, thus reducing blood flow and stimulating the formation of thrombus. Vasopressin is associated with a high rate of cardiac complications and is no longer the drug of choice for pharmacologic hemostasis.
- Octreotide, a long-acting analog of somatostatin, causes selective splanchnic vasoconstriction without cardiac complications when given by IV infusion and is currently the drug of choice as an adjunct to endoscopy (Savides & Jensen, 2000).
- Transcatheter embolization using angiography to identify and embolize a bleeding artery may also be used. Substances such as coils, Gelfoam, cyanoacrylate glue, clots, and polyvinyl alcohol may be used. Ischemia or infarction may occur if collateral circulation is inadequate.
- Mechanical tamponade with the use of Ewald, Cantor, Minnesota, Sengstaken-Blakemore, or Linton-Nachlas tubes to apply direct pressure to bleeding sites may be used as a last-resort measure. Although balloon therapy provides initial tamponade 85% to 98% of the time, there is a 30% rate of serious complications and up to a 60% rate of rebleeding after deflation (Savides & Jensen, 2000).

8. **Identify pharmacologic therapy commonly used in the treatment of GI tract bleeding.**

Pharmacologic therapy is used to treat underlying conditions that cause GI tract bleeding and as an adjunct to management of bleeding. IV histamine-receptor antagonists are commonly used, but there is no evidence that they stop or prevent rebleeding. However, oral omeprazole (Prilosec), a proton pump inhibitor, significantly decreased recurrent bleeding for peptic ulcers that were not actively bleeding (Zuckerman, 1999). Stress ulcers are treated with a combination of sucralfate, histamine-receptor antagonists, and antacids. Metoclopramide (Reglan) may be used to decrease nausea, vomiting, and gastric stasis (Savides & Jensen, 2000).

Histamine-receptor antagonists inhibit the action of histamine on the receptor sites of the parietal cells by competing for the sites. They reduce the amount and concentration of gastric secretions. Examples include ranitidine (Zantac), cimetidine (Tagamet), nizatidine, and famotidine (Pepcid). Common side effects include headache, dizziness, diarrhea, and constipation (Bucher & Melander, 1999).

Antacids work by chemical neutralization of hydrochloric acid. By increasing the stomach's pH, antacids decrease the erosion of the stomach and duodenum by gastric acid. Long-term use of antacids may lead to metabolic alkalosis, increased serum sodium levels (sodium bicarbonate antacids), hypercalcemia and renal impairment (calcium carbonate antacids), constipation, phosphate depletion (aluminum-containing antacids), diarrhea, and hypermagnesemia (magnesium-containing antacids). Administration of antacids and histamine blockers should be staggered to allow for maximum absorption of both drugs.

9. What are the indications and types of surgical procedures for upper GI tract bleeding?

Indications for surgery are persistent bleeding after medical treatment, presence of neoplasm or malignancy, perforation of obstruction, and recurrence of ulcers.

Surgical interventions range from oversewing the ulcer site to gastric resection. Billroth I or II procedures involve partial resection of the stomach. Intractable ulcer disease and bleeding may be treated with a total gastrectomy. Vagotomy may be done in conjunction with or separate from these operations. Vagotomy reduces gastric secretions by eliminating vagal stimulation to the stomach.

Several surgical options exist to create portal-systemic shunts. Placement of a transjugular intrahepatic portosystemic shunt device can also be used to reduce portal hypertension seen with esophageal varices.

10. Identify six nursing diagnoses appropriate for Mr. Jones.
- Fluid volume deficit related to vomiting, active bleeding, and decreased circulatory volume
- Altered tissue perfusion related to hypotension, decreased oxygen transport, increased oxygen demand, and metabolic acidosis
- Pain (acute abdominal) related to disruption of the mucosal barrier of GI tract (Alspach, 1998)
- Anxiety related to fear of death, hemorrhage, and unfamiliar procedures
- Altered nutrition: less than body requirements related to prolonged NPO status and NGT suction
- Knowledge deficit related to risk factor control (smoking, alcohol, stress management, and acetylsalicylic acid intake), medications, and treatments

11. What is the incidence of *H. pylori* infection in gastritis and duodenal ulcer?

H. pylori, first identified in 1984, is found in 90% to 100% of duodenal ulcers and 70 to 90% of gastric ulcers (Bucher & Melander, 1999). It is recognized as the major cause of environmental (nonautoimmune) gastritis and peptic ulcer (Fennerty, 1994).

12. What is the treatment of choice for *H. pylori* infection?

H. pylori eradication therapy usually consists of bismuth and two antibiotics. Eight tablets of bismuth with tetracycline 2 g and metronidazole 750 mg daily for 2 weeks have been recommended treatment. Current therapy may substitute omeprazole, amoxicillin, or clarithromycin for the previously mentioned antibiotics. These newer antibiotics have high rates of eradication and are better tolerated. Antibiotics may also be prescribed without bismuth. Recurrence of ulcers after healing is less than 10%, and reinfection rates are 1% to 2% per year after treatment (Fennerty, 1994).

GASTROINTESTINAL BLEEDING

References

Alspach, J. G. (1998). *American Association of Critical-Care Nurses: Core curriculum for critical care nursing* (5th ed.). Philadelphia: Saunders.

Bucher, L., & Melander, S. (1999). *Critical care nursing.* Philadelphia: Saunders.

Eastwood, G. L. (1998). Gastrointestinal bleeding. In Stein, J. H. (Ed.), *Internal medicine.* St Louis: Mosby.

Fennerty, M. B. (1994). *Helicobacter pylori. Archives of Internal Medicine, 154,* 721-727.

Gawlinski, A., & Hamwi, D. (Eds.) (1999). *Acute care nurse practitioner clinical curriculum and certification review.* Philadelphia: Saunders.

Savides, T. K., & Jensen, D. M. (2000). Severe gastrointestinal hemorrhage. In Shoemaker, W. C., Ayres, S. M., Grenvik, A., & Holbrook, P. R. (Eds.), *Textbook of critical care* (4th ed.). Philadelphia: Saunders.

Thelan, L. A., Lough, M. E., Urden, L. D., & Stacy, K. M. (1998). *Critical care nursing: diagnosis and management* (3rd ed.). St Louis: Mosby.

Zuckerman, G. R. (1999). GI bleeding: principles of diagnosis and management. In Irwin, R. S., Cerra, F. B., & Rippe, J. M. (Eds.), *Intensive care medicine* (4th ed.). Philadelphia: Lippincott-Raven.

CHAPTER 17

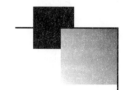

ACUTE PANCREATITIS

Ann H. White, CNA, RN, MBA, PhD

CASE PRESENTATION

Jan, a 43-year-old woman, came to the emergency department (ED) with acute abdominal pain. This pain had been present for approximately 2 days but had increased in severity over the last 6 hours. The pain was localized to the upper-left abdominal quadrant with some radiation to the back. She had vomited three times in the last 6 hours with no relief of pain. Jan's brother, who accompanied her to the ED, reported that Jan drinks heavily and has a history of intravenous (IV) drug use. Her brother reported that she no longer uses IV drugs but has continued to drink at least a fifth of hard liquor a day. Jan admitted to having a past problem with alcohol and drug use but stated she is now "clean." Jan agreed to having blood drawn for analysis, including blood alcohol and drug screening tests.

Vital signs and laboratory results obtained in the ED were as follows:

BP	134/76 mm Hg	Respirations	24 breaths/min
HR	68 bpm	Temperature	38.6° C (101.4° F) (tympanic)

A complete blood count (CBC) revealed the following:

Na^+	141 mmol/L	Amylase	505 U/L
K^+	3.0 mmol/L	AST (SGOT)	307 U/L
WBCs	$11 \times 10^3/mm^3$	Lipase	519 U/L
RBCs	$11 \times 10^6/mm^3$	LDH	891 U/L
Total protein	4.9 g/dl	Glucose	266 ml/dl
Hgb	12.3 g/dl	Blood alcohol	205 mg/dl
Hct	52%	Mg^{++}	1.3 mg/dl
Albumin	2.4 g/dl	Ca^{++}	7.3 mg/dl
Alkaline phosphatase	120 U/L		

Drug screening results are pending.

Arterial blood gas (ABG) measurements were as follows:

pH	7.35	HCO_3^-	25 mmol/L
P_{CO_2}	33 mm Hg	Base excess	1
P_{O_2}	90 mm Hg	Sao_2	91%

After a 2-hour stay in the ED, Jan reported increased pain in the upper-left abdominal quadrant. She vomited 100 ml of brown liquid. Her vital signs were as follows:

BP	90/60 mm Hg	Respirations	28 breaths/min
HR	100 bpm	Temperature	39.4° C (103° F) (tympanic)

On physical examination, her abdomen was tender, with guarding in all abdominal quadrants, and bowel sounds were hypoactive. A nasogastric tube was inserted, and an IV line was started in the ED. Jan was transferred to the intensive care unit (ICU) with a preliminary diagnosis of acute pancreatitis. The following orders accompanied Jan to the ICU:

1. IV infusion of 0.45% normal saline solution (NSS) with 20 mEq of potassium in each bag to run at 125 ml/hr
2. Daily CBC, amylase and lipase levels, and basic metabolic profile 20
3. ABG measurements in the morning
4. Morphine sulfate 3 mg IV push q2h prn for severe pain
5. Nothing by mouth (NPO) (no ice chips)
6. Nasogastric tube to intermittent suction
7. Two sets of blood cultures if not done in the ED
8. Gentamicin (Garamycin) 80 mg IV piggyback q8h after blood for cultures is drawn

Jan's laboratory results after the first 24 hours in the ICU are listed next. CBC results were the following:

Na^+	139 mmol/L	Alkaline	139 U/L
K^+	3.2 mmol/L	phosphatase	
WBCs	$14.6 \times 10^3/mm^3$	Amylase	575 U/L
RBCs	$3.82 \times 10^6/mm^3$	AST (SGOT)	436 U/L
Total protein	4.6 g/dl	Lipase	789 U/L
Hgb	10.3 g/dl	LDH	798 U/L
Hct	42%	Glucose	203 ml/dl
Albumin	2.2 g/dl	Mg^{++}	1.3 mg/dl
		Ca^{++}	7.8 mg/dl

Drug screening results were negative. ABG results were the following:

pH	7.22	HCO_3^-	10 mmol/L
P_{CO_2}	26 mm Hg	Base excess	6
P_{O_2}	84 mm Hg	Sao_2	80%

Additional orders received included the following:

1. Change IV infusion to 0.45% NSS with 30 mEq of potassium and 9 mEq of magnesium in each IV bag to run at 125 ml/hr.
2. Administer oxygen at 2 L via nasal cannula.
3. Repeat basic metabolic profile 20 and ABG measurements in the morning.

Jan's heart monitor revealed a normal sinus rhythm with a prolonged QT interval. Jan's pain subsided after 72 hours, bowel sounds were heard, and she was started on a clear liquid diet. After 24 hours without pain, Jan was transferred to a medical-surgical unit.

ACUTE PANCREATITIS

Questions

1. Discuss the pathophysiology of acute pancreatitis.
2. Describe the classic assessment findings that support a diagnosis of acute pancreatitis. Relate Jan's history and physical assessment findings to this description.
3. Compare and contrast interstitial and necrotizing acute pancreatitis.
4. Jan requested pain medication. What should be the initial nursing actions?
5. Discuss the appropriateness of administering gentamicin (Garamycin) to patients with acute pancreatitis.
6. Discuss significant diagnostic studies that assist in confirming or in monitoring the progress of acute pancreatitis. Relate the diagnostic studies completed on Jan to this discussion.
7. Discuss the dietary management of a patient with acute pancreatitis. What is the purpose of the nasogastric tube and the NPO status?
8. List the nursing diagnoses, outcomes, and interventions appropriate for a patient with acute pancreatitis.
9. Identify complications of acute pancreatitis. Based on the change in vital signs, laboratory data, and history, which complication has most likely occurred in this case study?
10. Discuss the prognosis for a patient with acute pancreatitis.
11. Discuss the psychosocial aspects of caring for a patient with acute pancreatitis.

ACUTE PANCREATITIS

Questions and Answers

1. **Discuss the pathophysiology of acute pancreatitis.**

   Acute pancreatitis is an "acute inflammatory process of the pancreas with variable involvement of other regional tissues or remote organs" (Banks, 1998). Acute pancreatitis is believed to result from the premature activation of pancreatic enzymes that cause autodigestion and major cellular destruction of the pancreas and surrounding gastrointestinal structures.

Most experts believe the initial injury is in the acinar cells. As a result of this cellular injury, pancreatic enzymes are released into the surrounding tissues, causing edema and inflammation. These enzymes damage the surrounding fat cells, which leads to the release of noxious agents that cause injury to additional more peripheral acinar cells. This begins a cycle that continues until medical assistance is sought (Banks, 1998).

Trypsin is believed to be the enzyme that is initially activated and begins the autodigestion process by releasing phospholipase A, elastase, and kallikrein (Thelan, Urden, Lough, & Stacy, 1998). With the release of these enzymes, pancreatic tissue and fat cell necrosis occurs with the release of free fatty acids. Kallikrein initiates the release of bradykinin and kallidin that cause a decrease in peripheral vascular resistance, vasodilation, and increased vascular permeability (Thelan et al, 1998).

Although premature activation of enzymes seems important in this process, recent research on the pathophysiology of acute pancreatitis indicates that other processes may be more important in the development of acute pancreatitis. One theory is that the release of activated polymorphonuclear leukocytes and their secretions may have more to do with the severity of the disease than the release of activated enzymes (Banks, 1998).

Several other theories have been proposed to explain the destruction of the pancreatic tissue, none of which are conclusive. Hennessey (1996) identifies six theories that have been proposed to explain how the autodigestion process begins. The following summarizes these theories:

- Certain substances act as cell toxins, which are believed to alter the metabolic processes of the acinar cells. The acinar cells are responsible for the production and release of pancreatic juice, which contains digestive enzymes. Normally, these enzymes are not activated until they reach the intestines. The hormone cholecystokinin (pancreozymin) stimulates the release of the enzymes through the pancreatic duct system to reach the intestine. Once in the intestine, trypsinogen is converted to trypsin, which activates the other pancreatic enzymes (Giuliano & Scott, 1999).
- Alcohol consumption has been closely associated with pancreatitis. Although the exact mechanism is unclear, alcohol may induce ischemia to the pancreatic tissues due to secondary hypertriglyceridemia (Giuliano & Scott, 1999). Another possible explanation for the high incidence of acute pancreatitis with alcohol ingestion is the relaxation or spasm of the sphincter of Oddi. This allows the release/reflux of duodenal contents or bile, which seem to activate the process (Banks, 1998).
- Ductal hypertension is another theory. This theory focuses on the obstruction in the release of pancreatic juices as a result of distal obstruction of the biliary ductal system. The distal obstruction is commonly caused by gallstones actually blocking the duct or by the resulting edema that forms as a gallstone passes. The resulting ductal hypertension may lead to the rupture of small ducts and the release of the enzymes.
- The bile reflux theory is that gallstone(s) may obstruct the flow of bile. As a result, the bile takes the path of least resistance, which is to

BOX 17-1	Drugs Associated with Acute Pancreatitis
DEFINITE Azathioprine Sulfonamides Ethacrynic acid Thiazide diuretics Tetracycline Valproic acid Furosemide Estrogens **PROBABLE** Chlorthalidone Procainamide	Methyldopa Iatrogenic hypercalcemia L-Asparaginase **EQUIVOCAL** Acetaminophen Isoniazid Rifampin Corticosteroids Propoxyphene

> back up into the pancreatic duct, leading to the activation of the enzymes. This is also referred to as the *common channel theory.* This theory is being challenged as an increasing number of patients who have pancreatitis but do not have this common channel are found.

- The duodenal reflux theory proposes that the duodenal contents back up into the pancreas. Because of activation on the pancreatic enzymes when they reach the intestines, autodigestion and cell damage begin.
- The final theory is the activation of intracellular protease. As a result, there is release of lysosomes that cross the acinar cell wall, activate the enzymes, and lead to release of these activated enzymes into the pancreatic and surrounding tissues.

Other factors that can lead to acute pancreatitis include the use of certain drugs such as thiazides, acetaminophen, tetracyclines, and estrogen-containing contraceptives (Box 17-1).

Surgical procedures including exploration of the common bile duct, pancreatic biopsy, and endoscopic retrograde cholangiopancreatography, may predispose the patient to the development of acute pancreatitis (Banks, 1998). Recent research has indicated that infectious agents and toxins may also cause acute pancreatitis (Hudak, Gallo, & Morton, 1998). Whatever the cause, the result is autodigestion and cellular damage in the pancreas and surrounding tissues. Once the cycle is begun, it is perpetuated by the cellular damage that causes cell destruction and death. This results in further release of pancreatic enzymes and destruction of more pancreatic cells as a result of autodigestion. The cycle continues until medical intervention interrupts it.

2. **Describe the classic assessment findings that support a diagnosis of acute pancreatitis. Relate Jan's history and physical assessment findings to this description.**

History taking should include gathering detailed information regarding gallbladder disease, recent abdominal surgical procedures, alcohol use, and prescription and over-the-counter medication use. Specific medications to inquire about include thiazides, acetaminophen, tetracyclines, and oral contraceptives containing estrogen. The patient should be asked about recent consumption of alcohol or a large meal with high levels of fat. A family history of pancreatic or gallbladder disease is of interest when completing the history (Elrod, 1996).

Classic assessment findings include abdominal pain that is almost always severe, persistent, and penetrating (Giuliano & Scott, 1999). Abdominal pain that differs in intensity usually is not associated with acute pancreatitis (Hennessey, 1996). The pain typically is located in the upper-left abdominal quadrant or may be in the midepigastric area and may radiate to the back or flank areas. The onset of pain may be directly associated with consumption of alcohol or a large meal with fatty foods. Patients experiencing pain associated with acute pancreatitis may prefer to sit up or lie in a fetal position to decrease the pain.

Physical assessment of the abdomen may include decreased or absent bowel sounds. The abdomen may be somewhat distended, guarded, and tender to palpation. This tenderness is noted more in the upper quadrants but may be present in all four abdominal quadrants. Ecchymotic areas may be noted in the flank and umbilical areas. Cullen's sign is an irregular hemorrhagic area around the umbilicus. Grey Turner's sign is a bluish discoloration of the abdominal flank or lower back area (Westfall, 1999a; Wright, 1997).

In addition, nausea and vomiting occur. Vomiting without a decrease in pain is considered a hallmark symptom of acute pancreatitis (Hennessey, 1996). Vomiting, along with the extensive third spacing, may lead to dehydration. As a result, the patient may have poor skin turgor and dry mucous membranes. With extensive loss of fluid, symptoms of hypovolemic shock may be seen (Banks, 1998).

Because the respiratory system may be seriously compromised by the development of acute pancreatitis, respirations and lung sounds must be monitored carefully. Assessment findings may include dyspnea, tachypnea, hypoxemia, diminished or absent breath sounds especially in the left base, and referred pain to the shoulder. Careful assessment of the respiratory status is required to prevent acute respiratory distress syndrome (ARDS), the most serious respiratory problem associated with acute pancreatitis.

An elevated temperature may also be indicative of acute pancreatitis. The elevated temperature, if present, is typically less than 39° C (102.2° F) (Hudak et al, 1998). Persistent temperature elevation may indicate complications, including infection or abscess formation.

Jan had several assessment findings that supported the diagnosis of acute pancreatitis. Her history of alcohol abuse is definitely a factor. Although alcohol abuse and acute pancreatitis are more commonly associated with men in their 50s, this does not preclude other patients from exhibiting this clinical picture. Jan also had the abdominal pain radiation associated with acute pancreatitis. She vomited without relief of pain, which further supports the diagnosis of acute pancreatitis. Jan's temperature was elevated. Diagnostic criteria for acute pancreatitis are listed in Table 17-1.

3. **Compare and contrast interstitial and necrotizing acute pancreatitis.**

With acute interstitial or acute edematous pancreatitis, there is edema in the surrounding tissues with minimal necrotizing of the fat tissue. Activated enzymes are released, causing cellular damage. Typical symptoms have been described in the previous answer. Necrotizing acute pancreatitis is considered the more serious form

TABLE *17-1* Diagnostic Criteria for Acute Pancreatitis	
Criteria	Pancreatitis
LABORATORY VALUE	**ELEVATED**
Serum analyses	Elevated
Serum isoamylase	Elevated
Urine analyses	Elevated
Serum lipase	Elevated
Serum triglycerides	Elevated or decreased
Hematocrit	Decreased
Sodium	Decreased or increased
Potassium	Decreased
Calcium	Decreased
Magnesium	Elevated
Glucose	Decreased
Albumin	May be elevated
WBC count	May be elevated
Bilirubin	May be elevated
BUN	May be elevated
Liver enzymes	May be elevated
Arterial blood gases	Hypoxemia and metabolic acidosis
RADIOGRAPHIC RESULTS	
Abdominal computed tomography	Evidence of damage to pancreas, infection, or pseudocyst
Ultrasonography	Evidence of damage to pancreas, infection, or pseudocyst
Magnetic resonance imaging	Evidence of damage to pancreas, infection, or pseudocyst
Abdominal and chest films	Evidence of pancreatic and lung involvement

and is characterized by necrosis of the pancreatic tissue with bleeding into the surrounding tissue. The patient may have all the symptoms of interstitial pancreatitis as well as Grey Turner's sign and Cullen's sign as described earlier. The bleeding into the tissue is thought to be the result of damage caused by circulating trypsin to the intravascular structures (Wright, 1997). Both signs are grave indications of the progression of the disease. The mortality rate with necrotizing acute pancreatitis may be as high as 50% (Smith, 1998).

4. Jan requested pain medication. What should be the initial nursing actions?

A call to the physician is the appropriate action to ensure that the most effective pain medication is given. Opiate analgesics (morphine) are widely used for the relief of acute pain. However, in this case, morphine may not be the drug of choice to manage pancreatic pain. Because morphine may cause biliary colic and spasms of the sphincter of Oddi, meperidine (Demerol) usually is ordered for a patient with acute pancreatitis. With more severe pain, hydromorphone (Dilaudid) may be administered parenterally (Banks, 1998). Experts in the care of patients with acute pancreatitis have reported in recent studies with morphine that patients achieve significant pain relief with minimal effect on the sphincter of Oddi (Hennessey, 1996).

Pain management is an important component of treating patients with the diagnosis of acute pancreatitis. Not only does the patient experience a great deal of discomfort, but severe pain also increases the metabolic activity in the body. This increase in metabolic activity further increases the release of pancreatic enzymes, which is detrimental because of the pathology occurring in the pancreas. The use of a patient-controlled analgesia pump or the scheduled use of analgesics every 2 to 3 hours has been suggested to maintain pain control (Hennessey, 1996).

5. **Discuss the appropriateness of administering gentamicin (Garamycin) to patients with acute pancreatitis.**

The use of antimicrobials in the treatment of mild to moderate forms of acute pancreatitis has not been supported by research findings or clinical trials. Antimicrobials are sometimes ordered if an infection is suspected or in severe cases of necrotizing acute pancreatitis (Hennessey, 1996). Typically, antimicrobials are ordered only once an infection has been confirmed through culture and sensitivity tests, when a computed tomographic (CT) scan has confirmed necrotizing pancreatitis, or when additional clinical symptoms (e.g., an elevation in temperature) are present. The initial antimicrobials of choice are imipenem (Primaxin), ciprofloxacin (Cipro), or cefotaxime (Claforan) (Giuliano & Scott, 1999).

6. **Discuss significant diagnostic studies that assist in confirming or in monitoring the progress of acute pancreatitis. Relate the diagnostic studies completed on Jan to this discussion.**

Specific laboratory studies to assist in confirming the diagnosis of acute pancreatitis include serum and urine amylase levels, isoamylase levels, serum lipase levels, CBC, basic metabolic profile 20 (electrolytes, blood glucose, liver enzymes, blood urea nitrogen [BUN]), ABGs, and culture and sensitivity tests of blood and any drainage.

Serum and urine levels of amylase are usually elevated. The serum amylase level is elevated within the first 24 to 48 hours after the onset of symptoms. However, many other disease processes can also cause an elevation, and this elevation may not reflect the extent of the disease process. Drugs can also elevate serum amylase levels. Common drugs that have been associated with elevations include meperidine, morphine, and codeine (Westfall, 1999b).

Isoamylase levels are more specific, but many laboratories are unable to perform these types of tests because they do not have the equipment required. Banks (1998) reported that an elevation in the isoamylase P_4 level is indicative of acute pancreatitis. Hennessey (1996) reported that a serum amylase level three times the normal level (60 to 160 Somogyi U/dl) in a patient with symptoms associated with acute pancreatitis confirms the diagnosis. Hennessey further reported that other enzyme levels, including trypsin, elastase, and phospholipase A, have not been found to be any more reliable than amylase and lipase. Serum lipase levels are also elevated during the first 24 to 48 hours of the onset of symptoms and remain elevated for 5 to 7 days. Lipase is found predominantly in the pancreas; however, other disease processes can cause this elevation.

Nonspecific abnormal laboratory findings include an elevated white blood cell count caused by the infection. The hematocrit may be elevated initially because of third-space fluid losses but later may decrease because of hemorrhaging. Sodium, potassium, calcium, and magnesium levels may be decreased because of vomiting, fluid shifts, and the saponification of fats. Calcium levels may also be decreased as a result of low levels of albumin. The calcium level may appear to be low because of the close association with albumin. Once the albumin level is corrected, the calcium level may return to normal (Giuliano & Scott, 1999). However, in severe cases of acute pancreatitis, the calcium level may be decreased and must be monitored carefully. The blood glucose level may be elevated if the islets of Langerhans are affected by the disease process and are unable to produce insulin. The BUN level may be elevated because of dehydration. Liver enzyme levels will also be elevated, and prothrombin time may be prolonged with concurrent biliary tract disease and liver involvement.

ABG determinations are imperative because of the respiratory compromise associated with acute pancreatitis. Blood for serial ABG measurements should be drawn to monitor development of metabolic acidosis and hypoxemia. Culture and sensitivity tests of the blood and any other drainage should be performed to gather information about the infectious process. The sensitivity will identify any antimicrobial therapy that must be started.

Radiologic testing that may be useful in the diagnosis of acute pancreatitis includes flat plates of the abdomen, ultrasound, CT scanning, or magnetic resonance imaging (MRI) with specific detail to the pancreas. Ultrasound, CT scanning, and MRI are commonly used today. Specific detail of the pancreas and surrounding structures involved may be well defined with the use of these radiologic tests. If the patient is obese, CT scanning and MRI are typically the tests of choice.

The final diagnostic tool to consider is an electrocardiogram or telemetry. If the patient with acute pancreatitis has a low calcium level, the cardiac rhythms must be monitored carefully. A low calcium level may lead to a prolonged QT interval, with the potential for R on T phenomenon and torsades de pointes or ventricular tachycardia. Correction of the calcium level should prevent the occurrence of arrhythmias (Giuliano & Scott, 1999).

7. **Discuss the dietary management of a patient with acute pancreatitis. What is the purpose of the NGT and the NPO status?**

The initial strategy of diet management is to minimize pancreatic secretions. It was believed that placing an NGT connected to suction should indirectly decrease the release of pancreatic secretions by preventing the release of secretin (Hennessey, 1996). Secretin must have an acid environment to be released. With the nasogastric suction removing gastric secretions, it was thought that the acid environment would not be created. However, recent clinical studies have not demonstrated this to be true. Today, nasogastric suction should be used only for patients with vomiting, gastric distension, ileus, or an altered mental status.

The patient will be assigned NPO (including no ice chips) status for a period of time until the pain subsides, bowel sounds are clearly present, and the serum amylase levels are normal. Diet intake should begin gradually; starting with clear liquids and progressing to more solid food based on patient tolerance. As the diet is advanced, fat, cholesterol, and triglycerides should be kept to a minimum. If an increase in pain develops, the patient should return to NPO status. An increase in pain indicates that enzymes have been released into the tissue and the resulting autodigestion has begun again. Returning to NPO status is an attempt to rest the pancreas and decrease or minimize pancreatic secretions.

Nutritional support is imperative during this time. The patient with acute pancreatitis requires aggressive therapy to meet metabolic and healing needs without stimulation of the pancreas. Total parenteral nutrition (TPN) should be considered for patients with moderate to severe pancreatitis. Composition of the TPN depends on the patient's clinical picture and laboratory values. Typically, an amino acid and glucose base is used with essential minerals and vitamins. Electrolyte replacement depends on the laboratory values. The inclusion of insulin in the TPN solution depends on the production of insulin by the pancreas and the blood glucose levels. Lipid preparations are not used for the patient with pancreatitis because their use will lead to an increase in the release of pancreatic enzymes (Banks, 1998).

8. List the nursing diagnoses, outcomes, and interventions appropriate for a patient with acute pancreatitis.

Elrod (1996) developed a nursing care plan for the patient with acute pancreatitis. Although specific nursing diagnoses must be identified based on the patient's clinical picture, this plan provides the basis for care. One additional nursing diagnosis has been added to complete the nursing care plan for a patient with acute pancreatitis. See Table 17-2 for nursing diagnoses, outcomes, and interventions.

9. Identify complications of acute pancreatitis. Based on the change in vital signs, laboratory data, and history, which complication has most likely occurred in this case study?

A common complication associated with acute pancreatitis is hypovolemic shock. If this complication occurs, it carries with it the potential to cause renal failure, pulmonary insult, electrolyte imbalances, pancreatic pseudocyst, and pancreatic abscess (Banks, 1998). All of these complications should be treated immediately.

Hypovolemic shock commonly occurs as a result of third spacing. Fluid shifts from the vascular system to the intraperitoneal and retroperitoneal spaces as a result of the injury to the abdominal structures from the activated enzymes. Banks (1998) also reported the release of kinins as a result of the inflammation. With the release of these kinins, there is vasodilation and increased capillary permeability. As a result, large amounts of plasma and protein leave the vascular system, adding to the potential for hypovolemic shock. Hypovolemia can be extensive, with as much as 4 to 6 L of fluid shifting into the abdomen with severe pancreatitis. Further loss of fluid in the vascular system results from decreased dietary intake of protein, thus affecting the oncotic pressure. Patients usually do not take anything by mouth and may experience vomiting, which also add to the loss of fluid in the vascular system. Without aggressive replacement therapy, renal failure may result because of hypoperfusion of the kidneys.

The inflammatory response in the pancreatic and surrounding tissues also leads to the release of agents such as myocardial depressant factor, histamine, and prostaglandin, which depress the myocardial tissue, cause vasodilation, and increase capillary permeability. With the release of these agents and the subsequent response, the body is unable to compensate for the decreased fluid volume, thus increasing the potential for hypovolemic shock (Giuliano & Scott, 1999).

Pulmonary complications are common with acute pancreatitis, including the development of atelectasis, acute lung injury, and pleural effusion. The most serious

TABLE 17-2	Nursing Diagnoses, Outcomes, and Interventions for Acute Pancreatitis	
Nursing Diagnoses	Outcome Criteria	Nursing Interventions
Fluid volume deficit causing hemodynamic instability related to fluid, plasma, albumin, and blood losses into peritoneum and retroperitoneal space, nausea and vomiting	Hemodynamic stability (blood pressure, pulse, central venous pressure; pulmonary arterial pressure, adequate peripheral circulation, urine output within normal limits	1. Monitor and record intake and output every hour. 2. Monitor and record central venous pressure and pulmonary arterial pressure. 3. Weigh patient daily. 4. Monitor vital signs every 1-2 hr. Assess peripheral circulation and level of consciousness. 5. Monitor laboratory values for abnormal hemoglobin and hematocrit, electrolyte imbalance (calcium, magnesium, potassium), and blood urea nitrogen and creatinine. 6. Monitor for signs of bleeding (hemorrhagic pancreatitis: Cullen's sign, Grey Turner's sign, increased abdominal girth). 7. Monitor for signs of hypocalcemia: Chvostek's sign, Trousseau's sign. 8. Monitor for signs of cardiac failure such as dyspnea, chest pain, edema. 9. Provide IV fluids; monitor for signs of fluid overload, such as shortness of breath, edema, abnormal breath sounds (crackles).
Altered comfort; pain related to obstruction of pancreatic duct and diminished blood supply and activation of pancreatic enzymes	Pain at tolerable level Vital signs stable	1. Assess patient's pain using a pain-rating scale; use pain rating to evaluate response to pain management interventions. 2. Provide analgesics as ordered and before activity or diagnostic procedures; remember to draw blood to determine amylase levels before giving first dose of analgesic to avoid false elevation in amylase. 3. Assist patient to assume a comfortable position to decrease pain. 4. Maintain bed rest and limit activities to reduce metabolic stress.

TABLE *17-2*	Nursing Diagnoses, Outcomes, and Interventions for Acute Pancreatitis—cont'd	
Nursing Diagnoses	**Outcome Criteria**	**Nursing Interventions**
		5. Administer humidified oxygen to avoid hypoxemia and help to decrease respiratory efforts.
		6. Eliminate oral intake and maintain nasogastric suction, if ordered, to decrease nausea and vomiting, thereby improving patient comfort.
		7. Provide alternative methods of pain control (i.e., back massage, guided imagery, and relaxation techniques).
High risk for ineffective breathing patterns related to abdominal distension and pain	Maintains an effective breathing pattern	1. Assess respiratory status every 2 hr.
		2. Maintain aggressive pulmonary hygiene.
		3. Monitor fluid volume.
		4. Place patient in semi-Fowler's position.
		5. Maintain effective pain management.
Impaired gas exchange related to inflammatory process and aggressive fluid therapy, respiratory distress syndrome, atelectasis, microemboli, pain, pleural effusion	Effective breathing patterns with adequate ventilation and oxygenation (Pao_2 and $Paco_2$ within normal limits) Absence of atelectasis Absence of reduction of pleural effusion, pulmonary edema, microemboli	1. Administer analgesics to relieve pain and allow adequate ventilation.
		2. Provide chest physiotherapy and reposition every 1-2 hr to prevent atelectasis.
		3. Provide oxygen therapy as ordered to prevent hypoxemia.
		4. Monitor chest x-ray films for presence of atelectasis, effusion, or edema.
		5. Perform respiratory assessments every 1-2 hr and note presence of tachypnea, dyspnea, or wheezing; identify presence of adventitious breath sounds and absence of normal breath sounds.
		6. Monitor arterial blood gas results for hypoxemia, hypercapnia, or acidosis.
High risk for tissue injury related to pancreatic inflammation, peritonitis, formation of pseudocyst, formation of abscesses, bleeding, formation of fistulas	Absence of resolution of peritonitis Absence of fever, pseudocyst, abscesses	1. Administer antibiotics as ordered if causative organism(s) has been identified.
		2. Monitor vital signs, especially increases in temperature, and monitor for increase in white blood cell count.

Continued

	Nursing Diagnoses, Outcomes, and Interventions	
TABLE *17-2*	for Acute Pancreatitis—cont'd	
Nursing Diagnoses	**Outcome Criteria**	**Nursing Interventions**
		3. Observe for signs of pseudocyst: upper abdominal pain, mass, tenderness, fever, deterioration, or no improvement in condition.
		4. Observe for signs of abscess: abdominal pain, distension, tenderness, fever, leukocytosis, tachycardia, and hypotension.
		5. Assess for paralytic ileus and fluid accumulation; auscultate bowel sounds every shift.
		6. Observe for respiratory distress resulting from ascites or abdominal mass; check breath sounds, presence of cough, sputum production, shallow breathing, elevated diaphragm, and fluid accumulation.
		7. Provide skin care for draining fistulas; use skin barrier to protect skin from pancreatic enzymes; monitor fistula output.

Alteration in nutrition and metabolic status related to pancreatic dysfunction with altered production of digestive enzymes, insulin, and glucagon; decrease or absence of oral intake; alcoholism; abnormal metabolism	Normal nutritional status
	Weight gain or maintenance
	Positive nitrogen balance
		1. Eliminate oral intake during acute phase of illness.
		2. Assess nutritional status and general appearance for the following:
		  a. Poor skin turgor
		  b. Lethargy
		  c. Anorexia
		  d. Dry, flaky, discolored skin
		  e. Sunken eyeballs
		  f. Decreased muscle mass and decreased muscular control
		  g. Tremors, twitching
		3. Monitor the following:
		  a. Serum amylase
		  b. Urine amylase
		  c. Lipase
		  d. Glucose
		4. Provide nutritional support as ordered.
		5. Monitor laboratory results to prevent complications of nutritional support.
		6. Provide oral care every 4-8 hr.
		7. Monitor nasogastric output.

TABLE *17-2*	Nursing Diagnoses, Outcomes, and Interventions for Acute Pancreatitis—cont'd	
Nursing Diagnoses	**Outcome Criteria**	**Nursing Interventions**
		8. Maintain ongoing assessment of nutritional status and therapy, including the following: a. Daily weights b. Intake and output c. Nutritional laboratory data (albumin, transferrin, total lymphocyte count) d. Nitrogen balance e. Altered mental status f. Skin turgor g. Muscle atrophy or weakness 9. Monitor fistula drainage and record output every shift.
Anxiety (patient or family) related to insufficient knowledge of disease process, treatment, and diagnostic procedures	Reduction in patient's or family's anxiety with information about disease process, treatment, and diagnostic procedures Patient and family participate in care planning process	1. Assess patient's or family's reason for and level of anxiety. 2. Provide information to patient and family about disease process, treatment(s), and diagnostic procedures. 3. Include patient and family in care planning process. 4. Evaluate reduction in patient's or family's anxiety.
Knowledge deficit related to change in lifestyle, care, and diet needs	Increased patient knowledge of disease and thus better compliance with treatment regimen	1. Develop client teaching plan. 2. Include significant others in plan. 3. Allow verbalization of concerns regarding care and change in lifestyle. 4. Return demonstration of information understood. 5. Encourage group support such as Alcoholics Anonymous.

pulmonary complication is ARDS. Factors that have an impact on the development of respiratory complications include splinting, minimal movement, and decreased coughing during episodes of severe pain. In addition, abdominal distension related to fluid shifting that leads to decreased diaphragmatic effort can also depress respirations (Giuliano & Scott, 1999). Seepage of pancreatic fluid can also result in the development of pleural effusion, typically on the left side (Thelan et al, 1998). Assessment findings indicating pulmonary complications include adventitious breath sounds, tachypnea, diminished breath sounds, and dyspnea.

Electrolyte imbalances include losses of sodium, potassium, calcium, and magnesium. Sodium and potassium loss is the result of third spacing and gastrointestinal losses with the NGT or vomiting. Hypocalcemia is a common electrolyte imbalance seen with acute pancreatitis. Calcium deficits may result from hypoalbuminemia. Careful review of the calcium and albumin laboratory values are necessary. Careful monitoring for neuromuscular irritability and prolonged QT intervals is required with hypocalcemia. Another concern is the development of hyperglycemia, which occurs when the pancreatic cells are no longer able to produce insulin.

A pancreatic pseudocyst is the development of necrotic pancreatic tissue, fluid, debris, enzymes, and blood encapsulated in a fibrous tissue (Banks, 1998). A pseudocyst usually resolves by itself but must be monitored through the use of a CT scan or MRI. The cyst may begin to obstruct abdominal structures, or it may rupture, leading to hemorrhagic shock. Assessment findings indicating the development of a pseudocyst include abdominal pain, nausea and vomiting, weight loss, and anorexia after the acute episode of pancreatitis has subsided.

Pancreatic abscesses may form in patients with acute pancreatitis (Banks, 1998). They usually develop 4 weeks after an episode and are the result of necrosis of tissue and translocation of gastrointestinal bacteria such as *Escherichia coli, Pseudomonas, Staphylococcus,* and *Klebsiella.* Assessment findings that indicate the formation of an abscess include an elevated temperature, abdominal pain, vomiting, and possibly a palpable mass in the abdomen. A pancreatic abscess typically requires a surgical procedure for incision and drainage. Antibiotic therapy may also be ordered.

Hematologic complications may result from altered levels of fibrinogen and factor VIII. These alterations are thought to be a result of the activation of certain enzymes in the pancreas. Based on Jan's clinical picture, her most likely complication is hypovolemic shock. However, with the elevation in temperature a possible source of infection must be considered.

10. Discuss the prognosis for a patient with acute pancreatitis.

One method to predict the outcome of an episode of acute pancreatitis is to use the guidelines established by Ranson in 1974 (Banks, 1998). Eleven criteria were identified by Ranson to help predict the prognosis for patients with pancreatitis. Five of the criteria are evaluated in the ED. The remaining six are evaluated during the first 48 hours after treatment is begun. See Box 17-2 for Ranson Criteria (Banks, 1998; Giuliano & Scott, 1999).

Box *17-2* Ranson Criteria

USE IN THE EMERGENCY DEPARTMENT
1. Age >55 yr
2. White blood cell count >16 × 10^3/mm^3
3. Blood glucose >200 mg/dl
4. Lactate dehydrogenase >350 U/L
5. AST (SGOT) >250 U/L

DURING THE FIRST 48 HOURS
1. Hematocrit decreases >10%
2. Blood urea nitrogen >5 mg/dl above baseline
3. Calcium levels <8 mg/dl
4. Arterial Po_2 <60 mm Hg
5. Base deficit increases >4 mmol/L
6. Estimated fluid sequestration >6000 ml

Patients with three or more of the criteria listed in Box 17-2 require supportive care. Patients with seven or more of the criteria are considered a medical challenge with an estimated 100% mortality (Giuliano & Scott, 1999). According to Hennessey (1996), the Ranson criteria are 96% accurate in predicting severity of the disease and mortality.

Another method to establish severity of the disease and the prognosis is use of the APACHE II (Acute Physiology and Chronic Health Evaluation) system (Fig. 17-1). A patient with eight or more points from Fig. 17-1 requires supportive care. The APACHE II system has the added advantage of being able to monitor the patient after the first 48 hours (Hennessey, 1996).

Based on the Ransom guidelines, Jan has 6 of the 11 criteria, including a blood glucose level of more than 200 mg/dl, lactate dehydrogenase (LDH) level more than 350 U/L, and AST level more than 250 U/L in the ED. After 24 hours, her calcium levels dropped below 8 mg/dl, hematocrit dropped more than 10 percentage points, and base deficit rose more than 4 mmol/L.

Based on the APACHE II system, Jan received a score of 9 points that included an elevated temperature, low potassium, high hematocrit, and chronic health problems. Both ratings indicate that Jan requires treatment in the ICU and must be monitored closely.

11. Discuss the psychosocial aspects of caring for a patient with acute pancreatitis.

Once a patient has experienced the pain of acute pancreatitis, that patient never wants to experience it again. If the acute pancreatitis is caused by consumption of alcohol, the patient must stop drinking alcohol to decrease the episodes of acute pancreatitis. Counseling of the patient and significant others must be encouraged and supported by the nursing staff.

With other causes of acute pancreatitis, such as biliary obstruction resulting from gallstones, patients usually have surgery to decrease the possibility of further episodes of acute pancreatitis. However, they must realize the need to be cautious regarding consumption of high-fat diets and alcohol.

PHYSIOLOGIC VARIABLE	+4	+3	+2	+1
1. TEMPERATURE—rectal (°C)	≥41°	39°–40.9°		38.5°–38.9°
2. MEAN ARTERIAL PRESSURE (mm Hg)	≥160	130–159	110–129	
3. HEART RATE (ventricular response)	≥180	140–179	110–139	
4. RESPIRATORY RATE (nonventilated or ventilated)	≥50	35–49		25–34
5. OXYGENATION: A-aDO$_2$ or PaO$_2$ (mm Hg) a. FIO$_2$ ≥ 0.5: record A-aDO$_2$	≥500	350–499	200–349	
b. FIO$_2$ < 0.5: record only PaO$_2$	--------	--------	--------	--------
6. ARTERIAL Ph	≥7.7	7.6–7.69		7.5–7.59
7. SERUM SODIUM (mmol/L)	≥180	160–179	155–159	150–154
8. SERUM POTASSIUM (mmol/L)	≥7	6–6.9		5.5–5.9
9. SERUM CREATININE (mg/100 mL) (Double point score for acute renal failure)	≥3.5	2–3.4	1.5–1.9	
10. HEMATOCRIT (%)	≥60		50–59.9	46–49.9
11. WHITE BLOOD COUNT (total/mm^3) (in 1000 sec)	≥40		20–39.9	15–19.9
12. GLASGOW COMA SCORE (GCS): Score = 15 minus actual GCS				
A Total ACUTE PHYSIOLOGY SCORE (APS) Sum of the 12 individual variable points				
Serum HCO$_2$ (venous: mmol/L) (Not preferred, use if no ABGs)	≥52	41–51.9		32–40.9

B AGE POINTS

Assign points to age as follows:

AGE (years)	POINTS
≤44	0
45–54	2
55–64	3
65–74	5
≥75	6

C CHRONIC HEALTH POINTS

If the patient has a history of severe organ system insufficiency or is immunocompromised, assign points as follows:

a. For nonoperative or emergency postoperative patients: 5 points

or

b. For elective postoperative patients: 2 points

DEFINITIONS: Organ insufficiency or immunocompromised state must have been evident prior to this hospital admission and conforms to the following criteria:

LIVER: Biopsy-proven cirrhosis and documented portal hypertension, episodes of past upper GI bleeding attributed to portal hypertension; or prior episodes of hepatic failure/encephalopathy/coma.

CARDIOVASCULAR: NY Heart Association Class IV.

RESPIRATORY: Chronic restrictive, obstructive, or vascular disease resulting in severe exercise restriction (e.g., unable to climb stairs or perform household duties); or documented chronic hypoxia, hypercapnia, secondary polycythemia, severe pulmonary hypertension (>40 mm Hg), or respirator dependency.

RENAL: Recurring chronic dialysis.

FIGURE 17-1 APACHE II Severity of Disease Classification System. (Reprinted from Sleisenger, B., & Fordtran, M. (1998). *Gastrointestinal and liver disease: Pathophysiology/diagnosis/management* [6th ed.]. Philadelphia: Saunders.)

LOW ABNORMAL RANGE

0	+1	+2	+3	+4
36°–38.4°	34°–35.9°	32°–33.9°	30°–31.9°	≤29.9°
70–109		50–69		≤49
70–109		55–69	40–54	≤39
12–24	10–11	6–9		≤5
<200 --------- PO_2 >70	--------- PO_2 61–70	---------	--------- PO_2 55–60	--------- PO_2 <55
7.33–7.49		7.25–7.32	7.15–7.24	<7.15
130–149		120–129	111–119	<110
3.5–5.4	3–3.4	2.5–2.9		<2.5
0.6–1.4		<0.6		
30–45.9		20–29.9		<20
3–14.9		1–2.9		<1
22–31.9		18–21.9	15–17.9	<15

IMMUNOCOMPROMISED: The patient has received therapy that suppresses resistance to infection (e.g., immunosuppression, chemotherapy, radiation, long-term or recent high-dose steroids) or has a disease that is sufficiently advanced to suppress resistance to infection (e.g., leukemia, lymphoma, AIDS).

APACHE-II SCORE
Sum of **A + B + C**

A APS points   —

B Age points   —

C Chronic Health points _____

Total APACHE-II SCORE _____

FIGURE 17-1, cont'd   For legend see opposite page.

Score	Date		
(Enter one score for each of the following categories listed below)	month day year **Time**		
		24-hr clock	

Verbal	Oriented	5	
	Confused	4	
	Inappropriate words	3	
	Incomprehensible sounds	2	
	None	1	
Motor	Obeys commands	6	
	Localizes pain	5	
	Flexion to pain	4	
	Decorticate movement	3	
	Extension to pain	2	
	None	1	
Eye	Spontaneous	4	
	To speech	3	
	To pain	2	
	None	1	
GCS total score			

Completed by _____   Date   month   day   year

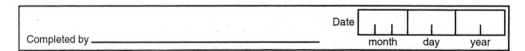

FIGURE 17-1, cont'd   APACHE II Severity of Disease Classification System.
(Reprinted from Sleisenger, B., & Fordtran, M. (1998). *Gastrointestinal and liver disease: Pathophysiology/diagnosis/management* [6th ed.]. Philadelphia: Saunders.)

Acute Pancreatitis

References

Banks, P. (1998). Acute and chronic pancreatitis. In M. Feldman, M. Sleisenger, & B. Scharschmidt (Eds.), *Gastrointestinal and liver disease* (pp. 809-838). Philadelphia: WB Saunders.

Elrod, R. (1996). Problems of the liver, biliary tract and pancreas. In S. Lewis, I. Collier, & M. Heitkemper (Eds.), *Medical surgical nursing* (pp. 1291-1295). St Louis: Mosby.

Giuliano, K., & Scott, S. (1999). Acute pancreatitis. In L. Bucher & S. Melander (Eds.), *Critical care nursing* (pp. 764-778). Philadelphia: Saunders.

Hennessey, K. (1996). Patients with acute pancreatitis. In J. M. Clochesy, C. Breu, S. Cardin, A. A. Whittaker, & E. B. Rudy (Eds.), *Critical care nursing* (pp. 1091-1104). Philadelphia: Saunders.

Hudak, C., Gallo, B., & Morton, P. (1998). *Critical care nursing: A holistic approach.* Philadelphia: Lippincott.

Smith, S. (1998). The gastrointestinal system. In J. Alspach (Ed.), *American Association of Critical-Care Nurses: Core curriculum for critical care nursing* (5th ed., pp. 674-687). Philadelphia: Saunders.

Thelan, L., Urden, L., Lough, M., & Stacy, K. (1998). *Critical care nursing.* St Louis: Mosby.

Westfall, U. (1999a). Gastrointestinal assessment. In L. Bucher & S. Melander (Eds.), *Critical care nursing* (pp. 692-704). Philadelphia: Saunders.

Westfall, U. (1999b). Gastrointestinal laboratory and diagnostic tests. In L. Bucher & S. Melander (Eds.), *Critical care nursing* (pp. 705-725). Philadelphia: Saunders.

Wright, J. (1997). Seven abdominal assessment signs every emergency nurse should know. *Journal of Emergency Nursing 23*(5), 446-450.

CHAPTER 18

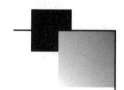

PERITONITIS

Lynn Rodgers, RNC, MSN, CCRN, CNRN, ACNP

CASE PRESENTATION

Ginny Graber, age 40 years, came to the emergency department (ED) with severe lower-left abdominal pain. The day before her admission, she felt nauseated and had abdominal distension, which she attributed to having had no bowel movement for 4 days. Mrs. Graber has diverticulosis and stated that she only has a bowel movement twice a week. She often takes a laxative, which she had done the day before her ED visit. She had no results from the laxative, was still quite nauseated, and had vomited one time. Her last menstrual period was 3 weeks ago. She is 165 cm (5 feet 6 inches) tall and weighs 74 kg (165 lb).

Physical Assessment

Mrs. Graber was lying on her back with her knees flexed. Her face was flushed, and she was quietly crying, obviously in great distress. Bowel sounds were absent. Her abdomen was slightly distended, firm, and rigid. Rebound tenderness existed over the lower-left abdominal quadrant, although her entire abdomen was painful to light palpation. Breath sounds were clear, but respirations were shallow. Mrs. Graber's diagnostic data were as follows:

BP	96/50 mm Hg lying; 84/46 mm Hg standing	Hct	48%
		Na$^+$	148 mmol/L
HR	112 bpm lying; 128 bpm standing	K$^+$	3.6 mmol/L
		Cl$^-$	107 mmol/L
Respirations	28 breaths/min	Creatinine	1.6 mg/dl
Temperature	38.7° C (101.6° F) (oral)	BUN	50 mg/dl
RBCs	3.8×10^6/mm^3	Amylase	60 U/L
WBCs	19,000/mm^3	HCG	Negative
Hgb	12.6 g/dl	Urinalysis	Normal findings

Immediate treatment included the following:

- Lactated Ringer's solution (LR) was started at 150 ml/hr via an 18-gauge intravenous (IV) catheter.
- Green fluid was aspirated from the nasogastric tube (NGT), which was connected to low continuous suction.

- Immediately after a Foley catheter was anchored, 100 ml of clear, dark urine was returned. Hourly urine specimens were obtained.
- A right subclavian triple-lumen central line was inserted. Initial central venous pressure (CVP) and right atrial pressure (RAP) were 1 mm Hg.
- Kidneys, ureters, and bladder x-ray (KUB) and upright chest x-ray examination showed free air under the diaphragm and good location of the CVP line. No pneumothorax was evident. Large distended intestinal loops were obvious.

Further treatment included the following:

- Morphine sulfate 1 to 2 mg IV push was given every 10 to 15 minutes, with a total of 14 mg given in the first 2 hours.
- Over the next 2 hours, 2000 ml of LR was infused. Breath sounds and orthostatic blood pressure (BP) changes were reevaluated every 15 to 30 minutes. Breath sounds remained clear, and orthostatic changes in BP were less than 6 mm Hg. Urine output was 45 to 50 ml/hr. CVP and RAP increased to 4 mm Hg.
- Clavulanic acid/ticarcillin 3.1 g IV partial fill was initiated immediately and then ordered every 6 hours.
- A consultation with the enterostomal therapist was held to assess and mark the patient's abdomen for stoma placement, to implement preoperative teaching, and to provide further emotional support to the patient and family.
- An exploratory laparotomy was performed, and the suspected ruptured diverticulum was confirmed. A temporary colostomy was created.

Surgical Intensive Care Unit

After an uneventful recovery room stay, Mrs. Graber was transferred to the surgical intensive care unit (SICU). She received LR at 125 ml/hr, oxygen 28% via Venturi mask, and morphine sulfate by a patient-controlled anesthesia pump. Her CVP readings were 6 to 8 mm Hg, and her urine output was 50 to 70 ml/hr. Her NGT remained at low suction. Her lower abdominal incision was well approximated without drainage. Her colostomy was brick red with only a small amount of serosanguineous fluid in the ostomy bag. She had no bowel sounds. Her blood urea nitrogen (BUN) and creatinine levels dropped to normal by the second postoperative day. Her white blood cell (WBC) count peaked at 21,000/mm^3 but also started to drop by the second postoperative day. She was transferred out of the SICU during the afternoon of her second postoperative day in stable condition.

PERITONITIS

Questions

1. What is the function of the peritoneum?
2. Discuss the pathophysiology and potential causes of peritonitis.
3. What are the clinical signs and symptoms of peritonitis?
4. Explain the abnormalities in Mrs. Graber's admission laboratory results.
5. What are the significant findings of the KUB and chest x-ray examinations?
6. What is the rationale for checking Mrs. Graber's BP in the lying and sitting positions?

7. Discuss the reason for initiating fluid resuscitation in the ED.
8. Discuss the rationale for the IV antibiotic chosen for Mrs. Graber.
9. Identify other possible diagnoses that were considered and ruled out for Mrs. Graber.
10. What interventions helped relieve Mrs. Graber's pain? Why?
11. Give the rationale for withholding pain medication immediately after Mrs. Graber's admission to the ED.
12. What is the prognosis for patients with peritonitis?
13. What are the primary nursing diagnoses for Mrs. Graber?
14. Do the signs and symptoms of peritonitis differ in elderly patients?
15. What other specific abdominal diagnostic tests could be done to confirm or rule out this or other diagnoses for abdominal pain?

PERITONITIS

Questions and Answers

1. What is the function of the peritoneum?

The peritoneum is the largest semipermeable serous membrane in the body. It is made up of the visceral peritoneum, which envelops the viscera, and the parietal peritoneum, which lines the outer walls of the abdominal cavity. As described by Markey (1999), the large folds of these peritoneal layers bind the abdominal contents together and contain the nerve, blood, and lymph supplies to these organs. Exchange of fluids and electrolytes occurs between the visceral and parietal peritoneal layers via these blood and lymph vessels. The peritoneal cavity is the potential space between these two membranes. It contains less than 50 ml of serous fluid secreted by the cells of the serosa that keep the two surfaces moist. This lubrication allows the organs within the abdominal cavity to slide freely against one another during peristalsis. In addition, the peritoneum will react to the presence of chemical or bacterial contaminates with a localized inflammatory reaction (Hirsch & Caswell, 1999).

2. Discuss the pathophysiology and potential causes of peritonitis.

According to McGill (1998), *peritonitis* is an inflammation of the peritoneum, resulting from bacterial or chemical invasion of the peritoneal cavity. Peritonitis may be classified as primary or secondary and as localized or diffuse, depending on the cause and the severity of the condition. Primary peritonitis is an acute bacterial infection that is not associated with a perforated viscus or organ. A bacterial infection originating in another area of the body and then transported to the peritoneum by the vascular system is typically the causative agent. Tuberculosis elsewhere in the body or alcoholic cirrhosis and ascites are examples of potential sources of primary peritonitis.

Another source of primary peritonitis is through peritoneal dialysis, especially patient-administered continuous ambulatory peritoneal dialysis (CAPD). Of those receiving CAPD, 60% to 70% will develop peritonitis in the first year of therapy.

Between 60% and 70% of cases are caused by gram-positive organisms such as *Staphylococcus aureus* and *Staphylococcus epidermidis,* 15% to 30% are caused by gram-negative organisms such as *Escherichia coli,* and only 5% to 10% are caused by fungi such as *Candida albicans* and are most common in immunosuppressed patients (Qadir & Cunha, 1998). Afthentopoulos, Passadakis, and Oreopoulos (1998) also described sclerosing peritonitis and sclerosing encapsulating peritonitis as extremely serious complications of CAPD with multifactorial causes.

Secondary peritonitis can occur with a perforation or rupture of the abdominal viscus, as in Mrs. Graber's case. Any abdominal organ, including any part of the gastrointestinal tract, gallbladder, pancreas, liver, ovary, or fallopian tube, may be involved. Bacteria from the ruptured organ and severe chemical reactions resulting from the released pancreatic enzymes, digestive fluids, and bile instigate the inflammatory insult. Initially, when the peritoneum is contaminated, macrophages, mast cells, eosinophils, and basophils are released from the visceral peritoneal mesentery. These inflammatory cells release prostaglandins and histamine, which results in a localized vascular dilation and increased capillary permeability. This allows movement into the peritoneal space of inflammatory serous fluid that is high in immunoglobulins, fibrin, complement, clotting factors, and chemotaxins such as leukotriene C_{5a} and B_4. This inflammatory exudate attracts phagocytic WBCs into the peritoneal cavity to begin destruction of bacteria. Fibroblastic inflammatory exudate coats the peritoneum and essentially isolates the inflammatory process by sealing off the abdominal contents from the contaminant.

If effective, these polymorphonuclear neutrophil leukocytes ingest or wall off the offending substances, resulting in a contained or localized peritonitis. If these attempts fail or if the contamination is continuous or massive, generalized peritonitis develops (Hirsch & Caswell, 1999). Generalized or diffuse peritonitis is a result of bacterial invasion into a large majority of the peritoneum. The tissues begin to swell, fibrous exudate develops, and adhesions may form. When the irritant is eliminated, these adhesions may or may not shrink and disappear. Diffuse peritoneal infection can affect the entire body and eventually can result in bacteremia or septic shock.

Infectious peritonitis can be caused by several different organisms; however, in Mrs. Graber's case, *E. coli* was the causative agent. Such organisms can also be the culprits if peritonitis results from a rupture of the appendix or from perforation caused by colonic obstruction, toxic megacolon, or traumatic intestinal injury. Pneumococcal peritonitis is a common occurrence in patients with pneumococcal pneumonia and should be suspected, especially during the winter months. Tuberculous peritonitis is slow to develop and heals, causing little or no pain. It should be suspected in patients at high risk for tuberculosis such as those who are infected with human immunodeficiency virus-. Gonococcal peritonitis can occur occasionally after massive gonococcemia. A vaginal swab for gonorrhea will help in establishing this diagnosis (Moran, 1999).

Chemical peritonitis occurs when the inflammation of the peritoneum results primarily from the caustic effects of some substance rather than from infection by an organism. Offending substances are gastric acid, pancreatic fluid, bile, or starch. There are also reports in the literature of peritoneal contamination resulting from peritoneal leakage of gastric nutritional feedings after percutaneous endoscopic gastrostomy (Haslam, Hughes, & Harrison, 1996). Although this complication is rare, occurring only in 1% of cases, Haslam et al. indicate that this can develop in the first 2 weeks after gastrostomy tube placement until a permanent fibrous tract between the skin and the gastric wall has formed.

3. What are the clinical signs and symptoms of peritonitis?

Hirsch and Caswell (1999) described the most common symptom reported in acute peritonitis, which is abdominal pain. Pain may be localized or diffuse, but the most intense pain has been reported in the area of the patient's primary gastrointestinal disorder. Referred pain to either the shoulder or thoracic areas is common. Movement often aggravates this pain. Rebound tenderness, muscular rigidity and spasm, and guarding of the abdomen are other major signs of irritation of the peritoneum. Often, the patient assumes a side-lying position with knees and hips flexed to decrease the peritoneal irritation. A history of low-grade fever is also common. Pain usually is followed by spikes of fever (=39.4° C [103° F]), chills, extreme weakness, and absolute exhaustion. Stein (1998) stated that a complete and thorough history and physical examination of the patient with abdominal pain should include type, onset, character, and distribution of pain; chronologic appearance of symptoms; and exact time, mode and acuteness of symptom onset.

Accumulation of serous fluid and inflammatory exudate in the peritoneal cavity results in ascites and abdominal distension. As more intravascular fluid enters the peritoneal cavity, the patient becomes volume depleted and dehydrated as evidenced by dry mucous membranes, poor skin turgor, thirst, tachycardia, orthostatic BP changes, and decreased urinary output. A shallow and rapid breathing pattern develops, decreasing diaphragm excursion and thereby lessening peritoneal irritation and pain. Paralytic ileus commonly occurs in the patient with acute peritonitis. Nausea, vomiting, inability to pass feces and flatus, and absence of bowel sounds are common findings. If a pelvic abscess does develop, diarrhea and urinary urgency may be present. Malaise, vomiting, and a generalized "toxic" ill appearance are usually seen in proportion to the severity of the peritonitis. Complications associated with peritonitis are hypovolemic shock, septicemia, organ failure, and mental confusion. Multisystem organ failure is the ultimate result of extensive peritonitis.

4. Explain the abnormalities in Mrs. Graber's laboratory results at admission.

Mrs. Graber's complete blood count revealed some important information. Her red blood cell count was $3.8 \times 10^6/mm^3$, which could indicate some blood loss. Her WBC count was elevated at $19,000/mm^3$, with a normal range being 5000 to $10,000/mm^3$. Her particular laboratory values are important in determining the severity of the infectious process. The hemoglobin level is important for determining the oxygen-carrying capacity of the blood. The normal range for women is between 12 and 16 g/dl. Mrs. Graber's hemoglobin result was 12.6 g/dl, which is within the lower limits of the normal range. The normal hematocrit for women is 40% to 48%. Mrs. Graber's result was 48%, which could indicate hemoconcentration resulting from a shift of fluid out of the intravascular space into the peritoneal cavity (Hirsch & Caswell, 1999).

Normal levels for serum creatinine are between 0.6 and 1.2 mg/dl for women. Mrs. Graber's level was elevated at 1.6 mg/dl. Initial vital signs indicated tachycardia and orthostatic hypotension, which are commonly seen in situations in which blood or volume loss occurs. Elevated creatinine levels could be caused by the resulting decrease in kidney function. Her urine output of 100 ml of clear, dark urine upon catheterization further indicates a decrease in her kidney perfusion. The BUN level is normally 7 to 18 mg/dl. Mrs. Graber's result of 50 mg/dl may indicate a serious condition. Several possible factors causing this condition could be gastrointestinal hemorrhage, shock, dehydration, and impaired renal function. Normal sodium levels are 135 to 148 mmol/L. Mrs. Graber's sodium level was 148 mmol/L, which may be increased because of dehydration, insufficient fluid intake, and a shift of intravascular fluid to the interstitial areas. Her potassium level was within the normal limits of 3.5 to 5 mmol/L but should be monitored closely for a decrease resulting from fluid loss and sodium conservation efforts by the kidney. Normal blood values for chloride are 98 to 106 mmol/L. Mrs. Graber's slightly elevated level of 107 mmol/L could possibly be caused by dehydration.

5. What are the significant findings of the KUB and chest x-ray examinations?

The significant radiographic findings that apply to acute abdominal pain are free intraperitoneal air and dilated loops of the intestine (McGill, 1998; Stein, 1998). Free intraperitoneal air can indicate perforation of a hollow viscus. In Mrs. Graber's case, a ruptured diverticulum was suspected. Dilated loops of the intestine can indicate a paralytic ileus, also commonly seen with a ruptured colon. A chest x-ray film was obtained after central line placement to rule out accidental pneumothorax, chest problems that could contribute to abdominal pain, and pneumonia, which can develop with peritonitis as a result of decreased lung excursion and possible bacteremia. Stein (1998) suggested that a patient should be kept in an upright position long enough for free air to collect beneath the diaphragm so it will show on the x-ray film.

6. What is the rationale for checking Mrs. Graber's BP in the lying and sitting positions?

Mrs. Graber's BP was checked in the lying and sitting positions to determine whether she had postural or orthostatic hypotension. According to Jones and Bucher (1999), when a person experiences blood or fluid loss that significantly affects total blood volume, BP will decrease as the patient sits and then stands. With a decrease in BP, there is also a compensatory increase in the heart rate to maintain a consistent cardiac output. A decrease in BP of 10 to 20 mm Hg or more and an increase in heart rate of 10 to 20 bpm or more with position changes is called a postural drop. Mrs. Graber's BP and heart rate did change significantly enough to warrant this diagnosis. Further monitoring of orthostatic hypotension would be indicated if blood and fluid losses increased or if the sitting position was contraindicated. Other significant measurements from the subclavian line were the initial CVP and RAP, which measure the pressure on the right side of the heart. Normal values are 0 to 8 mm Hg. Mrs. Graber's low reading of 1 mm Hg could indicate a decrease in blood volume and a "dry" condition intravascularly (Rice, 1997).

7. Discuss the reason for initiating fluid resuscitation in the ED.

Mrs. Graber was obviously volume depleted, as evidenced by the assessment changes discussed. The CVP and RAP were initially 1 mm Hg, were 4 mm Hg after 2000 ml of IV fluids, and were 6 to 8 mm Hg while she was in the SICU. Mrs. Graber's hypotensive state needed to be corrected as soon as possible to prevent hypovolemic shock. The treatment of choice for hypotension resulting from a volume deficit is to correct the volume problem rather than constrict the vasculature (Gawlinski, McCloy, Caswell, and Quinones-Baldrich, 1999).

8. Discuss the rationale for the IV antibiotic chosen for Mrs. Graber.

IV antibiotics should be administered as soon as possible preoperatively once the diagnosis of peritonitis is established because the time that antibiotics are started is the biggest determinant of successful treatment (Barie et al, 1997). Selection of antibiotics for peritonitis is based on severity, etiology, and practitioner preference, but the antibiotic chosen must be effective for colonic aerobes and anaerobes. For mild to moderate peritonitis, second-generation cephalosporins such as cefuroxime or third-generation penicillins such as ampicillin/sulbactam are suggested. For severe peritonitis, broad-spectrum penicillins such as piperacillin or ticarcillin or aminoglycosides such as gentamicin with metronidazole for anaerobic bacteria are recommended (Hirsch & Caswell, 1999). A single antibiotic with effectiveness against both aerobes and anaerobes was selected for Mrs. Graber. Thus clavulanic acid/ticarcillin (Timenti) was administered. Antibiotics should be continued throughout the preoperative, operative, and postoperative periods. If the patient is afebrile, has a normal leukocyte count, and has a band count of less than 3%, the chance of recurrent sepsis after discontinuation of antibiotic therapy is virtually zero (Howard & Simmons, 1995). With these criteria, antibiotics may be discontinued as early as the fourth postoperative day. If the patient does not meet these criteria, postoperative antibiotics are continued for a minimum of 7 to 10 days.

9. Identify other possible diagnoses that were considered and ruled out for Mrs. Graber.

A brief review of Mrs. Graber's laboratory work and symptoms in the ED indicated that other possible diagnoses needed to be ruled out. These included bowel obstruction, appendicitis, pancreatitis, peptic ulcer, urinary tract stones, ectopic pregnancy, and ovarian cyst (Ferri, 1999).

Mrs. Graber had severe lower-left abdominal pain, nausea, vomiting, and abdominal distension. She had a history of diverticulosis and frequent laxative use. Assessment revealed that she was doubled over in acute pain, her face was flushed, and she was crying. Bowel sounds were absent, and the abdomen was slightly distended, firm, and rigid. Rebound tenderness was noted over her lower-left abdominal quadrant with her entire abdomen painful to light tough. Her respirations were shallow.

All of the aforementioned signs and symptoms, including a WBC count greater than $15,000/mm^3$, seemed to indicate appendicitis or possible bowel obstruction. The only symptom that possibly negated a diagnosis of appendicitis was that the severe pain and rebound tenderness were on the side opposite to the appendix.

Acute pancreatitis is another possible cause for her symptoms. Certainly, the symptoms of nausea, vomiting, elevated temperature, tachycardia, hypovolemia, and hypotension are similar in both diseases, but the location of pain is a key difference. Pancreatic pain is usually felt in the epigastric region or the upper-left abdominal quadrant. Abdominal rigidity usually indicates a late sign of pancreatitis, which does not correspond to Mrs. Graber's history. Mrs. Graber's serum amylase level was 60 U/L, which is normal and, thus, ruled out pancreatitis. Amylase levels are significantly increased in patients with pancreatitis within 3 to 6 hours after the onset of pain.

Peptic ulcer could also be another consideration because of the sudden onset of constant intense pain. The pain with peptic ulcer is more generalized and has a tendency to be affected by food intake. Signs of hemorrhagic shock that occur with bleeding peptic ulcers were also present. However, lack of blood in the NGT drainage and the lack of history ruled out this diagnosis.

The last diagnosis to be considered is a genitourinary complication, such as an ectopic pregnancy, ovarian cyst, or urinary tract stone. The human chorionic gonadotropin test in this case was negative, which rules out a possible pregnancy; the urinalysis was normal, which rules out urinary tract stones. Ultrasonography or an abdominal computed tomographic (CT) scan could have diagnosed an ovarian cyst, but ovarian cysts generally do not result in absent bowel sounds.

10. What interventions helped relieve Mrs. Graber's pain? Why?

Initially, an NGT was inserted, and green drainage was aspirated. This drainage could be irritating to a ruptured diverticulum and even more irritating to the peritoneum. Decompressing the stomach may also decrease intraabdominal pressure and thus decrease pain. Insertion of a Foley catheter can also relieve intraabdominal pressure. Morphine sulfate 1 to 2 mg IV push was given at 10- to 15-minute intervals for a total of 14 mg within the first 2 hours of appearance of symptoms. The position of comfort Mrs. Graber assumed also helped decrease intraabdominal pressure (Hirsch & Caswell, 1999).

11. Give the rationale for withholding pain medication immediately after Mrs. Graber's admission to the ED.

Obtaining an accurate assessment of Mrs. Graber's pain required that all pain medications be withheld. The identification of the exact location of the most severe pain is very important in diagnosing her condition. Pain medication would have masked the signs and symptoms of pain, wasted valuable time, and possibly led to an erroneous diagnosis (Bynum, 1998). When the diagnosis was confirmed, pain medication was given, and other steps were taken to reduce Mrs. Graber's pain.

12. What is the prognosis for patients with peritonitis?

Intraabdominal infections are associated with significant mortality and morbidity despite the powerful antibiotics made available over the past 35 years. Survival is most strongly associated with the body's response to the peritoneal contamination rather than the medical interventions performed. Studies indicate mortality of 30% to 50%. The risk of death is increased in patients whose peritonitis develops after surgery or trauma compared with patients with peritoneal infection at admission. Mortality is also increased in patients requiring more than one surgical intervention or when intervention is delayed more than 24 hours after presentation. The type of surgical procedure performed does not influence the mortality rate, nor does better drainage of the peritoneal cavity. Prognosis depends on the cause of peritoneal inflammation, the amount of time the infection has been present, the body's immunologic response to the infection, the extent of surgical intervention, and body systems involved. Fluid and electrolyte resuscitation, antibiotic therapy, and surgical repair of any perforated viscus are still the most important interventions to prevent death (Hirsch & Caswell, 1999).

13. What are the primary nursing diagnoses for Mrs. Graber?

According to Cox et al (1997), the following nursing diagnoses are most applicable in Mrs. Graber's situation:

- Alteration in comfort, pain, and anxiety
- High risk for infection
- Fluid volume deficit: actual
- Alteration in tissue perfusion
- Anxiety
- Body image disturbance
- Ineffective patient and family coping

14. Do the signs and symptoms of peritonitis differ in elderly patients?

According to a study by Watters, Blakslee, Roderick, and Redmond in the *Canadian Journal of Surgery* (1996), patients who were 65 years of age or older were three times more likely to have generalized peritonitis than younger patients. These findings are consistent with the hypothesis that the biologic features of peritonitis differ in elderly patients. Impaired local peritoneal responses can result in less localized and less severe abdominal pain, leading to the development of generalized peritonitis by the time treatment is pursued. Because pain is not intense, older patients may delay in seeking medical assistance. Such delays may be attributed to difficulties leaving home, fear of hospitalization, alterations in usual symptoms, diminished perception of symptoms, or diminished ability to express them effectively. In addition, elderly patients do not always develop a significant febrile response to peritonitis. To further complicate the diagnosis, WBC counts do not always rise in elderly patients in response to infection, although an elevation in immature leukocyte numbers or a shift to the left does occur (Stanley, 1996).

15. What other specific abdominal diagnostic tests could be done to confirm or rule out this or other diagnoses for abdominal pain?

McGill (1998) and Hirsch and Caswell (1999) concluded that the following diagnostic tests can be useful for the diagnoses listed when developing differential diagnoses for abdominal pain.

- *Chest x-ray film:* can indicate the presence of free air, pleural effusion, pneumonia, or bibasilar atelectasis that may infer inflammatory disease
- *Abdominal ultrasound:* can indicate abdominal masses such as abscesses or tumors, gallbladder disease, pancreatitis, abdominal fluid or free air, ectopic pregnancy, or uterine and ovarian disease
- *Abdominal series:* can indicate free air under the diaphragm, bowel obstruction or ileus, organ displacement, a space-occupying lesion, or air within the colon
- *CT scan with contrast:* can indicate with great specificity most diagnoses although it is expensive and requires exposure to radiation
- *Radionuclide scan:* can isolate difficult-to-locate abdominal abscesses

PERITONITIS

References

Afthentopoulos, I. E., Passadakis, P., & Oreopoulos, D. G. (1998). Sclerosing peritonitis in continuous ambulatory dialysis patients: One center's experience and a review of the literature. *Advances in Renal Replacement Therapy, 5*(3), 157-167.

Barie, P. S., Voel, S. B., Dellinger, E. P., Rotstein, D., Solomkin, J. S., Yang, J. L., & Baumgartner, T. F. (1997). A randomized, double-blind clinical trial comparing cefepime plus metronidazole with imipenem-cilastatin in the treatment of complicated intra-abdominal infections. *Archives of Surgery, 132*(12), 1294-1302.

Bynum, T. (1998). Abdominal pain. In J. H. Stein (Ed.), *Internal medicine* (5th ed., pp. 2030-2035). St Louis: Mosby.

Cox, H. C., Hinz, M. D., Lubno, M., Newfield, S. A., Ridenour, N. A., Slater, M. M., & Sridaroment, K. L. (1997). *Clinical applications of nursing diagnosis* (3rd ed.). Philadelphia: FA Davis.

Ferri, F. (1999). *Ferri's clinical advisor.* St Louis: Mosby.

Gawlinski, A., McCloy, K., Caswell, D., & Quinones-Baldrich, W. J. (1999). Cardiovascular disorders. In A. Gawlinski & D. Hamwi (Eds.), *Acute care nurse practitioner: Clinical curriculum and certification review* (pp. 136-294). Philadelphia: WB Saunders.

Haslam, N., Hughes, S., & Harrison, R. F. (1996). Peritoneal leakage of gastric contents, a rare complication of percutaneous endoscopic gastrostomy. *Journal of Parenteral and Enteral Nutrition, 20*(6), 433-434.

Hirsch, C. G., & Caswell, D. (1999). Gastrointestinal disorders. In A. Gawlinski & D. Hamwi (Eds.), *Acute care nurse practitioner: Clinical curriculum and certification review* (pp. 618-722). Philadelphia: WB Saunders.

Howard, R. J., & Simmons, R. L. (Eds.). (1995). *Surgical infectious diseases* (3rd ed.). Norwalk, CT: Appleton & Lange.

Jones, K. M., & Bucher, L. (1999). Shock. In L. Bucher & S. Melander (Eds.), *Critical care nursing* (pp. 1010-1035). Philadelphia: WB Saunders.

Markey, D. W. (1999). Gastrointestinal anatomy and physiology. In L. Bucher and S. Melander (Eds.), *Critical care nursing* (pp. 675-691). Philadelphia: WB Saunders.

McGill, J. M. (1998). Diseases of the peritoneum, mesentery, and omentum. In J. H. Stein (Ed.), *Internal medicine* (5th ed., pp. 2247-2252). St Louis: Mosby.

Moran, J. (1999). Gonorrhea. In R. E. Rackel (Ed.), *Conn's current therapy.* Philadelphia: Saunders.

Qadir, M. T., & Cunha, B. A. (1998). Penicillium peritonitis in a patient receiving continuous ambulatory peritoneal dialysis. *Heart & Lung, 27*(1), 67-68.

Rice, V. (1997). *Shock: A clinical syndrome.* Aliso Viejo, CA: American Association of Critical-Care Nurses.

Stanley, M. (1996). Sepsis in the elderly. *Critical Care Nursing Clinics of North America, 8*(1), 1-6.

Stein, J. H. (1998). *Internal medicine* (5th ed.). St Louis: Mosby.

Stone, R. (1996). Primary care diagnosis of acute abdominal pain. *The Nurse Practitioner, 21*(12), 19-31.

Watters, J. M., Blakslee, J. M., Roderick, J. M., & Redmond, M. L. (1996). The influence of age on the severity of peritonitis. *Canadian Journal of Surgery, 39*(2), 142-146.

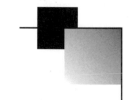

CHAPTER *19*

ESOPHAGEAL VARICES

Linda K. Evinger, RN, MSN, C-OGNP

CASE PRESENTATION

Joseph Hubert, age 59 years, was brought to the emergency department (ED) with complaints of dizziness, dyspnea, restlessness, and anxiety. Mr. Hubert currently works as an accountant for a large firm. He is married and has two children living at home. He reported a 2-day history of hematemesis with some bright red blood and large amounts of "coffee-grounds" colored emesis. Mr. Hubert denied any recent or chronic illnesses and was unable to remember if anyone in his family had ever had problems with gastrointestinal tract bleeding. He did admit to drinking six to eight alcoholic beverages almost every day for the past 7 years. Initial assessment revealed cool and clammy skin, a distended abdomen with hyperactive bowel sounds, and tachycardia.

Current vital signs and laboratory results are as follows:

BP	92/60 mm Hg	AST (SGOT)	950 U/L
HR	120 bpm	ALT (SGPT)	1000 U/L
Respirations	28 breaths/min	Alkaline phosphatase	165 U/L
Temperature	36.9° C (98.3° F) (oral)	Total bilirubin	2.5 mg/dl
Ammonia	60 µg/dl	Albumin	2.3 g/dl
Glucose	87 mg/dl	PT	26 sec
LDH	500 U/L	PTT	85 sec

Three hours after arriving in the ED, Mr. Hubert was admitted to the intensive care unit (ICU) with an intravenous infusion of normal saline. Two units of packed red blood cells were administered. Twenty units of vasopressin (Pitressin) in 100 ml of 5% dextrose in water (D5W) were given intravenously over 20 minutes. A continuous infusion of vasopressin 0.4 U/min was then initiated. Sublingual nitroglycerin was added to the medication regimen. Diagnostic endoscopy, immediately preceded by a saline lavage, was scheduled for the following day. Endoscopy revealed a large esophageal varix (1.5 cm) above the gastroesophageal junction. Only a small amount of bright red blood was observed, so sclerotherapy was performed. A solution of 5% ethanolamine oleate was given by intravariceal injection. Mr. Hubert's condition remained stable after sclerotherapy and he was transferred to a medical floor. Subsequent sclerotherapy sessions were scheduled on a weekly basis for 4 weeks.

ESOPHAGEAL VARICES

Questions

1. Define and discuss the pathophysiology of esophageal varices and portal hypertension.
2. What do Mr. Hubert's laboratory tests indicate about his current health status?
3. Explain how Mr. Hubert's history and laboratory results relate to portal hypertension.
4. Discuss the clinical manifestations of esophageal varices.
5. Identify the diagnostic procedures and nursing implications for esophageal varices.
6. Compare and contrast the treatment options and nursing implications for esophageal varices.
7. Discuss the rationale for Mr. Hubert's vasopressin therapy, management of side effects, and nursing concerns.
8. Identify the relevant nursing diagnoses for Mr. Hubert while he is in the ICU.
9. Discuss the patient/family teaching indicated for Mr. Hubert.
10. What special nursing considerations are prompted by Mr. Hubert's past drinking pattern?
11. Discuss the psychosocial aspects of the care of Mr. Hubert and his family.

ESOPHAGEAL VARICES

Questions and Answers

1. **Define and discuss the pathophysiology of esophageal varices and portal hypertension.**

Anderson (1998) defines *varix* as "a tortuous dilated vein" (p. 1694) and *esophageal varices* as "a complex of longitudinal tortuous veins at the lower end of the esophagus, enlarged and swollen as the result of portal hypertension" (p. 588). Clochesy, Breu, Cardin, Whittaker, and Rudy (1996, p. 1063) define *portal hypertension* as "increased hydrostatic pressure within the portal venous system." Blood enters the liver through the hepatic artery and the portal vein. The liver is a highly vascular organ that normally offers little resistance to splanchnic blood flow.

Alcohol is oxidized to aldehyde by the liver. This change results in permanent hepatocellular damage. Excessive and chronic consumption of alcohol causes an increase of smooth endoplasmic reticulum in the cells of the liver. This stimulates an increased production of cholesterol that accumulates in the liver. Mitochondria swell, which leads to increased inflammation, fibrosis, and necrosis of the cells of the liver (Altman, 1999).

This chronic injury to the liver leads to irreversible scarring. The scarring and regeneration nodules that develop result in a distortion of the vascular bed, which leads to portal hypertension (Altman, 1999). In an attempt to compensate, the liver develops collateral circulation connecting the portal veins to other organs. This effort is inefficient and results in venous backflow into the spleen, esophagus, stomach, and intestines. Varices form in the esophagus (McEwen, 1996). According to Alspach (1998), collateral vessels form in the esophagus, rectum, stomach, duodenum, peritoneum, and retroperitoneum. With an increase in portal venous pressure greater than 10 mm Hg, the collateral vessels distend with blood, thus causing enlargement and the formation of varices. Varices usually develop in the esophagus or the upper portion of the stomach. Bleeding typically occurs when the pressure exceeds 12 mm Hg (Alspach, 1998). Esophageal varices occur in up to 75% of those with cirrhosis (Elrod, 1996, chap. 41). Variceal bleeding occurs more often in patients who have more severe liver dysfunction and also in those who have large varices or have varices with red signs, which are considered to be varices on varices (Burroughs & Patch, 1999).

2. What do Mr. Hubert's laboratory tests indicate about his current health status?

Mr. Hubert has advanced liver disease. He experienced blood loss resulting in hypovolemia, which decreased the hemoglobin level and hematocrit and elevated the white blood cell (WBC) count, platelet count, and blood urea nitrogen (BUN) level. His sodium and potassium levels were decreased because of the vomiting. His ammonia level was elevated because the diseased liver was unable to convert ammonia to urea for excretion. Lactate dehydrogenase (LDH), aspartate aminotransferase (AST), and alanine aminotransferase (ALT) levels were elevated because enzymes and end products are released into the blood with the destruction of liver cells. The alkaline phosphatase level was increased because of biliary obstruction. The albumin level was low because of impaired liver synthesis. The bilirubin level was elevated because of the liver's inability to conjugate bilirubin, and the prothrombin time (PT) was longer because of diminished synthesis of prothrombin by the liver.

3. Explain how Mr. Hubert's history and laboratory results relate to portal hypertension.

Portal hypertension is the primary cause of esophageal varices. The esophageal varices caused the symptoms experienced by Mr. Hubert. Hematemesis is bloody emesis that is either bright red color, indicating fresh bleeding, or a dark, "coffee-grounds" color, indicating that blood has been in the stomach where gastric juices have had a chance to act on it. The blood loss accounts for his dizziness, dyspnea, restlessness, tachycardia, and anxiety. Mr. Hubert's admission of long-term heavy alcohol intake implies cirrhosis as a cause for the portal hypertension. It also suggests liver disease as a cause for the abnormal laboratory test results indicated in question 2. Abdominal distension may be explained by ascites from liver disease. The cool and clammy skin is a sign of shock.

Portal hypertension is the cause of esophageal varices. The varices, by rupturing, then cause hypovolemia, resulting in a decreased hemoglobin level and hematocrit and an increased BUN level, WBC count, and platelet count. The vomiting contributes to the decreased sodium and potassium levels. Increased ammonia, LDH, alkaline phosphatase, AST, ALT, and total bilirubin levels; increased PT; and a decreased albumin level also are common in advanced liver disease. The calcium level is low because of the decreased albumin level and because 50% of the total calcium is protein bound.

4. Discuss the clinical manifestations of esophageal varices.

A common symptom of ruptured esophageal varices is hematemesis, which may be bright red or "coffee-grounds" in color. Patients may also report hematochezia (Younossi, 1996, p. 300). Giacchino and Houdek (1998) state that no abdominal pain is considered a classic sign that helps differentiate esophageal varices from bleeding ulcers. Hematochezia (blood in the feces) of bright red or maroon color can occur. Sometimes, patients report signs and symptoms of blood loss, which include dizziness, dyspnea, restlessness, and anxiety. Hypotension, tachycardia, decreased level of consciousness, decreased urinary output, and shock may also be seen (Younossi, 1996, p. 301).

5. Identify the diagnostic procedures and nursing implications for esophageal varices.

Endoscopy is used in the diagnosis of esophageal varices. Once the patient's condition is hemodynamically stable, gastric lavage may be performed to improve visualization before endoscopy. The patient should be reassured that the endoscopy procedure is safe and informed that gagging may occur but that medication will be given to minimize the gagging response. Usually, about 5 minutes before endoscopy is begun, the patient is given a medication such as lorazepam, meperidine, or midazolam for sedation. An endoscope or gastroscope is used because it has a fiberoptic light source that enables a clear view of the upper gastrointestinal tract. The patient is instructed to lie on the left side. A rubber mouthpiece is inserted to protect the patient's teeth. The endoscope is inserted into the esophagus and then into the stomach and duodenum. Complications of endoscopy include aspiration, perforation of the esophagus, and rupture of the varices (Clochesy et al, 1996).

6. Compare and contrast the treatment options and nursing implications for esophageal varices.

Endoscopic Injection Sclerotherapy

Injection sclerotherapy is used to treat active bleeding. Sclerotherapy is currently considered the treatment of choice for an acute episode of bleeding from esophageal varices (Clochesy et al, 1996; McEwen, 1996). Sclerosing agents vary, but sodium morrhuate is used most often in the United States. An intravariceal injection, which delivers the agent directly into the lumen of the varix, causes a thrombus to form in the vein and this in turn stops the bleeding. The number of injections is based on the patient, extension of the bleeding area, and effect of the sclerosing agent on the varices. Injections every 2 to 3 months may be necessary for some patients. During sclerotherapy, the patient is kept lying on the left side with the head of bed elevated to 30 degrees to reduce the risk of aspiration. General anesthesia may not be recommended because of the liver disease and the resulting inability to metabolize the anesthetic agents. The nurse must closely monitor the patient's respiratory status during and after the procedure. Mortality is less than 1%, but complications occur in 10% to 15% of patients. Complications include ulceration of the esophagus, mucosal sloughing, esophageal perforation, stenosis of the esophagus, variceal bleeding, venous embolism, esophageal spasm resulting in substernal chest pain, fever, aspiration pneumonia, and an allergic reaction to the sclerosant (Clochesy et al, 1996).

Endoscopic Band Ligation

A more recent development in treatment options is ligation of the varices using the endoscope. Results are favorable, and the procedure may produce fewer complications and therefore better survival rates (Koff, 1996, p. 630). Bands are used to prevent or control bleeding. The bands are small and tight and thrombose the varix. Because no chemical agent is needed, the complications associated with the sclerotherapy chemicals are avoided (Clochesy et al, 1996). A study comparing ligation of esophageal varices and drug therapy found greatly improved bleeding rates only in those who had ligation of their varices (Burroughs & Patch, 1999).

Intravenous Vasopressin (Pitressin)

Vasopressin, somatostatin, and octreotide have all been used to reduce blood flow to the gut and decrease portal flow and pressure. When vasopressin is used, there is often a loading dose of 20 U in 50 ml of D5W given for 30 minutes; then a maintenance dose ranging from 0.1 to 0.5 U/min is begun. No more than 0.9 U/min is considered safe. The vasopressin dosage must be tapered over at least 24 hours when discontinuation is chosen (Altman, 1999). The critical care nurse must continuously monitor the patient's electrocardiogram and blood pressure. Side effects include myocardial infarction, arrhythmias, bradycardia, hypertension, decreased cardiac output, abdominal cramps, and coronary artery vasoconstriction. Concurrent administration of nitroglycerin may help decrease the side effects of vasopressin therapy (Clochesy et al, 1996).

Balloon Tamponade

Balloon tamponade is another method sometimes used to control the bleeding. Several types of tubes may be used for balloon tamponade therapy. The Sengstaken-Blakemore tube is a triple-lumen tube in which one lumen is for gastric aspiration, one is for inflating the esophageal balloon, and one is for inflating the gastric balloon. Another type is the Minnesota tube, which has one additional lumen for aspiration of the esophagus. A third type is the Linton-Nachlas tube, a triple-lumen tube in which one lumen is for gastric aspiration, one is for esophageal aspiration, and the other is for inflation of a large gastric balloon. Balloon inflation puts pressure on the varices, which will stop the blood flow (Altman, 1999, chap. 36). Initially, the tip of the balloon is inserted into the stomach and inflated and clamped. The tube is then withdrawn until resistance is felt, causing pressure to be exerted at the gastroesophageal junction. An external traction source may be used via a helmet or the foot of the bed (McEwen, 1996). Traction must be monitored carefully and is believed to be uncomfortable for the patient. If bleeding still is not controlled, the esophageal balloon is inflated with pressure from 25 to 40 mm Hg. Tissue damage can occur in only a few hours. The esophageal balloon should not be left inflated for more than 72 hours. Confirmation of the gastric balloon port below the gastroesophageal junction is done by x-ray examination (Clochesy et al, 1996). Evaluation of the bleeding status of the varices should be done during the deflation time, and the nurse must be prepared for rebleeding and hematemesis. For deflation, the esophageal balloon is deflated first to prevent airway occlusion by displacement of the tube upward. Major complications of balloon tamponade are upper airway obstruction caused by deflation or rupture of a balloon(s), pulmonary aspiration, and esophageal rupture. Scissors should be kept at the bedside to facilitate immediate removal of the tube by cutting the lumens if airway obstruction occurs. Suction may be applied above the most proximately located balloon to reduce the possibility of aspiration. Symptoms of esophageal rupture include sudden onset of upper abdominal or back pain, which is accompanied with a sudden drop in blood pressure. The naris used for the tube insertion needs to be protected to prevent necrosis (Clochesy et al, 1996). Once the balloons are deflated, they are usually left in place from 6 to 24 hours.

Portosystemic Shunt

Management of bleeding varices inevitably begins with pharmacologic agents and sclerotherapy. For patients with uncontrolled bleeding, a portosystemic shunt may be considered (Altman, 1999). The purpose of the surgery is to divert blood flow away from the liver and toward the systemic circulation. Shunts are categorized as selective, nonselective, or partial. Partial shunts allow the most effective preservation of portal blood flow (McEwen, 1996). Although rebleeding is usually avoided, the long-term survival rates are not good because of the patient's compromised status before surgery. Problems seen with selective shunts include shunt thrombus, inadequate variceal decompression, and possible redevelopment of high- and low-pressure pathways. Nonselective shunts have been associated with more occurrences of postoperative hepatic encephalopathy (McEwen, 1996).

Transjugular Intrahepatic Portosystemic Shunt

The transjugular intrahepatic portosystemic shunt is a fairly recent approach to treatment of variceal bleeding and portal hypertension. Catheterization of the hepatic vein is done, preferably through the right internal jugular vein. Using fluoroscopy, the clinician directs a needle into a branch of the portal vein along an intrahepatic tract. The intrahepatic tract is dilated, and a stainless steel stent holds it open. The stent is delivered via a balloon catheter (Clochesy et al, 1996). The procedure allows a portosystemic shunt to be placed entirely within the liver. The risks include puncture site bleeding, hematoma formation, reactions to the contrast medium, fever, bacteremia, encephalopathy, transient renal failure, subendocardial myocardial infarction, vascular injury, bile duct trauma, and stent stenosis or thrombosis (Altman, 1999). Alspach (1998) identifies a rebleeding rate of only 20% in the first year after the procedure.

7. **Discuss the rationale for Mr. Hubert's vasopressin therapy, management of side effects, and nursing concerns.**

Vasopressin (Pitressin) is a synthetic antidiuretic hormone that was first used clinically in 1968. It is a vasoconstrictor that lowers portal venous pressure, thereby reducing venous blood flow. The lowered portal venous pressure subsequently lowers pressure in the collateral circulation, which reduces bleeding (Clochesy et al, 1996). Side effects include coronary vasoconstriction, myocardial infarction, cardiac arrhythmias, bradycardia, elevated blood pressure, decreased cardiac output, and abdominal cramps (Altman, 1999). Nitroglycerin may be given to lessen the cardiac effects (Clochesy et al, 1996). Mr. Hubert must be advised to report any changes or concerns immediately to the nurse.

A study completed by Avgerinos and Nevens (1997) found somatostatin to be superior to placebo in managing esophageal bleeding. Altman (1999) reported that somatostatin's more limited effects result in fewer side effects.

Octreotide, an analog of somatostatin, may also be used (Giacchino & Houdek, 1998).

Propranolol, a β-blocker, is sometimes used in the management of esophageal varices. Studies have yielded conflicting results regarding its efficacy (Clochesy et al, 1996). Trevillyan and Carroll (1997) report that propranolol may be used to prevent the first episode of bleeding and to manage bleeding episodes.

8. Identify the relevant nursing diagnoses for Mr. Hubert while he is in the ICU.

Relevant nursing diagnoses include the following:

- Altered bowel elimination: diarrhea
- Altered cardiac output: decreased
- Altered comfort: acute pain, nausea, and vomiting
- Altered family processes
- Altered nutrition: less than body requirements
- Altered role performance
- Altered thought processes
- Altered tissue perfusion: gastrointestinal, cerebral, cardiovascular, peripheral
- Disturbance in self-concept: body image, self-esteem (long-term or situational)
- Fear
- Fluid volume deficit
- High risk for altered oral mucous membranes
- High risk for ineffective breathing pattern
- High risk for infection due to invasive procedures
- High risk for injury: suffocation
- High risk for aspiration
- Ineffective individual coping
- Powerlessness
- Self-care deficit
- Sleep pattern disturbance

9. Discuss the patient/family teaching indicated for Mr. Hubert.

Teaching areas include those related to procedures, treatments, medications, expectations of therapies, nutrition, alcohol abuse, the ICU, and lifestyle changes.

10. What special nursing considerations are prompted by Mr. Hubert's past drinking pattern?

In regard to Mr. Hubert's history of heavy alcohol use, the nurse must discuss the amount of alcohol intake and treatment strategies for elimination of alcohol. Family considerations are of utmost importance in this area. The nurse must offer emotional and psychologic support to Mr. Hubert related to his fears of not surviving and his treatment regimen.

11. Discuss the psychosocial aspects of the care of Mr. Hubert and his family.

Mr. Hubert and his family may or may not have acknowledged that he has a drinking problem. Acknowledging the drinking problem, the problems associated with his health, and the impact of these problems on the family will affect family dynamics. Common emotions Mr. Hubert and/or his family may experience are guilt and anger. It is natural for an individual and his family to grieve the loss of health and other secondary losses. Mr. Hubert may have difficulty changing his drinking behavior if his family does not support him. Family members must be evaluated for possible codependence and appropriate referrals made. Alcoholism has an impact on the entire family, not only the spouse, so consideration of the children is important.

ESOPHAGEAL VARICES

References

Alspach, J. G. (Ed.). (1998). *American Association of Critical-Care Nurses: Core curriculum for critical care nurses* (5th ed.). Philadelphia: Saunders.

Altman, M. (1999). Hepatic disorders. In L. Bucher & S. Melander (Eds.), *Critical care nursing* (pp. 36-1–36-18). Philadelphia: Saunders.

Anderson, K. N. (Ed.). (1998). *Mosby's dictionary* (5th ed.). St Louis: Mosby.

Avgerinos, A., & Nevens, F. (1997). Early administration of somatostatin and efficacy of sclerotherapy in acute oesophageal variceal bleeds: The European acute bleeding oesophageal variceal episodes (above) randomized trial. *Lancet, 350,* 1495-1499.

Burroughs, A. K., & Patch, D. (1999). Primary prevention of bleeding from esophageal varices (WWW document). URL http://www.hepatitis-central.com/hcv/liver/prevention/varices.html.

Clochesy, J. M., Breu, C., Cardin, S., Whittaker, A. A., & Rudy, E. B. (1996). *Critical care nursing* (2nd ed.). Philadelphia: Saunders.

Elrod, R. (1996). Nursing role in management: Problems of the liver, biliary tract, and pancreas. In S. M. Lewis, I. C. Collier, & M. M. Heitkemper (Eds.), *Medical-surgical nursing* (4th ed., pp. 1258-1308). St Louis: Mosby.

Giacchino, S., & Houdek, D. (1998). Ruptured varices! Act fast. *RN, 61*(5), 33-36.

Koff, R. S. (1996). Liver. In J. Noble (Ed.), *Textbook of primary care medicine* (2nd ed., pp. 614-634). St Louis: Mosby.

McEwen, D. R. (1996). Management of alcoholic cirrhosis of the liver. *AORN Journal, 64,* 209-226.

Trevillyan, J., & Carroll, P. J. (1997). Management of portal hypertension and esophageal varices in alcoholic cirrhosis. *American Family Physician, 97,* 1851-1859.

Younossi, Z. M. (1996). Acute upper gastrointestinal bleeding. In R. E. Rakel (Ed.), *Saunders manual of medical practice* (pp. 300-301). Philadelphia: Saunders.

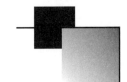

CHAPTER 20

ADRENAL CRISIS

Anne G. Denner, MS Biology, BSN

CASE PRESENTATION

Jim Catt, age 42 years, was admitted to the intensive care unit (ICU) after surgery for a ruptured appendix. His history revealed that he has type I diabetes (formerly called *IDDM* or *insulin-dependent diabetes mellitus*). On his admission to the ICU, Mr. Catt's skin was cool and pale and had a slight bronze color. His pedal and tibial pulses were present bilaterally but faint. Breath sounds were clear but slightly diminished bilaterally.

Mr. Catt had taken prednisone 5 mg three times daily for the past 3 weeks for treatment of a presumed bout with ulcerative colitis.

After returning from surgery at 3:45 PM, he received an intravenous (IV) infusion of 0.5 normal saline (NS) at 100 ml/hr, cefazolin sodium (Ancef) 1 g every 6 hours, and gentamicin (Garamycin) 70 mg every 8 hours.

Postoperative laboratory values and vital signs immediately after surgery at 4 PM were as follows:

BP	126/80 mm Hg	Na$^+$	140 mmol/L
HR	80 bpm	K$^+$	5.0 mmol/L
Respirations	18 breaths/min	Cl$^-$	100 mmol/L
Temperature	37.0° C (100° F)	Glucose	128 mg/dl

The next morning, however, Mr. Catt complained of feeling so tired and weak that he was almost unable to stand up to urinate. At 6 AM, his vital signs were as follows:

BP	90/60 mm Hg lying;	Respirations	24 breaths/min
	65/36 mm Hg standing	Temperature	38.3° C (101° F)
HR	120 bpm		

Blood was sent to the laboratory for electrolyte analysis, and a bolus of 200 ml of 0.5 NS was administered. After this bolus at 6:20 AM, his vital signs were as follows:

BP	90/60 mm Hg
HR	130 bpm
Respirations	20 breaths/min

Laboratory results included the following:

Na⁺	136 mmol/L	Glucose	60 mg/dl
K⁺	6 mmol/L	HCO₃⁻	20 mmol/L
Cl⁻	90 mmol/L		

A second physical assessment of Mr. Catt at this time revealed vague abdominal pain and nausea. He noted that this was not the first time he had experienced these symptoms. He recalled having had these same feelings about a month ago but thought it was the "flu" or a part of his ulcerative colitis. His incision was checked for hemorrhage but was found to be dry and intact. An immediate electrocardiogram showed sinus tachycardia and peaked T waves. At 7 AM, another set of electrolyte measurements was ordered in addition to a cortisol level. One ampule of 50% dextrose in water was given, and Mr. Catt's IV infusions were changed to 5% dextrose in water at a rate of 200 ml/hr.

The 7 AM laboratory results included the following:

Na⁺	122 mmol/L	Glucose	66 mg/dl
K⁺	6.8 mmol/L	HCO₃⁻	18 mmol/l
Cl⁻	88 mmol/L	Cortisol	2.6 mg/dl

Mr. Catt was given dexamethasone (Decadron) 4 mg IV as a bolus with an additional 4 mg given every 8 hours until completion of the cosyntropin test. Laboratory data and vital signs at 3 PM were as follows:

BP	110/70 mm Hg	K⁺	5.5 mmol/L
HR	100 bpm	Cl⁻	98 mmol/L
Respirations	20 breaths/min	Glucose	150 mg/dl
Temperature	38.3° C (101° F)	HCO₃⁻	22 mmol/L
Na⁺	135 mmol/L		

A rapid screening test using cosyntropin (Cortrosyn) was ordered. Serum cortisol levels measured at 30, 60, and 90 minutes were 2.2, 2.6, and 2 mg/dl, respectively. The serum aldosterone level at 90 minutes was 2 ng/dL, and the plasma adrenocorticotropic hormone (ACTH) level was 294 pg/ml.

Mr. Catt's feelings of fatigue soon began to subside, medications was regulated to oral dosages within 5 days, and he was discharged.

ADRENAL CRISIS

Questions

1. Mr. Catt has just experienced an adrenal crisis. What are the precipitating factors that have caused his short-term situation? Describe the pathophysiologic mechanisms involved in the precipitation of an adrenal crisis.
2. What are the characteristic signs and symptoms of an adrenal crisis?
3. Differentiate primary adrenal insufficiency from secondary adrenal insufficiency.

4. Describe the components of the axis involving the hypothalamus, anterior pituitary, and the adrenal cortex. What major secretions are produced by each component, and what is the secretion's effect on the other components of the axis (i.e., stimulate or inhibit)?

5. The adrenal cortex secretes both glucocorticoids and mineralocorticoids. Describe the controlling mechanism of the primary mineralocorticoid aldosterone. How did this mechanism affect Mr. Catt's 7 AM electrolyte values?

6. Describe the physiologic functions of endogenous cortisol in the body. Which functions were not being performed as evidenced by Mr. Catt's 6:20 AM and 7 AM laboratory results and vital signs?

7. What other hormones have been shown to interact with the renin-angiotensin-aldosterone system (RAAS) and control aldosterone levels and functions? What other hormones interact with cortisol to affect its physiologic function? What are the effects?

8. Define the stimulation test and the suppression test. Describe the mechanism used in Mr. Catt's diagnosis. Compare the normal hormone values involved in the hypothalamohypophysial adrenal axis with Mr. Catt's values.

9. Discuss how the diagnosis of Addison's disease is made.

10. What are the goals of treatment for adrenal crisis?

11. What are the primary nursing considerations for patients with adrenal crisis?

12. Identify potential medications for the future treatment of Mr. Catt's Addison's disease. What are their functions and potential adverse reactions?

13. What concepts regarding his disease should Mr. Catt know before leaving the hospital? List the critical events that might precipitate another crisis.

ADRENAL CRISIS

Questions and Answers

1. Mr. Catt has just experienced an adrenal crisis. What are the precipitating factors that caused his short-term situation? Describe the pathophysiologic mechanisms involved in the precipitation of an adrenal crisis.

An adrenal crisis requires some type of trigger or stressor such as surgery, trauma, or infection (Balducci-Silano & Maclaren, 1996). Mr. Catt had several factors contributing to his present situation. He evidently had undiagnosed borderline Addison's disease, yet had been medicated with prednisone. Prednisone masked and treated the Addison's disease for a few weeks, and its withdrawal helped precipitate the adrenal crisis. Obviously, the stress of the ruptured appendix and resultant surgery were major precipitating factors. In addition, alcohol withdrawal is another precipitating factor. Increased levels of both glucocorticoids (primarily cortisol) and mineralocorticoids (primarily aldosterone) are needed for the body to adapt to the stress (Bucher & Melander, 1999).

Corticotropin-releasing hormone (CRH) from the hypothalamus eventually prompts release of ACTH from the anterior pituitary gland. ACTH then stimulates release and synthesis of cortisol from the adrenal cortex. Cortisol mobilizes amino acids from skeletal muscle and generally enhances the liver's capacity for gluconeogenesis (Griffin & Ojeda, 1996).

The autonomic nervous system's craniosacral outflow also responds to stressors by causing release of norepinephrine and epinephrine, which stimulate hepatic glycogenolysis, lipolysis, and gluconeogenesis (Griffin & Ojeda, 1996). These catecholamines also cause vasoconstriction, which in the kidney, probably initiates release of renin, stimulating the RAAS. Antidiuretic hormone (ADH, also called *vasopressin*), is released from the hypothalamus and posterior pituitary during periods of stress. Both aldosterone and ADH attempt to conserve water and electrolytes to sustain a sufficient vascular volume (Griffin & Ojeda, 1996).

When the adrenal glands are unable to produce sufficient quantities of the needed hormones, fluid and electrolyte imbalances, decreased plasma glucose levels, and hypotension lead to the potentially life-threatening situation of adrenal crisis (McCance & Huether, 1998).

2. What are the characteristic signs and symptoms of an adrenal crisis?

Severe hypotension and vascular collapse are the hallmarks of the addisonian crisis (Bucher & Melander, 1999). Symptoms usually present in patients with adrenal insufficiency are weakness, fatigue, and anorexia. In addition, gastrointestinal symptoms such as nausea, vomiting, abdominal pain or cramping, and diarrhea are often present (Bucher & Melander, 1999).

Hypoglycemia, hyponatremia, hypovolemia, and hyperkalemia that occur in primary insufficiency contribute to the symptoms just described. Other symptoms include malaise, personality changes, arthralgias, and myalgias. With primary insufficiency, presenting symptoms might include salt craving, coagulopathies, weight loss, vitiligo, and a history of acquired immunodeficiency syndrome or recent surgery.

In patients with chronic adrenal insufficiency, hyperpigmentation in the buccal mucosa, skin creases, and nonexposed skin areas may be noted. The hyperpigmentation is caused by excess plasma ACTH levels in the absence of cortisol, the endogenous negative feedback factor for the hypothalamus (Hadley, 2000).

It has been shown that a portion (the first 13 amino acids) of the ACTH molecule is identical to melanocyte-stimulating hormone (MSH). MSH normally increases skin pigmentation. Hadley (2000) also states that the heptapeptide sequence (-Met-Glu-His-Phe-Arg-Try-Gly-) is probably responsible for the melanotropic activity of ACTH.

Patients with secondary insufficiency do not necessarily have the hallmark signs of hyponatremia, hypovolemia, and hyperkalemia because the secretion of mineralocorticoid is not significantly affected. Additional symptoms often seen with secondary adrenal insufficiency include cold intolerance and hair loss as a result of hypothyroidism. Patients with secondary adrenal insufficiency will also lack the hyperpigmentation seen with the primary insufficiency. In the case of secondary insufficiencies, the entire anterior pituitary may be hypofunctioning, producing a variety of symptoms (Bucher & Melander, 1999).

3. Differentiate primary adrenal insufficiency from secondary adrenal insufficiency.

Adrenal insufficiency may be primary or secondary. Primary insufficiency usually occurs from a progressive destruction of the adrenal gland. Primary insufficiency is uncommon but results in a deficiency of both glucocorticoids and mineralocorticoids. Clinical signs may not by evident until 90% of the gland has been destroyed

(Rubin & Farber, 1999). Primary insufficiency may be caused by an autoimmune or idiopathic atrophy. Adrenal autoantibodies appear in 50% to 70% of patients who have idiopathic atrophy (Rubin & Farber, 1999). As is the case with most autoimmune diseases, Addison's disease is more common in adult women and children (Rubin & Farber, 1999).

Although tuberculosis is a rare cause of Addison's disease in the United States and Europe, it is still a major cause in Japan (Rubin & Farber, 1999). Other causes for primary insufficiency include leukemia, amyloidosis, histoplasmosis and sarcoidosis, hemorrhage from trauma, anticoagulation therapy and sepsis, metastasis, and a congenital absence of the ACTH response (Rubin & Farber, 1999). Drugs account for a small number of cases of adrenal crisis. Ketoconazole (Nizoral) and aminoglutethimide (Cytadren) may decrease steroid production, whereas phenytoin (Dilantin), barbiturates, and rifampin (Rifadin) cause increased steroid degradation. Each, then, may contribute to an adrenal crisis.

Adrenal hemorrhage leading to adrenal insufficiency is seen as a side effect of medical intervention. Patients receiving anticoagulant therapy (i.e., patients with acute myocardial infarction receiving anticoagulant therapy) may have concomitant adrenal hemorrhage. The incidence of adrenal hemorrhage from patients with sepsis is variable but is seen more commonly in children with severe meningococcal (Waterhouse-Friderichsen syndrome) or pneumococcal septicemia (McCance & Huether, 1998).

Secondary renal insufficiency is usually associated with glucocorticoid deficiency and results from an abnormality in the hypothalamohypophysial-adrenal axis function (Hadley, 2000). Secondary insufficiency is associated with reduced or absent ACTH secretion. A common cause of reduced or suppressed ACTH production is prolonged steroid administration for diseases of a nonendocrine origin (Zoorob & Cender, 1998). Other causes of secondary insufficiency include pituitary tumors and infarction, hypophysectomy, irradiation of the pituitary gland, and infection.

Aldosterone deficiency is uncommon in secondary adrenal insufficiency because aldosterone's release in the body is in response to the RAAS. With normal levels of aldosterone, fluid and electrolyte imbalances are not usually seen with secondary adrenal insufficiency. Exogenous suppression of the hypothalamohypophysial-adrenal axis is generally classified as a secondary adrenal insufficiency. One source noted that 30% of patients in one ICU took steroids or had a condition requiring glucocorticoids (Zoorob & Cender, 1998).

Two rare types of familial hypocortisolism are adrenoleukodystrophy and adrenomyeloneuropathy (Balducci-Silano & Maclaren, 1996).

The two types of insufficiency are differentiated using stimulation and suppression tests, which are discussed in question 8. Primary insufficiency is more serious because of the endogenous lack of a portion of the checks and balances of the negative feedback system.

4. **Describe the components of the axis involving the hypothalamus, anterior pituitary, and the adrenal cortex. What major secretions are produced by each component, and what is the secretion's effect on the other components of the axis (i.e., stimulate or inhibit)?**

The hypothalamus produces CRH, which stimulates release of ACTH from the anterior pituitary or adenohypophysis. ACTH is derived from a much larger molecule called *proopiomelanocortin* (POMC). Included in the fragments cleaved from POMC are ACTH, MSH, β-endorphin, and β-lipotropin (Thelan, Urden, Lough, & Stacy, 1998). ACTH specifically stimulates the middle region of the adrenal cortex. This region is called the *zona fasciculata* and secretes mainly glucocorticoids. The inner zone, called the *zona reticularis,* is also stimulated somewhat by ACTH, but the zona reticularis secretes only the relatively weak adrenal sex steroids (Hadley, 2000).

ACTH, then, stimulates the zona fasciculata of the adrenal cortex to secrete glucocorticoids, the primary one being cortisol or hydrocortisone. Cortisol accounts for about 95% of the glucocorticoid activity, but the other 5% is stimulated by cortisone and corticosterone. The glucocorticoids provide negative feedback to the hypothalamus and anterior pituitary to inhibit the production of CRH and ACTH, respectively (Thelan et al, 1998). This is typical of the negative feedback pattern shown by many other hormones.

5. **The adrenal cortex secretes both glucocorticoids and mineralocorticoids. Describe the controlling mechanism of the primary mineralocorticoid aldosterone. How did this mechanism affect Mr. Catt's 7 AM electrolyte values?**

Aldosterone is the primary mineralocorticoid secreted by the outer layer of the adrenal cortex, the zona glomerulosa. Although three different mineralocorticoids are secreted by the adrenal cortex, the most important one is aldosterone, which accounts for about 95% of the mineralocorticoid activity (Thelan et al, 1998). The other major mineralocorticoid of the adrenal cortex is 11-deoxycorticosterone (Bucher & Melander, 1999). Aldosterone plays an important role in the maintenance of extracellular fluid volume and electrolyte balance. It helps maintain control of blood pressure as a result of the RAAS. The RAAS is stimulated when the body perceives a decrease in normal plasma volume. This decrease in plasma volume is detected by the renal afferent arterioles, which stimulate the juxtaglomerular (JG) cells of the juxtaglomerular apparatus (JGA) in the kidney to secrete renin. The JGA consists of JG cells and special chemoreceptor cells of the distal convoluted tubule called the macula densa (Hadley, 2000). Renin converts a plasma protein called *angiotensinogen* to angiotensin I. The angiotensin I (nonactive form) is converted to angiotensin II by an angiotensin-converting enzyme found in the lungs. Angiotensin II is one of the most powerful vasoconstrictors known. Not only does angiotensin II cause vasoconstriction, it also stimulates the adrenal cortex to produce aldosterone. The aldosterone causes increased reabsorption of sodium and its accompanying expansion of the extracellular fluid compartment (Thelan et al, 1998).

Mr. Catt's 7 AM laboratory results were as follows:

Na^+	122 mmol/L	Cl^-	88 mmol/L
K^+	6.8 mmol/L	HCO_3^-	18 mmol/L

Two mechanisms have complicated the situation. Mr. Catt already had borderline primary adrenal insufficiency or Addison's disease. Note that multiple autoimmune diseases are not uncommon in these patients. Mr. Catt's diseases include type I diabetes, Addison's disease, and ulcerative colitis (Balducci-Silano & Maclaren, 1996).

Because of lack of aldosterone, Mr. Catt is hyponatremic. Aldosterone maintains sodium levels and normally does so at the expense of the intracellular cation potassium. This is why, in the absence of aldosterone, hyperkalemia results. Recall that the sodium-potassium pump is necessary for the transport of those ions. Note that the anions chloride and bicarbonate are also reduced to maintain the normal state of a neutral charge. Mr. Catt is also experiencing an abnormal anion gap. This is calculated by subtracting total known contributing anions from cations, which, in this case, gives $122 + 6.8 - (88 + 18) = 23$. When potassium is used, any value over 15 is probably abnormal (Bullock, 1996).

6. Describe the physiologic functions of endogenous cortisol in the body. Which functions were not being performed as evidenced by Mr. Catt's 6:20 AM and 7 AM laboratory results and vital signs?

In 1936, Hans Selye published his paper "A Syndrome Produced by Diverse Nocuous Agents." This syndrome was later referred to as the general adaptation syndrome (GAS). GAS is characterized by three stages: (1) an initial alarm reaction, (2) resistance, and finally, (3) exhaustion (Hadley, 2000). These actions describe the sympathoadrenal system's response to stress. Much of the response is brought about by an increase in circulating catecholamines. However, adrenal glucocorticoids are also essential for the body's response to stress (Hadley, 2000).

Glucocorticoids are produced by the zona fasciculata of the adrenal cortex under the regulation of ACTH from the anterior pituitary (Hadley, 2000). Under normal stimuli, cortisol is released in a diurnal pattern, with peaks in the morning and dips in the evening. Stress alters this secretion rhythm. Glucocorticoids affect carbohydrate, lipid, and protein metabolism. Glucocorticoids increase free fatty acids and amino acid release from tissues. Its action is antagonistic to insulin, and excessive secretion of glucocorticoids predisposes persons to diabetes mellitus.

Glucocorticoids also have an effect on reproduction and the nervous system. They are important in the fetal period in imprinting for the fetus (Hadley, 2000).

Cortisol probably suppresses the inflammatory reaction by inhibiting release of mediators of inflammation such as kinins, histamine, and prostaglandins. Cortisol also decreases proliferation of T lymphocytes and killer cell activity and decreases the production of complement. It stimulates appetite, decreases serum calcium, sensitizes the arterioles to the effects of the catecholamines, and increases the glomerular filtration rate (Czerwiec & Cutler, 1996). The effect on the arterioles helps to maintain the blood pressure.

Cortisol assists in the maintenance of normal excitability of the myocardium and central nervous system and helps maintain emotional stability and personality. Cortisol also aids in insulin production to counterbalance the glucocorticoid-induced effects of hyperglycemia (Czerwiec & Cutler, 1996).

When the body is exposed to a stressful situation, the hypothalamus senses this stress and secretes CRH. CRH promotes release from the anterior pituitary gland of ACTH, which then stimulates the release of cortisol by the adrenal cortex. Cortisol aids in the body's adaptation to stress in three ways. First, cortisol increases glycogenesis in hepatic tissue. Second, cortisol inhibits the release of kinins, which participate in the antiinflammatory response. Third, cortisol augments the release of catecholamines from the adrenal medulla and increases blood pressure.

Mr. Catt experienced the classic signs of acute adrenal insufficiency (crisis), which include hypotension, dehydration, weakness, and tachycardia. The cardiovascular system was affected by lack of cortisol in that it has lost its vascular tone, as evidenced by orthostatic hypotension. Mr. Catt's blood pressure dropped to 65/36 mm Hg when he stood up. Although his urine osmolality was unavailable, he was probably dehydrated because of lack of aldosterone. In addition, even though Mr. Catt had type I diabetes, his glucose level was only 60 mg/dl because of the low cortisol level.

Rubin and Farber (1999) stated that because of the vagueness of the symptoms of early acute adrenal insufficiency, a high degree of suspicion would be required to make an early diagnosis. They added that orthostatic hypotension and tachycardia are almost always present. The hypotension is caused by the loss of responsiveness of the vascular system to the catecholamines, whereas the tachycardia is produced in response to the loss of vascular fluids and a drop in cardiac output. This loss stems from aldosterone deficiency, which leads to fluid and electrolyte loss, especially sodium.

7. What other hormones have been shown to interact with the RAAS and control aldosterone levels and functions? What other hormones interact with cortisol to affect its physiologic function? What are the effects?

Research has confirmed that atrial natriuretic hormone (ANH) is also important in the regulation of aldosterone and sodium and water metabolism (Griffin & Ojeda, 1996). ANH is produced by the atrial cardiocytes and is a polypeptide hormone with 28 amino acids. It produces diuresis and sodium loss (natriuresis) by inhibiting aldosterone and inhibiting release of renin and ADH from the posterior pituitary. Finally, it relaxes vessels, possibly by antagonizing angiotensin II (Hadley, 2000).

Cortisol has "permissive action" with many other hormones. *Permissive action* is a term used in endocrinology to indicate that a hormone "just has to be present in the vicinity for another hormone to carry out its action." This is the role of cortisol with the catecholamines. Cortisol's absence leads to vascular collapse and death. It is essential for synthesis within the sympathetic nerve terminals and for reuptake from the cleft. Cortisol also decreases the rate of degradation by catechol-*O*-methyltransferase. In addition, cortisol's action on fat mobilization is really its effect on the ability of catecholamines to mobilize fats. Again, cortisol seems to be necessary for the activation of enzymes involved in lipid mobilization (Hadley, 2000).

There is also neural regulation and regulation by certain vitamins and antioxidants (Capponi & Rossier, 1996). In addition, a relatively new potential regulator has been isolated from human pheochromocytoma tumor and is called *adrenomedullin*. It is described as a hypotensive polypeptide (Capponi & Rossier, 1996).

8. Define the stimulation test and the suppression test. Describe the mechanism used in Mr. Catt's diagnosis. Compare the normal hormone values involved in the hypothalamohypophysial-adrenal axis with Mr. Catt's values.

Dynamic tests of endocrine function provide information beyond that obtained from measurements of single hormones or even of hormone pairs. These tests are based on either stimulation or suppression of endogenous hormone production. The ultimate functional test of endocrine function is to demonstrate a normal response in target tissues to physiologic or stressful stimuli in vivo.

Stimulation tests are used when hypofunctioning is suspected. A tropic hormone is administered to test the capacity of a target gland to increase hormone secretion. Response is measured in plasma as an increased concentration of target hormone. One example is when ACTH is given intramuscularly (IM) or IV when the adrenal cortex is malfunctioning.

Suppression tests are used to assess suspected hyperfunctioning. They also determine whether the feedback mechanism is intact. A hormone or other inhibitory compound is administered, and suppression of the target substance is measured. For example, dexamethasone is used to assess hyperfunctioning of the pituitary in the secretion of ACTH.

Several problems exist with this type of testing, including the age of the person, the need for several subsequent stimulation tests to elicit a normal response, and the inherent rhythmicity of cycles. In addition, many drugs might interfere with the dynamic testing.

There are several types of stimulation tests available for use to test the hypothalamohypophysial-adrenal axis. These tests are the cosyntropin (Cortrosyn) test and a prolonged ACTH stimulation test, which involves collection of a 24-hour urine sample. During this test, the patient who was in a crisis situation is treated with dexamethasone, which does not interfere with the stimulation test. The single-dose metyrapone test is useful when secondary adrenal insufficiency is strongly suspected. Metyrapone is an inhibitor of the enzyme needed to convert 11-deoxycortisol to cortisol (Pagana & Pagana, 1998).

Initial diagnosis of Mr. Catt's problem involves administration of an ACTH stimulation test or cosyntropin, which is a synthetic derivative of ACTH. It should rapidly stimulate cortisol and aldosterone production. During the procedure, blood is drawn to determine a base level of cortisol. ACTH and aldosterone can also be measured. Then 0.25 mg of cosyntropin is injected IV or IM. Repeat samples of blood are drawn at 30, 60, and 90 minutes to determine the diagnosis.

A normal response to ACTH should increase plasma cortisol to at least 6 mg/dl above the baseline. The normal morning level of cortisol is 5 to 23 mg/dl or 138 to 635 nmol/L. The normal value for aldosterone is 0.015 µg/dl or 15 pg/dl. Values for ACTH range from 9 to 52 pg/ml or 2 to 11.5 pmol/L (Pagana & Pagana, 1998). Mr. Catt's cortisol and aldosterone levels are too low, and his ACTH level is too high, indicating a diagnosis of at least acute adrenal insufficiency.

9. Discuss how the diagnosis of Addison's disease is made.

Mr. Catt's diagnosis of Addison's disease is now at least a tempting one for the following reasons. He already has type I diabetes, and he has been treated for ulcerative colitis. Both of these diseases are autoimmune in nature. It is common for patients to have multiple endocrinopathies, especially if they are of the autoimmune type. Mr. Catt fails to fit one aspect of this syndrome, however; he is male, and many individuals with multiple endocrine disorders are female.

However, look at some of his laboratory values and presenting signs. His response to the ACTH stimulation test was indicative of an adrenal-deficient state. The question is whether it was only temporary, truly acute, and induced by the 15 mg of prednisone per day for 3 weeks or whether the prednisone actually was masking the onset of true primary insufficiency. According to Pagana and Pagana (1998), when the ACTH level exceeds 250 pg/ml (as does Mr. Catt's), primary adrenal insufficiency or Addison's disease is suspected. When the rapid ACTH test results are abnormal, a longer ACTH test should be performed for a conclusive diagnosis.

Mr. Catt's pale bronze skin tone indicates primary adrenal insufficiency. This hyperpigmentation, caused by excess ACTH, accompanies primary states but does not accompany the secondary states or those induced by exogenous steroid administration. Also, Mr. Catt's sodium level was extremely low. This indicates that he was having an addisonian crisis of the primary type. It could also be concluded that Mr. Catt had an exacerbation of ulcerative colitis at the same time he was slowly developing Addison's disease.

Generally, more than 80% of the adrenal gland must be destroyed before the onset of symptoms of Addison's disease. Sometimes, the hyperpigmentation appears before other symptoms appear (Saladin, 1998). The knuckles, knees, elbows, and mucous membranes are the first areas affected by the hyperpigmentation. The patient then complains of fatigue, weakness, irritability, anorexia, and depression.

10. What are the goals of treatment for adrenal crisis?

There are three main goals for treatment of the patient with adrenal crisis. The first goal is replacement of fluid volume and correction of electrolyte imbalances. This may require IV administration of as much as 5 L of fluid in the first 12 to 24 hours. Hyperkalemia often responds to volume expansion and glucocorticoid replacement (Czerwiec & Cutler, 1996). Medications should be administered to reestablish high blood levels of the adrenal steroids as the second goal. Hormonal replacement may be dexamethasone (Decadron) 4 mg IV bolus, then 4 mg every 8 hours until the quick ACTH test can be completed. Another common treatment is hydrocortisone (Solu-Cortef) 100 mg IV push as a bolus with a continuous infusion of hydrocortisone over the next 24 hours. In Mr. Catt's case, fludrocortisone (Florinef) should also be given as a single daily dose of 0.05 to 0.30 mg. The third goal is identification and correction of the underlying illness that leads to increased stress. Once Mr. Catt recovers from his ruptured appendix and the Addison's disease becomes stabilized, the insulin regimen can be readjusted.

Complications seen with glucocorticoid therapy are delayed wound healing, hyperglycemia, metabolic acidosis, and fluid retention (Zoorob & Cender, 1998).

11. What are the primary nursing considerations for patients with adrenal crisis?

One nursing diagnosis for the patient in adrenal crisis is fluid volume deficit and electrolyte imbalance. The patient may experience as much as 20% depletion of fluid volume during the crisis. The severity of fluid depletion makes restoration of fluid and electrolyte balance the primary goal (Bucher & Melander, 1999).

During the acute phase of the illness, the severity of symptoms associated with the illness makes emotional support and a calm attitude valuable in helping reduce stress. Once the crisis is over, knowledge deficit of the disease process and long-term care becomes a nursing diagnosis priority (Alspach, 1998). Exploring the role of stress in precipitating a crisis and identifying ways to avoid emotional and physical stress should occur. Knowledge regarding long-term corticosteroid use is also critical. Medication doses must not be missed, and during times of extreme stress, the patient should also consult the heath care provider for possible supplemental doses and should be encouraged to wear a Medic-Alert bracelet (Lavin, 1993).

12.   Identify potential medications for the future treatment of Mr. Catt's Addison's disease. What are their functions and potential adverse reactions?

Hydrocortisone succinate (Solu-Cortef) is a glucocorticoid that has effects similar to cortisol (Zoorob & Cender, 1998). It is also antiinflammatory and immunosuppressive. At high dosages, it has mineralocorticoid effects. The initial dose is 100 to 300 mg IV as a bolus, and then 100 mg every 8 hours in a continuous infusion is often prescribed. The main side effects include vertigo, headache, fluid and electrolyte disturbances, hypertension, congestive heart failure, and impaired wound healing. There may also be a tendency for a cushingoid appearance (Bucher & Melander, 1999).

Cortisone acetate (Cortone) is also used in the treatment of adrenal crisis. It is given as an individualized dosage of 50 mg IV every 12 hours. Its actions are the same as those of hydrocortisone.

Dexamethasone (Decadron) is used during the cosyntropin test. It is given as a 4 mg IV bolus and then 4 mg IV every 8 hours until the test is complete. Its side effects are the same as those of hydrocortisone (Bucher & Melander, 1999).

Fludrocortisone (Florinef) is used as a mineralocorticoid. It increases sodium reabsorption in renal tubules and potassium and hydrogen excretion. Its side effects include increased blood volume, edema, and hypertension. It may precipitate congestive heart failure, headaches, and weakness (Thelan et al, 1998).

13.   What concepts regarding his disease should Mr. Catt know before leaving the hospital? List the critical events that might precipitate another crisis.

Mr. Catt's instructions should include the signs and symptoms of insufficiency. His awareness of these facts is essential if he is to cope with Addison's disease and the other chronic diseases he has. Patients must adjust their dosage for mild illnesses and must maintain regular contact with their physicians. Patients also must inform all their health care professionals about their disease. Patients with Addison's disease should wear a Medic-Alert bracelet. Mr. Catt should obtain and carry with him a traveling kit containing cortisone acetate, prednisone, or deoxycorticosterone acetate for self-injection, and 100-mg vials of hydrocortisone for emergency administration by a physician (Lavin, 1993).

Mr. Catt should have a firm understanding of what type of stressors could potentially precipitate another episode of adrenal crisis. One example is a visit to a dental office. Other stressors include surgery, cold, fever, flu, or even emotional stress. Patients should consult their health care provider if any questions or concerns arise.

ADRENAL CRISIS

References

Alspach, J. G. (Ed.). (1998). *American Association of Critical-Care Nurses: Core curriculum for critical care nursing* (5th ed.). Philadelphia: Saunders.

Balducci-Silano P. L., & Maclaren, N. K. (1996). Autoimmunity and the adrenal cortex. *Current Opinion in Endocrinology and Diabetes, 3*(3), 212-219.

Bucher, L. & Melander, S. (Eds.). (1999). *Critical care nursing.* Philadelphia: Saunders.

Bullock, B. L. (1996). *Pathophysiology: Adaptations and alterations in function* (4th ed.). Philadelphia: Lippincott.

Capponi, A. M., & Rossier, M. F. (1996). Regulation of aldosterone secretion. *Current Opinion in Endocrinology and Diabetes, 3*(3), 248-257.

Czerwiec, F. S., & Cutler, G. B.(1996). Modern approach to corticosteroid replacement therapy. *Current Opinion in Endocrinology and Diabetes, 3*(3), 239-246.

Griffin, J. E., & Ojeda, S. R. (1996). *Textbook of endocrine physiology* (3rd ed.) New York: Oxford University Press.

Hadley, M. E. (2000). *Endocrinology* (4th ed.). Upper Saddle River, NJ: Prentice Hall.

Lavin, N. (1993). *Manual of endocrinology and metabolism* (2nd ed.). Boston: Little, Brown.

McCance, K. L., & Huether, S. E. (1998). *Pathophysiology—The biologic basis for disease in adults and children* (3rd ed.). St Louis: Mosby.

Pagana, K., & Pagana, T. (1998). *Manual of diagnostic and laboratory tests.* St Louis: Mosby.

Rubin, E., & Farber, J. L. (1999). *Pathology* (3rd ed.). Philadelphia: Lippincott-Raven.

Saladin, K. S. (1998). *Anatomy & physiology: The unity of form and function.* Boston: WCB/McGraw-Hill.

Thelan, L., Urden, L., Lough, M., & Stacy, K. (1998). *Critical care nursing: Diagnosis and management* (3rd ed.). St Louis: Mosby.

Zoorob, R. J., & Cender, D. (1998). A different look at corticosteroids. *American Family Practice, 58*(2), 443-450.

CHAPTER 21

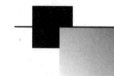

SYNDROME OF INAPPROPRIATE SECRETION OF ANTIDIURETIC HORMONE

Colleen R. Walsh, RN, MSN, ONC, ACNP-C

CASE PRESENTATION

Mrs. Carrie Lewis, a 77-year-old white woman, was transported to the emergency department (ED) by the local emergency medical service unit after falling at home. She was alert and oriented to time, place, and person and complained of severe right hip pain. Radiographs taken in the ED revealed a comminuted right femoral neck fracture, and an orthopedic consultation was obtained. Because of Mrs. Lewis's history of chronic airflow limitation as a result of long-standing asthma, it was believed that total hip arthroplasty (THA) performed under spinal anesthesia would allow for early ambulation and lessen the chances that she would develop significant pulmonary problems after surgery. In addition, early ambulation would also protect her from developing complications of immobility such as deep vein thrombosis (DVT), pulmonary thromboembolism, and skin breakdown from prolonged bed rest. Her medical workup in the ED included a chest radiograph, electrocardiogram (ECG), complete blood count (CBC), metabolic profile (Chem 7), and pulse oximetry. The results obtained were as follows.

The chest x-ray film did not show evidence of acute pulmonary processes although the diaphragm was slighted flattened consistent with longstanding asthma.

The ECG showed normal sinus rhythm with a rate of 84 without evidence of ischemia or axis deviation.

The CBC showed the following:

| WBCs | 9400/mm^3 | Hgb | 12.1 g/dl |
| RBCs | 3.9×10^6/mm^3 | Hct | 39% |

Chem 7 results were as follows:

Glucose	92 mg/dl	K$^+$	4.2 mmol/L
BUN	18 mg/dl	CO$_2$	37 mmol/L
Creatinine	1.1 mg/dl	Cl$^-$	97 mmol/L
Na$^+$	130 mmol/L	Pulse oximetry	94% with room air

Vital signs were as follows:

BP	134/78 mm Hg	Respirations	18 breaths/min
Pulse	84 bpm	Temperature	37° C (98.6° F)

Home medications included albuterol (metered-dose inhaler) as needed for her asthma, ibuprofen as needed for arthritis, and paroxetine (Paxil) 20 mg/day orally, which was started 10 days before admission for treatment of situational depression caused by the death of her husband 6 months previously. She denied any food or medicine allergy.

Mrs. Lewis was taken from the ED to the operating room, where she underwent successful right THA. She tolerated the procedure well, and after an uneventful course in the postanesthesia care unit, she was transferred to the orthopedic unit in stable condition. Per the THA clinical pathway, Mrs. Lewis had an intravenous (IV) solution of 5% dextrose in half-normal saline (D5½NS) at 100 ml/hr running into a peripheral line, a Hemovac drain to self-suction from the right hip incision, bilateral thigh-high elastic stockings with sequential compression devices, and an abduction pillow between her legs. She was also given a morphine sulfate patient-controlled analgesia (PCA) pump with a basal rate of 1 mg/hr with an as-needed dose of 1 mg every 10 minutes.

On postoperative day 1, Mrs. Lewis was lethargic and confused to time and place but oriented to person, and it was believed that she was having an adverse reaction to the morphine sulfate, which was discontinued. She was slightly more alert later in the day and was able to be out of bed to the chair as per the clinical pathway. She was slightly nauseous with decreased oral intake, and her IV infusion rate was increased to 125 ml/hr. During the evening, her physical assessment revealed pulmonary inspiratory and expiratory wheezes with rhonchi and the physician was notified. Pulse oximetry revealed arterial blood oxygen saturation (Sao_2) of 89% with room air, and nebulized aerosol treatments with albuterol were ordered. These did not relieve her wheezes and her Sao_2 continued to be 88% despite the addition of 2 L of oxygen via nasal cannula. She was transferred to the intensive care unit (ICU) for monitoring of her acute exacerbation of asthma.

Intensive Care Unit

On admission to the ICU, she was given ventilatory assistance with a 40% face mask, and blood was immediately drawn for testing. The data revealed the following:

Na^+	116 mmol/L	Glucose	126 mg/dl
K^+	3.5 mmol/L	Creatinine	0.8 mg/dl
Cl^-	86 mmol/L	Hgb	9.1 g/dl
BUN	9 mg/dl	Hct	27%

Immediate serum and urine osmolality tests were ordered and revealed the following:

Serum osmolality	243 mOsm/kg
Urine osmolality	541 mOsm/kg (serum osmolality + 100)

A pulmonary artery (Swan-Ganz) catheter was inserted to measure fluid and cardiac status. IV fluids were changed to 3% sodium chloride at 150 ml/hr. Furosemide (Lasix) 80 mg IV push was given. Mrs. Lewis then received demeclocycline (Declomycin) 250 mg four times daily. She remained confused and lethargic, but her respiratory wheezes improved after three albuterol treatments and her Sao_2 improved to 95%.

Twenty-two hours later, laboratory data were as follows:

Na^+	132 mmol/L	Serum osmolality	275 mOsm/kg
K^+	3.2 mmol/L	Urine osmolality	400 mOsm/kg (serum
Cl^-	98 mmol/L		osmolality + 100)

At this time, her IV infusion was changed to 5% dextrose in normal saline at 50 ml/hr. Over the next 24 hours, Mrs. Lewis was weaned off the oxygen; was alert and oriented to time, place, and person; and had the following vital signs:

BP	130/78 mm Hg	Respirations	20 breaths/min
Pulse	100 bpm	Temperature	37.3° C (99.2° F)

A fluid restriction of 1200 mg/day was prescribed. The demeclocycline was continued, and furosemide 40 mg twice daily was started. After 2 days, she was transferred back to the orthopedic unit, where she continued to recover from her THA, and on postoperative day 9, she was transferred to a rehabilitation center, where she remained symptom free and eventually returned home independent in all activities of daily living.

SYNDROME OF INAPPROPRIATE SECRETION OF ANTIDIURETIC HORMONE

Questions

1. Define syndrome of inappropriate secretion of antidiuretic hormone (SIADH).
2. Describe the role of ADH in water regulation.
3. Explain the pathophysiology associated with SIADH.
4. Identify the common symptoms associated with SIADH.
5. Explain the effects of SIADH on the major organs.
6. Discuss laboratory studies that are pertinent in diagnosing and treating SIADH.
7. Identify the common causes of SIADH.
8. Discuss why elderly patients are more prone to developing SIADH.
9. Discuss the medical management of SIADH.
10. Discuss the pharmacologic treatment for SIADH.
11. Describe the role that hemodynamic monitoring would have in the treatment of patients with SIADH.
12. Discuss the factors that contributed to the development of SIADH in Mrs. Lewis.
13. Identify pertinent nursing diagnoses for Mrs. Lewis.
14. Discuss the nursing care required for Mrs. Lewis.

SYNDROME OF INAPPROPRIATE SECRETION OF ANTIDIURETIC HORMONE

Questions and Answers

1. **Define syndrome of inappropriate antidiuretic hormone secretion (SIADH).**

SIADH is a group of symptoms that occurs when antidiuretic hormone (ADH, arginine vasopressin) is secreted in the presence of low plasma osmolality. A decrease in plasma osmolality normally inhibits ADH production and secretion. SIADH is characterized by fluid retention, dilutional hyponatremia, hypochloremia, concentrated urine, and lack of intravascular volume depletion (Konick-McMahon, 1999a). SIADH is characterized by normal to increased blood volume in normoproteinemic, nonedematous, hyponatremic patients with normal renal and endocrine function (Narins, Faber, & Krishna, 1998).

2. **Describe the role of ADH in water regulation.**

ADH regulates the body's water balance. It is synthesized in the hypothalamus and stored in the posterior pituitary gland. When released into the circulation, it acts on the kidney's distal tubules and collecting ducts, increasing their permeability to water. This decreases urine volume because more water is being reabsorbed and returned to the circulation. Two mechanisms control ADH release. The first mechanism is serum osmolality (the concentration of electrolytes and other osmotically active particles). When serum osmolality increases, osmoreceptors in the hypothalamus are stimulated, resulting in increased secretion of ADH. Water is reabsorbed, which dilutes the serum and lowers the osmolality.

The second mechanism controlling the release of ADH is blood volume. Baroreceptors in the left atrium are sensitive to changes in pressure. When blood volume rises, pressure on the baroreceptor increases. This stimulus prevents ADH release, so urine output increases and blood volume returns to normal levels. Conversely, a drop in pressure triggers ADH release. The kidney then conserves fluid, and this increases blood volume (Huether & Tomkey, 1998).

If too much ADH is released, SIADH results. If not enough ADH is released at the appropriate time, diabetes insipidus (DI) results. DI decreases water reabsorption and results in elevated serum osmolality and a low urine osmolality (Bennett, 1999; Konick-McMahon, 1999a).

3. **Explain the pathophysiology associated with SIADH.**

In SIADH, ADH continues to be released in the presence of below-normal serum osmolality, when normally its secretion is inhibited. This results in a simultaneous urine osmolality that is more than that of serum. Dilutional hyponatremia occurs from an increase in tubular reabsorption of water. The retention of water leads to expanded plasma volume. This increase in extracellular fluid causes an increase in the glomerular filtration rate and increases renal excretion of sodium (Baker, Defersor, & Hardwick, 1999; Konick-McMahon, 1999a). The expansion of the plasma volume also inhibits the release of renin and aldosterone (Huether &

Tomkey, 1998). Aldosterone is a mineralocorticoid that is released by the adrenal cortex in the presence of angiotensin II. It directly regulates sodium balance because of the sodium-water relationship. Because sodium in solution exerts osmotic pressure (water-pulling effect), water follows low sodium in physiologic proportional amounts. As a result of this sodium-water relationship, aldosterone secretion also indirectly regulates water balance. The primary target tissue for aldosterone is the renal tubular epithelium. Aldosterone secretion is stimulated by a series of events that occurs in response either to decreased sodium levels in the extracellular fluid or to an increased sodium load in the renal tubular fluid (Foster, 1999; Huether, 1998a).

Renin acts enzymatically on the inactive plasma protein angiotensin I. Angiotensin I is further decreased by angiotensin-converting enzyme, which seems to be produced in the lung and secreted into the blood. The converting enzyme catalyzes the reaction in which angiotensin I is changed to angiotensin II (Huether, 1998b).

Angiotensin II causes vasoconstriction of many blood vessels and increases selective blood flow to the kidney. If serum sodium concentration is low and blood volume is above normal, the efferent arteriole is constricted. Efferent arteriolar constriction causes the effective filtration pressure in the glomerulus to be raised, which increases glomerular filtration and urinary output. If serum sodium levels are low and blood volume is normal or low, angiotensin II causes constriction of the afferent arteriole. Blood flow to the glomerulus is then diminished, and effective filtration pressure is low, which decreases glomerular filtration and urinary output. This action preserves vascular volume while restoring the sodium concentration. At the same time, angiotensin II stimulates the release of the aldosterone from the adrenal cortex (Huether, 1998b; Huether & Tomkey, 1998).

Aldosterone exerts its effects primarily on the distal convoluted tubules of the nephrons. The major effect is the reabsorption of filtered sodium in exchange for excretion of potassium. This effect appears to be mediated via indirect activation of the sodium-potassium pumps in the tubular epithelial membranes. Osmotic water reabsorption passively occurs at the same time in response to sodium reabsorption. This response constitutes a physiologic coping mechanism during volume depletion or sodium depletion states (Peshman, 1996).

The release of aldosterone is inhibited in SIADH because of the expansion of plasma volume; therefore potassium levels may fluctuate because the secretion of potassium is influenced by aldosterone. When the kidney under the influence of aldosterone reabsorbs sodium, potassium is usually secreted. However, the aldosterone secretion and sodium reabsorption are inhibited in SIADH. Therefore potassium secretion will be diminished and potassium levels may increase; hypokalemia is rare (Brown, 1996).

Hypochloremia is also caused by inhibition of aldosterone secretion. Aldosterone indirectly regulates chloride homeostasis through its effect on sodium. Aldosterone causes sodium to be actively reabsorbed by renal tubular epithelium, and chloride follows passively because of the electrical attraction of cations and anions. However, in SIADH, sodium is not being reabsorbed into the circulation but is being secreted into the urine. According to the sodium-chloride relationship, chloride will not be reabsorbed, which leads to hypochloremia (Huether, 1998a).

The differential diagnosis between hyponatremia caused by SIADH and a modest decrease in serum sodium is that in the latter, sodium is conserved so that the urine sodium level should be less than 10 to 15 mmol/day. In contrast, in SIADH, the urine sodium level is high because of natriuresis (Peshman, 1996).

4. Identify the common symptoms associated with SIADH.

Early symptoms of SIADH include headache, weakness, anorexia, muscle cramps, and weight gain. As the serum sodium level decreases, the patient experiences personality changes, hostility, sluggish deep tendon reflexes, nausea, vomiting, diarrhea, and oliguria. Confusion, lethargy, and Cheyne-Stokes respirations herald impending crisis. When the serum sodium level drops below 110 mmol/L, seizures, coma, and death may occur (Abrams, Beers, & Berkow, 1999; Konick-McMahon, 1999a).

The severity of the symptoms is directly related to the serum sodium levels and underlying medical conditions that may have precipitated the SIADH (Narins et al, 1998). The rapidity in the decline of the sodium levels also influences the presentation of symptoms, with more severe, life-threatening symptoms occurring with a rapid decline in the sodium level (Konick-McMahon, 1999a; Narins et al, 1998).

5. Explain the effects of SIADH on the major organs.

The central nervous, cardiac, and respiratory systems are affected by water intoxication. The primary cause of cerebral edema, the central nervous system effect, is the shift of the intracellular fluid, leading to symptoms of increased intracranial pressure. With the rapid depletion of serum sodium in hypotonic hyponatremias, brain cells exhibit compensatory changes in cell volume by exporting solutes (sodium, potassium, and organic acids) and inactivating osmoles (Narins et al, 1998). The neurologic findings in SIADH are consistent with water intoxication or free water in the vascular system. As a result of serum dilution of sodium by the excess free water, the osmolality of the serum decreases. The brain, which has a higher osmolality, attracts and draws water from the serum into the brain cells, causing cerebral edema (Konick-McMahon, 1999a).

Alterations in cardiac output are associated with the hyponatremia and increased circulating intravascular volume. The patient will experience weight gain without evidence of edema, and the patient's blood pressure and pulse may be elevated in response to the increased circulating volume as well as elevated pressure in neck veins (Konick-McMahon, 1999a). Respiratory assessment findings may include crackles in the lungs as a result of fluid volume excess and central nervous system suppression of the natural respiratory drive. Hypoxemia has been associated with worse outcomes in patients with SIADH because hypoxemia is an underlying cause of SIADH in critically ill patients (Clinician Reviews, 1999). Gastrointestinal tract involvement is again related to the hyponatremia and is manifested by nausea, vomiting, and diarrhea (Konick-McMahon, 1999a). Renal manifestations of SIADH include decreased urine output related to the effects of ADH on the kidney to conserve water (Konick-McMahon, 1999a).

6. Discuss laboratory studies that are pertinent in diagnosing and treating SIADH.

Many laboratory values are helpful in diagnosing SIADH. The most important concept for the practitioner to remember is that adrenal, renal, and thyroid disorders that often manifest as SIADH must be excluded (Konick-McMahon, 1999b).

Thyroid function and cosyntropin stimulation tests can be used to determine whether these are the cause of the hyponatremia (Okuda, Kurokawa, & Papadakis, 1999). The serum sodium level is decreased to less than 130 mEq/L, as is the serum osmolality (<280 mOsm/kg). The serum osmolality (normally 285 to 285 mOsm/kg) can be calculated using the following formula (Okuda et al, 1999):

$$Osmolality = 2(Na^+ mmol/L) + Glucose mmol/L + BUN mmol/L$$

The urine osmolality is inappropriately elevated (>150 mOsm/kg). The blood urea nitrogen (BUN) level is usually less than 10 mg/dl with a low plasma uric acid level of less than 4 mg/dl (Okuda et al, 1999). This not only is dilutional in nature but also results from increased urea and uric acid clearances in response to the volume-expanded states (Okuda et al, 1999). Chloride levels are also below normal in proportion to the serum sodium. Urine-specific gravity is increased with very concentrated urine. Urine osmolality can be greater than 100% of the serum osmolality. Another diagnostic test, plasma ADH, will demonstrate elevated levels (Litwack, 1998). Specific tests may be ordered to diagnose the underlying cause of SIADH.

7. Identify the common causes of SIADH.

Almost any physiologic abnormality can result in SIADH. The important goal of treatment is to correct the SIADH and then identify any underlying disease process.
Specific body system causes are as follows.

Central Nervous System

Central nervous system causes include head trauma, intracranial hemorrhage, encephalitis, brain tumors, Guillain-Barré syndrome, brain abscess, nonhemorrhagic cerebral vascular accident (Cooke, Latif, Huch, & Wall, 1998; Litwack, 1998; Konick-McMahon, 1999b).

Cardiovascular System

Hypotension, hypovolemia, and redistribution of plasma into the interstitial space all trigger baroreceptor-mediated release of arginine vasopressin (Narins et al, 1998). Congestive heart failure can also trigger baroreceptors in the right atrium (Epstein, 1998), and decreased left atrial filling pressure stimulates ADH release (Litwack, 1998).

Pulmonary System

Chronic pulmonary diseases such as asthma and emphysema can cause SIADH. Any pulmonary process, such as bacterial or fungal pneumonias, tuberculosis, lung abscesses, cystic fibrosis, or infiltrative disease that results in hypoxemia, can initiate SIADH (Clinician Reviews, 1999; Konick-McMahon, 1999b; Narins et al, 1998; Okuda et al, 1999). Prolonged positive-pressure ventilation has also been implicated in the development of SIADH (Litwack, 1998; Narins et al, 1998).

Renal/Hepatic Causes

Hypoproteinemic states such as cirrhosis and nephrosis can stimulate release of ADH, and these disorders limit the excretion of free water (Narins et al, 1998). Chronic renal insufficiency and renal failure cause the glomerular filtration rate to fall, and the absolute volume of filtrate reaching the distal sites decreases (Narins et al, 1998). As renal function decreases, the maximal amount of free water that can be excreted also decreases, and even minimal increases in water intake may lead to hyponatremia (Narins et al, 1998). Hyponatremia without hypoosmolality can occur with elevated triglyceride levels, genitourinary irrigations, or azotemia (Konick-McMahon, 1999b).

Hematologic/Oncologic Causes

Primary neoplasms are often the cause of SIADH. Oat cell carcinoma of the lung, duodenal carcinoma, pancreatic cancer, thymoma, head and neck cancers, and lymphoma are the usual neoplastic diseases that trigger SIADH (Ferlito, Rinaldo, & Devaney, 1997; Konick-McMahon, 1999b). It is believed that these neoplasms secrete ADH from the tumor cells independently from the adrenal-pituitary axis.

Psychogenic Causes

Psychogenic polydipsia can occur in psychiatric patients who consume large volumes of water, often exceeding 10 L/day. Normal intravascular volume is maintained through the renal secretion of sodium (Okuda et al, 1999). This is not true in SIADH and can be corrected with water restrictions, but patients will have low serum sodium levels with suppressed ADH levels (Okuda et al, 1999).

Pharmacologic Therapy

Many drugs have been identified as contributing directly or indirectly to the development of SIADH. These drugs can be divided into two categories: those that stimulate ADH production and those that potentiate ADH action (Okuda et al, 1999).

Drugs That Increase ADH Production

- *Antidepressants:* tricyclic antidepressants, monoamine oxidase inhibitors, imipramine, desipramine, clomipramine, fluoxetine, and paroxetine (Konick-McMahon, 1999b; Monmany, Vasquez, Rodriguez, & Domingo, 1999; Okuda et al, 1999)
- *Antineoplastics:* cyclophosphamide, vincristine, and vinblastine (Konick-McMahon, 1999b; Okuda et al, 1999)
- *Neuroleptics:* thiothixene, thioridazine, fluphenazine, haloperidol, and trifluoperazine (Okuda et al, 1999)

Drugs That Potentiate ADH Action

- *Miscellaneous:* tolbutamide, carbamazepine, morphine sulfate, chlorpropamide, cyclophosphamide, nonsteroidal antiinflammatory drugs, and somatostatin (Konick-McMahon, 1999b; Okuda et al, 1999).

Surgical Procedures

Postoperative hyponatremia is caused by surgical stress, which stimulates ADH secretion in most patients. This promotes water retention for up to 5 days after surgery, leading to SIADH (Lane & Allen, 1999). Women are more often affected than men because of their smaller intravascular fluid volumes and sex-related hormonal factors (Lane & Allen, 1999). Premenopausal women can demonstrate symptoms of SIADH with serum sodium levels as high as 128 mmol/L, whereas postmenopausal woman do not usually exhibit symptoms until the serum sodium level reaches 120 mmol/L, although this varies depending on the rapidity of the change in sodium levels (Lane & Allen, 1999).

The risk of hyponatremia is especially significant in women receiving routine infusions of isotonic dextrose. After surgery, patients metabolize glucose almost immediately, so these isotonic solutions are in effect hypotonic (Lane & Allen,

1999). Volumes of isotonic solutions as low as 3 to 4 L over 2 days may cause convulsions, respiratory arrest, permanent brain damage, and death in women who were healthy before admission (Lane & Allen, 1999).

The postoperative setting is especially conducive to the development of SIADH. Pain, narcotics, hypoxemia, hypotension, and positive-pressure ventilation all increase the risk of SIADH (Konick-McMahon, 1999b; Litwack, 1998; Narins et al, 1998).

Four major clinician-mediated factors have been identified as contributing to SIADH: (1) failing to recognize those patients at high risk, (2) confusing early symptoms of hyponatremia with postoperative sequelae, (3) disregarding the dangers of routine infusions of hypotonic solutions, and (4) attributing serious neurologic symptoms of hyponatremic encephalopathy to other conditions such as stroke (Lane & Allen, 1999). Patients at risk for developing SIADH should be identified before surgical procedures and appropriate monitoring instituted.

8. Discuss why elderly patients are more prone to developing SIADH.

The incidence of adverse drug reactions (ADRs) increases with age. Until recently, elderly persons, especially those with multiple medical problems, have been excluded from most clinical drug trials (Pollock, 1999). That has left a gap in the literature concerning the actual causes of ADRs, but several theories have been postulated: drug metabolism via the cytochrome P450 isoenzyme pathway may be slower in elderly persons; the elderly person's homeostatic mechanisms may be decreased; the anticholinergic properties of many medications may lead to increased thirst with increased water intake; and catecholamine activity encourages the release of ADH (Pollock, 1999).

Another factor that possibly contributes to the development of SIADH is the polypharmacy required by elderly patients to control chronic disease (Pollock, 1999). The use of thiazide diuretics is known to increase the risk of development of SIADH (Narins et al, 1998). A careful patient history and review of the medications patients take may help alert clinicians to the possibility of SIADH. Because of the prevalence of orthopedic injuries in many patients with SIADH, many resulting from hyponatremic encephalopathy, it is recommended that elderly patients with acute orthopedic injuries be screened for hyponatremia (Ayus & Arieff, 1999).

9. Discuss the medical management of SIADH.

The primary treatment of mild SIADH is fluid restriction to reverse hyponatremia (Epstein, 1998; Ferri, 1998; Konick-McMahon, 1999b; Narins et al, 1998). The amount of fluid restriction is driven by the severity of the hyponatremia. As serum sodium levels return to normal, fluid intake may be increased to equal urine output plus insensible loss. Sodium intake should be increased by no more than 1 to 2 mmol/L/hr or 10 to 20 mmol/L/day (Konick-McMahon, 1999b). Too-rapid correction can lead to seizures, coma, and death (Narins et al, 1998).

If the SIADH is thought to be drug related, the drug responsible must be identified and stopped (Pollock, 1999). If the drug identified is an antidepressant, the drug should be stopped and the hyponatremia should be corrected. The drug may then be restarted at a lower dosage with frequent monitoring of electrolyte levels (Monmany et al, 1999; Pollock, 1999).

Hypertonic IV fluids should be initiated if there are neurologic symptoms suggesting cerebral edema (Konick-McMahon, 1999b; Narins et al, 1998). A 3% saline solution causes water to be excreted from the cells and reduces the brain cell edema. Extreme caution is needed when using this hypertonic solution because rapid infusion can cause cerebral osmotic demyelination syndrome (Lane & Allen, 1999; Litwack, 1998). Serum sodium levels should be monitored at least every 2 hours (Lane & Allen, 1999). Once the sodium level returns to normal, a normal saline solution (0.9% NaCl) should be used with a potassium replacement to prevent hypokalemia (Litwack, 1998). A high-sodium diet can also be ordered to increase the sodium levels (Konick-McMahon, 1999b). The calculations for volume and infusion rate correction are as follows (Konick-McMahon, 1999b):

Volume of 3% saline = 0.6 × Weight (kg) ×
(Desired Na - Current Na)/3 mmol/L

Infusion rate = Volume of 3% saline rate of correction/
(Desired Na - Current Na)

10. Discuss the pharmacologic treatment for SIADH.

The standard drug therapy for SIADH includes use of furosemide (Lasix) and demeclocycline (Declomycin). Lithium carbonate can also be used if ADH antagonism is needed (Konick-McMahon, 1999b; Narins et al, 1998). Furosemide is used to reduce the circulating intravascular volume by producing diuresis. Because large volumes of urine will be excreted, electrolytes, especially potassium, should be monitored closely (Litwack, 1998).

Demeclocycline also may be used. Demeclocycline is a tetracycline derivative that interferes with ADH's antidiuretic action and causes nephrogenic DI. The normal dose is 1 g given in four divided doses daily. This drug has the potential for nephrotoxic side effects; therefore it is imperative that electrolyte levels, especially BUN and creatinine, be monitored closely. Patients with cirrhosis have a higher risk of developing renal compromise if given demeclocycline (Narins et al, 1998).

11. Describe the role that hemodynamic monitoring would have in the treatment of patients with SIADH.

An arterial line would be helpful in monitoring the patient's blood pressure on an ongoing basis to evaluate cardiac output and peripheral resistance. A pulmonary artery (Swan-Ganz) catheter could be used to evaluate the ability of the heart to handle volume changes. The right atrial pressure measures preload (pressure generated at the end of diastole), which reflects the volume delivered to the heart. Because a change in the right atrial filling pressures is one of the precipitating factors in the development of SIADH, this would be an important measurement to track (Epstein, 1998). The pulmonary capillary wedge pressure measures afterload (resistance to ejection after systole), another important measure of volume status. Many of these patients already have pulmonary artery catheters in place for monitoring of the underlying disease process that stimulated the development of SIADH. In that case, monitoring the trends is an important nursing consideration.

12. Discuss the factors that contributed to the development of SIADH in Mrs. Lewis.

Mrs. Lewis had many factors that caused her to develop SIADH. The following are the major contributors:

- Mrs. Lewis's age of 73
- Her preoperative sodium level of 130 mmol/L, which was not investigated or corrected before surgery
- Her history of asthma
- The use of an isotonic/hypotonic IV solution of D5½NS over several days because of her nausea and vomiting
- The use of morphine sulfate PCA, which her postoperative confusion was attributed to but again, not fully investigated
- The recent addition of paroxetine, which can cause hyponatremia (usually within 10 days after the start of therapy), to her medication regimen (Monmany et al, 1999)
- Mrs. Lewis's acute episode of bronchospasms secondary to her asthma, which resulted in hypoxemia

13. Identify pertinent nursing diagnoses for Mrs. Lewis.

- Fluid volume excess related to a compromised regulatory mechanism and intravenous fluid overload
- Altered thought processes related to cerebral edema
- Alteration in nutrition: less than body requirements related to anorexia, nausea, vomiting
- High risk of injury related to confusion and post operative THA status
- Knowledge deficit related to diagnosis and treatment
- Impaired physical mobility related to THA
- Self-care deficits: partial in bathing, dressing, and toileting related to post-operative status and confusion
- Potential for neurovascular compromise related to THA
- Impaired gas exchange related to bronchospasms secondary to asthma
- Anxiety related to hospitalization and discontinuation of antidepressant/antianxiety medication (Cox et al, 1997)

14. Discuss the nursing care required for Mrs. Lewis.

Continual assessment of Mrs. Lewis's condition is imperative. Vital signs should be monitored closely, with physical assessment data correlating with the hemodynamic parameters being monitored. Neurologic assessment should be done hourly during the critical part of the disease process. Serum sodium levels should be obtained at least every 2 hours during hypertonic saline infusions (Konick-McMahon, 1999b). Seizure precautions should be instituted. Accurate hourly measurement of intake and output, including Hemovac drainage, provides valuable information on volume status. Daily weighing is important in assessing fluid status.

Because nutrition may be a problem, skin protection should be incorporated into the care plan. The elastic stockings and sequential compression devices should be removed three times daily for skin care and inspection. Good oral hygiene is important because the patient will have fluid restrictions. Preventing nausea and vomiting with use of antiemetics is helpful because electrolyte balance will be difficult to maintain.

As part of the THA critical pathway, abduction of Mrs. Lewis's legs with an abduction pillow should be maintained at all times to prevent hip dislocation. She should not sit with her hips flexed greater than 60 degrees, and an elevated toilet seat should be obtained. Mrs. Lewis should be turned to her affected side to prevent dislocation of her prosthesis because her body weight will act as a splint to prevent dislocation.

Prevention of DVT is a major component of the care for Mrs. Lewis. The low-molecular-weight heparin should be administered as ordered, and careful monitoring of the bleeding studies is essential. Mrs. Lewis should be assisted with her active and passive range-of-motion exercises, including dorsiflexion and circumduction of both her feet, and quadriceps and gluteal setting exercises. She should receive assistance to get out of bed to the chair. Physical and occupational therapy consultations should be obtained to assist with procurement of assistive devices.

Patient teaching should be an ongoing part of nursing care. The nurse should work with Mrs. Lewis and her family to ensure that they understand the treatment plan, the rationale for the plan, and the expected outcomes (Cox et al, 1998). One of the most important aspects of Mrs. Lewis's teaching is to instruct her to notify other physicians, especially dentists, that she has an artificial hip joint. Prophylactic antibiotics should be given before any dental work, including cleaning, to prevent infection of the new joint from oral bacteria.

SYNDROME OF INAPPROPRIATE SECRETION OF ANTIDIURETIC HORMONE

References

Abrams, W. B., Beers, M. H., & Berkow, R. *Merck Manual of Geriatrics.* (1999). Water and electrolyte disorders [WWW document]. URL http://www.merck.com/pubs/mm_geriatrics/3x.htm.

Ayus, J. C., & Arieff, A. I. (1999). Chronic hyponatremic encephalopathy in postmenopausal women: Association of therapies with morbidity and mortality. *Journal of the American Medical Association 281,* 2299-2304.

Baker, K., Defersor, R., & Hardwick, R. (1999). Endocrine assessment. In L. Bucher & S. D. Melander (Eds.). *Critical care nursing* (pp. 612-642). Philadelphia: WB Saunders.

Bennett, M. (1999) Fluid and electrolytes N205 nursing care of the adult I [WWW document]. URL http://www.indstate.edu/nurs/mary/fluid98/outlinee.htm.

Brown, D. (1996). Patients with disorders of neurohypophysis, thyroid and adrenals. In J. M. Clochesy, C. Breu, S. Cardin, A. A. Whittaker, & E. B. Rudy (Eds.). *Critical care nursing* (2nd ed., pp. 1122-1136). Philadelphia: WB Saunders.

Clinician Reviews. (1999). In house—Treating hyponatremia is a narrow path. *Clinician reviews 9*(9),111-121.

Cooke, C. R., Latif, K. A., Huch, K. M., & Wall, B. M. (1998). Inappropriate antidiuresis and hyponatremia with suppressible vasopressin in Guillain-Barré syndrome. *Journal of American Nephrology 18*(1), 71-78.

Cox, H. C., Hinz, M. D., Lubno, M. A., Newfield, S. A., Ridenour, N. A., Slater, M. M., & Sridaromont, K. L. (1997). *Clinical applications of nursing diagnosis: Adult, child, women's, psychiatric, gerontic, and home health considerations* (3rd ed.). Philadelphia: FA Davis.

Epstein, M. (1998). Disorders of sodium balance. In Stein, J. H. (Ed.). *Internal medicine* (5th ed., pp. 816-825). St Louis: Mosby.

Ferlito, A., Rinaldo, A., & Devaney, K. O. (1997). Syndrome of inappropriate antidiuretic hormone secretion associated with head and neck cancers: Review of the literature. *Annals of Otology, Rhinology and Laryngology 106*(10), 878-883.

Ferri, F. (1998). Endocrinology. In F. Ferri (Ed.). *Practical guide to the care of the medical patient* (5th ed., pp. 310-385). St Louis: Mosby.

Foster, J. D. (1999). Syndrome of inappropriate antidiuretic hormone secretion (SIADH) [WWW document]. URL http://www.emedicine.com/emerg/topic784.htm.

Huether, S. E. (1998a). The cellular environment: Fluids and electrolytes, acids and bases. In K. A. McCune & S. E. Huether (Eds.). *Pathophysiology: the biological basis for disease in adults and children* (3rd ed., pp. 82-113). St Louis: Mosby.

Huether, S. E. (1998b). Alteration of renal urinary tract function. In K. A. McCune & S. E. Huether (Eds.). *Pathophysiology: the biological basis for disease in adults and children* (3rd ed., pp. 1244-1272). St Louis: Mosby.

Huether, S. E., & Tomkey, D.(1998). Alterations of hormonal regulation. In K. A. McCance & S. E. Huether (Eds.). *Pathophysiology: the biological basis for disease in adults and children* (3rd ed., pp. 656-706). St Louis: Mosby.

Konick-McMahon, J. (1999a). Diabetes insipidus and syndrome of inappropriate antidiuretic hormone. In L. Bucher & S. D. Melander (Eds.). *Critical care nursing* (pp. 643-654). Philadelphia: WB Saunders.

Konick-McMahon, J. (1999b). Fluid, electrolyte, and acid-base abnormalities. In P. Logan (Ed.). *Principles of practice for the acute care nurse practitioner* (pp. 226-235). Stamford, CT: Appleton & Lange.

Lane, N., & Allen, K. (1999). Hyponatremia after orthopaedic surgery: Ignorance of the effects of hyponatremia is widespread-and damaging. *British Medical Journal 318*(7195), 1363-1364.

Litwack, L. (1998). The endocrine system. In J. G. Alspach (Ed.). *American Association of Critical-Care Nurses:* Core curriculum for critical care nursing (5th ed., pp. 565-600). Philadelphia: WB Saunders.

Monmany, J., Vasquez, G., Rodriguez, J., & Domingo, P. (1999). Syndrome of inappropriate secretion of antidiuretic hormone induced by paroxetine. *Archives of Internal Medicine 159*(17), 2089-2090.

Narins, R. G., Faber, M. D., & Krishna, G. G. (1998). Disorders of water balance. In J. H. Stein (Ed.). *Internal medicine* (5th ed., pp. 805-816). St Louis: Mosby.

Okuda, T., Kurokawa, K., & Papadakis, M. A. (1999). Fluid and electrolyte disorders. In L. M. Tierney, S. J. McPhee, & M. A. Papadakis (Eds.). *Current medical diagnosis and treatment* (38th ed., pp. 838-862). Stamford, CT: Appleton & Lange.

Peshman, P. (1996). Renal physiology. In J. M. Clochesy, C. Breu, S. Cardin, A. A. Whittaker, & E. B. Rudy (Eds.). *Critical care nursing* (2nd ed., pp. 871-891). Philadelphia: WB Saunders.

Pollock, B. G. (1999). Adverse reactions of antidepressants in elderly patients. *The Journal of Clinical Psychiatry 605*, 4-7.

CHAPTER 22

DIABETIC KETOACIDOSIS

Anne G. Denner, MS Biology, BSN

CASE PRESENTATION

Brady Wilson, a 39-year-old, 63-kg (140-lb) African-American man, was admitted to the hospital with diabetic ketoacidosis (DKA). After arrival at the emergency department, he had multiple episodes of vomiting. Mr. Wilson said he had been vomiting for the past 2 days and admitted to skipping several doses of insulin recently. He mentioned that he had feverish feelings at home and reported an occasional cough.

Mr. Wilson's assessment revealed pain throughout all abdominal quadrants, with "cramping" reported in all four abdominal quadrants. He was extremely lethargic and difficult to arouse at times. He complained of severe thirst. His skin was extremely dry. An electrocardiogram showed a sinus tachycardia at 120 bpm. His lungs were clear bilaterally, but respirations were deep and rapid. There was an acetone smell to Mr. Wilson's breath.

Mr. Wilson denied alcohol and illicit drug use and could recall no drug or food allergies. He did report that his father and two aunts have type I diabetes.

Mr. Wilson's psychosocial history revealed the following pertinent information. He works part-time as a janitor and intends to start a second job but only for 2½ hours a week. He stated, "I'm on a fixed income, and my medicine runs out sometimes." During the past year, Mr. Wilson had been admitted to the hospital with the diagnosis of DKA on March 2, June 29, and November 8. In addition, he had failed to keep his follow-up appointments on July 18 and November 23. Mr. Wilson's diagnostic data were as follows:

BP	124/80 mm Hg	Respirations	32 breaths/min
HR	122 bpm	Temperature	35.8° C (96.3° F)

Hematologic studies showed the following:

Hgb	14.6 g/dl	Phosphorus	6.8 mg/dl
Hct	58%	Acetone	Moderate
Cl^-	95 mmol/L	Na^+	126 mmol/L
Creatinine	4.9 mg/dl	AST (SGOT)	248 U/L
Cholesterol	338 mg/dl	K^+	5.3 mmol/L
BUN	52 mg/dl	CK	34/35 IU/L
Ca^{++}	8.8 mmol/L	LDH	38 U/L
Glucose	560 mg/dl	Alkaline phosphatase	132 U/L

Arterial blood gas values were as follows:

pH	7.19	Sao_2	98% (room air)
Pco_2	20 mm Hg	HCO_3^-	7.5 mmol/L
Po_2	100 mm Hg		

Urine tests showed the following:

Specific gravity	1.015	Nitrates	0
Glucose	4+	Leukocytes	Few
Ketones	4+	RBCs	Many

Mr. Wilson's home medications were 16 U of 70/30 insulin in the morning and 12 U of 70/30 insulin in the evening.

DIABETIC KETOACIDOSIS

Questions

1. The hormones involved in intermediary metabolism, exclusive of insulin, that can participate in the development of DKA are epinephrine, glucagon, cortisol, growth hormone, and thyroid hormone. Describe first the pertinent physiology of each hormone and then how each participates in the development of DKA.
2. What is insulin's function in the body? What is the most significant basic defect in the development of DKA? Describe the interplay of factors necessary for the development of DKA.
3. List the classic signs and symptoms of DKA.
4. What is an anion gap? Calculate Mr. Wilson's anion gap. Why is the anion gap important to calculate and follow in the treatment of DKA?
5. Mr. Wilson's pH of 7.19 indicates severe acidosis. Discuss Mr. Wilson's arterial blood gas values in regard to acid-base balance.
6. Discuss the possibility of an infection in Mr. Wilson's case and the effect sepsis or infection would have on a diabetic patient.
7. What are the goals of treatment for patients with DKA?
8. Identify Mr. Wilson's abnormal laboratory values and describe the treatment modalities used with a patient with DKA in regard to these values.
9. What are the major complications associated with DKA and its treatment?
10. Review Mr. Wilson's history and laboratory values to determine the complications of diabetes to which Mr. Wilson is most predisposed?
11. Mr. Wilson's current insulin regimen is 16 U of 70/30 insulin in the morning and 12 U of 70/30 insulin in the evening. Discuss Mr. Wilson's insulin coverage and its adequacy. Include the essential aspects of intensive insulin therapy.
12. What nursing considerations are important in planning Mr. Wilson's discharge?

DIABETIC KETOACIDOSIS

Questions and Answers

1. **The hormones involved in intermediary metabolism, exclusive of insulin, that can participate in the development of DKA are epinephrine, glucagon, cortisol, growth hormone, and thyroid hormone. Describe first the pertinent physiology of each hormone and then how each participates in the development of DKA.**

Catecholamines, cortisol, glucagon, and growth hormone (GH) are insulin counter-regulatory hormones. They antagonize insulin by increasing glucose production.

Glucagon is produced by the α cells of the pancreas. Glucagon increases blood glucose by stimulating glycogenolysis and glyconeogenesis in the liver. Glucagon is also an antagonist to insulin.

The catecholamines (adrenaline, or epinephrine [E], and noradrenaline, or norepinephrine [NE]) are secreted by the adrenal medulla and by adrenergic nerve fibers. E and NE are important mobilizers of stored energy (Alspach, 1998). They mobilize lipid from adipose cells and glucose from extrahepatic sources. E, NE, and glucagon favor the synthesis of glucose by the liver by promoting release of fatty acids, promoting gluconeogenesis, and inhibiting β oxidation of fatty acids (Hadley, 1996).

In the physiologically intact animal, catecholamines inhibit insulin secretion by stimulating β-adrenergic receptors. This tends to accentuate the metabolic actions of catecholamines.

These three hormones oppose the anabolic effects of insulin and activate the enzyme systems for lipolysis and glycogenolysis (Hadley, 1996). They also promote gluconeogenesis of amino acids; therefore, if there is little or no insulin, the catecholamines and glucagon effectively increase the glucose level, using the uncontrolled mechanisms described earlier.

Glucocorticoids are produced by the adrenal cortex under the stimulation of adrenocorticotropic hormone (ACTH), which is produced by the anterior pituitary gland (adenohypophysis). The main glucocorticoid in the human is cortisol. Cortisol's action on intermediary metabolism is best understood if its action is applied in response to stresses such as starvation, disease, or other stimuli that cause significant amounts of ACTH to be secreted (Hadley, 1996). Under these circumstances, cortisol first affects the body's stores of fat. As fat becomes depleted, protein is selected as the next source of energy for the body. The action of glucocorticoids on glucose-6-phosphatase is necessary to provide necessary levels of glucose for the brain.

Cortisol protects the organism against glycogen breakdown until protein wastage is so far advanced that hypoglycemia ensues. At that time, glucagon and the catecholamines stimulate glycogenolysis to ensure sufficient glucose for the central nervous system (brain and spinal cord).

The interaction of these hormones results in a hyperglycemia that is commonly called *steroid diabetes*.

Similar mechanisms, if not countered by insulin, will increase the glucose level as seen in DKA. Consider the importance of these diabetogenic mechanisms when the patient with diabetes has an infection or inadvertently omits insulin injections.

GH, which is secreted by the anterior pituitary, has a role in intermediate metabolism because some of its actions are carried out by insulin-like growth factors. GH is diabetogenic, but its mode of action is not known (Hadley, 1996). It is stimulatory to insulin secretion but has also been shown to reduce the sensitivity of insulin in the peripheral tissues (Hadley, 1996).

Increased insulin secretion may be indirect and caused by the hyperglycemia resulting from reduced glucose uptake by the peripheral tissues. GH promotes growth in that it stimulates transport of amino acids into the cell, incorporation of amino acids into protein, and inhibition of gluconeogenesis.

It has been determined clinically that there is an inverse relation between insulin responsiveness and GH levels. That is, with high exogenous GH dosages or in acromegaly, one would expect to find a relative glucose intolerance and an insulin resistance.

The last hormones affecting the body's use of glucose are the thyroid hormones. The thyroid hormones (triiodothyronine [T_3] and tetraiodothyronine or thyroxine [T_4]) are produced in response to thyroid-stimulating hormone (TSH) secreted by the anterior pituitary. The stimulus for TSH is thyrotropin-releasing hormone, which is produced by the hypothalamus. T_3 is the primary thyroid hormone involved in intermediary metabolism. Its main function is focused on respiratory oxygen consumption. At physiologic levels, T_3 is thought to regulate oxygen consumption indirectly by stimulating outward flow of sodium ions. Some dose-dependent net catabolic and anabolic effects on the organism are caused by the thyroid hormones. At lower dosages, T_3 favors anabolism and growth in general, as well as lipogenesis and protein synthesis. At higher levels, the effects are catabolic and lead to higher heat production, increased adenosine triphosphate generation, and depletion of cellular forms of energy. In patients with thyrotoxicosis, one could anticipate high levels of glucose as a result of T_3's stimulatory effect on gluconeogenesis and glycogenolysis (Hadley, 1996). In addition, increased lipolysis will increase glycerol and fatty acid fragments, which can effectively raise glucose levels. All these factors, working together and in the absence of insulin, cause DKA to develop.

These same factors may result in the insulin resistance seen in patients with severe DKA. Even low-dose insulin treatment in patients with DKA results in circulating levels of insulin 4 to 15 times higher than normal. Factors contributing to insulin resistance include high levels of free fatty acids, the presence of high concentrations of counterregulatory hormones, acidosis, and even the hydrogen ion itself. It appears that acidosis interferes with insulin action not only by affecting hormone receptor action but also by inhibiting glycolysis at the 6-phosphofructokinase step.

Other endocrine conditions associated with glucose intolerance include primary hyperaldosteronism, carcinoid tumors, and prolactinomas.

2. **What is insulin's function in the body? What is the most significant basic defect in the development of DKA? Describe the interplay of factors necessary for the development of DKA.**

The β cells of the pancreas synthesize insulin. Insulin lowers the blood glucose and may cause hypoglycemia if elevated levels are present by increasing uptake of glucose by muscle, adipose tissue, and liver. It also decreases release of glucose from the liver and increases facilitated diffusion of glucose and related sugars (galactose and xylose) into muscle and adipose tissue. Finally, it increases glycogen formation in liver and muscle by increasing the activity of glycogen synthesis (Hadley, 1996).

Insulin is a protein-sparing hormone. It increases amino acid uptake by muscle and synthesis of proteins from amino acids, especially in the liver. Insulin decreases protein catabolism and is called *anabolic* because it increases transfer of glucose from blood to the tissues (Griffin & Ojeda, 1996).

Insulin increases fatty acid transport across cell membranes. It decreases lipolysis in adipose and liver tissue and facilitates formation of triglycerides from fatty acids.

The absolute or relative lack of insulin is the most significant basic defect in the development of DKA. The person with DKA is most often a known diabetic, usually one with type I diabetes mellitus, who has failed to administer sufficient insulin either because of noncompliance or lack of education. Usually, the patient has omitted insulin during a mild gastrointestinal upset. Occasionally, there is a relative lack of hormones because of increases in some of the counterregulatory hormones. The cause for a relative lack of insulin should be determined, even in cases of known noncompliance such as Mr. Wilson's. Common causes of relative decreases include sepsis and myocardial infarction. Other causes might include infections of the sinuses, teeth, urinary bladder, and gallbladder and perirectal abscesses. In addition, endocrine disorders such as Cushing's syndrome, acromegaly, thyrotoxicosis, and pheochromocytoma may lead to a relative lack of insulin (Bucher & Melander, 1999).

3. List the classic signs and symptoms of DKA.

Any person of any age who is seen with the following symptoms should be suspected of having diabetes and DKA: hyperglycemia, ketosis, altered mental status ranging from drowsiness to coma, weight loss, blurred vision, thirst, excessive urination, enuresis, abdominal pain, nausea, or vomiting (Bucher & Melander, 1999). Other symptoms include tachycardia, orthostatic hypotension, tachypnea, and Kussmaul's respiration. Included also are weakness, anorexia, poor skin turgor, and dry mucous membranes.

The final diagnosis of DKA can be made with the following laboratory values (Bucher & Melander, 1999):

Glucose	>350 mg/dl	Anion gap	High
pH	<7.30	Ketones	Positive
HCO_3^-	Low		

Some signs of DKA result from the effect that DKA has on hemoglobin function. The molecule 2,3-diphosphoglycerate (2,3-DPG) regulates the functional activity of hemoglobin. Decreased levels of 2,3-DPG increase the affinity of hemoglobin to oxygen, and the hemoglobin is unable to supply oxygen to the cells. One factor that decreases the level of 2,3-DPG is an inadequate supply of phosphate. Therefore the combination of acidosis and dehydration results in inadequate perfusion of peripheral tissues. If the phosphate level is low, phosphate administration is required during the treatment of DKA (Bucher & Melander, 1999). Phosphate enables 2,3-DPG levels to be restored and normalizes hemoglobin function.

4. **What is an anion gap? Calculate Mr. Wilson's anion gap. Why is the anion gap important to calculate and follow in the treatment of DKA?**

The normal anion gap is 12 to 14 mmol/L (Thelan, Urden, Lough, & Stacy, 1998). It is a calculation to determine the presence or absence of substances contributing to the negatively charged group of ions in the body (Bullock, 1996). These primarily include chloride and bicarbonate but normally may also include albumin. Other substances that can contribute to the anion population include lactic acid as in sepsis or shock, phosphates and sulfates as with kidney failure, and metabolic byproducts of ingested substances such as aspirin and antifreeze. However, in the case of DKA, the main contributors to the anion gap are the ketoacids, including β-hydroxybutyric acid and acetoacetic acid.

Several estimations of the anion gap can be made. One formula for the anion gap is as follows:

$$Na^+ - (Cl^- + HCO_3^-)$$

Substituting Mr. Wilson's laboratory values reveals the following:

$$126 - (95 + 7.5) = 23.5$$

Note that the normal anion gap should not be greater than 12.

Mr. Wilson's anion gap is dangerously high, and it must be observed closely during treatment. The proper treatment will allow narrowing of the anion gap to within normal limits.

5. **Mr. Wilson's pH of 7.19 indicates severe acidosis. Discuss Mr. Wilson's arterial blood gas values in regard to acid-base balance.**

The Pco_2 is calculated as follows:

$$6 \text{ mmol/L} \times 1.5 = 9 + 8 = 17 \text{ mm Hg}$$

Mr. Wilson's calculated Pco_2 of 17 mm Hg is not equal to the last two numbers of the pH value of 7.07; therefore Mr. Wilson's disturbance is probably not a pure or simple metabolic acidosis (Bullock, 1996). However, if an acid-base map is used to plot Mr. Wilson's values of pH of 7.07 and actual Pco_2 of 14 mm Hg, these data are consistent with simple metabolic acidosis (Stein, 1998).

It is not uncommon for persons to have mixed disturbances (Bucher & Melander, 1999). Persons with DKA often have a combination of two or three separate types of acid-base disorders. They may have the anion gap acidosis caused by excretion of β-hydroxybutyrate dehydrogenase and acetoacetate until there is volume depletion and there can be no more excretion. If patients are able to maintain some oral intake, they may develop a hyperchloremic non–anion gap acidosis (Bullock, 1996). Finally, they may also have developed a lactic acidosis due to dehydration and poor perfusion.

The data given here are insufficient to determine the cause of Mr. Wilson's possible mixed acidosis. A blood lactate value (normal is about 1.8 mmol/L or 18 mg/dl) or acetoacetate value might be helpful for positive confirmation (Stein, 1998).

6. **Discuss the possibility of an infection in Mr. Wilson's case and the effect sepsis or infection would have on a diabetic patient.**

Mr. Wilson may have some type of acute inflammation in progress. He felt feverish for a few days. The fever could just be a result of the dehydration (Alspach, 1998). If, indeed, Mr. Wilson did have an infection, neither the infection nor its source could be confirmed because of inadequate laboratory data (no differential available). Plausible sites that must be investigated include the teeth and sinuses. The lungs were clear, but it is possible to have crackles in a dehydrated state (Alspach, 1998). No bowel hyperactivity or other gastrointestinal problems were noted. In addition, there were few white cells in the urine, which probably ruled out kidney or bladder infections. He could have had pancreatitis, but again, there was no increased amylase value that could help verify that possibility. In addition, there was no tenderness or rebound over the abdomen. However, some of his other enzyme levels (aspartate aminotransferase and alkaline phosphatase) were elevated, which could indicate generalized inflammatory responses or tissue degradation. The elevated alkaline phosphatase could, however, be indicative of obstructive liver disease. Again, no laboratory data were present to validate that.

7. **What are the goals of treatment for patients with DKA?**

According to Bucher and Melander (1999), the goals of managing DKA include improvement of circulatory volume and tissue perfusion, a decrease in blood glucose levels, correction of electrolyte imbalances, and prevention of complications.

Fluid replacement should be started immediately for patients with DKA. These patients are dehydrated and hypovolemic and have fluid deficits of 5 to 8 L or more. Therefore a rapid expansion of intravascular volume is imperative. This can be accomplished by an initial infusion of 1 to 2 L of ½ normal saline or normal saline in the first 1 to 2 hours. For adults, the amount given is determined by the amount of dehydration. In general, this is about 1 to 2 L in the first 1 to 2 hours.

Insulin administration protocols vary from hospital to hospital. The goal of insulin therapy is to reverse the absolute or relative lack of insulin. It may include constant or intermittent infusions and subcutaneous or intramuscular boluses. Constant infusion rates result in a smoother metabolic improvement and are associated with a decreased potential for hypoglycemic reactions. Many regimens of administration exist, but one includes a modest 10-U dose of regular or lispro insulin intravenous (IV) push. Lispro insulin has actions similar to those of regular insulin. Future doses may be given via a piggyback line through an infusion pump. Mixing 100 U of regular insulin in 100 ml of saline results in a solution that minimizes medication errors because the rate on the pump is the actual number of units being infused per hour. The blood glucose level should drop between 75 and 100 mg/dl/hr. Subcutaneous insulin can be given when Mr. Wilson begins to eat and should be given 30 minutes before IV insulin is discontinued (Bucher & Melander, 1999).

The main electrolyte replacement concerns potassium. The patient often is seen, as was Mr. Wilson, with hyperkalemia. The potassium level represents extracellular potassium and only indirectly reflects intracellular potassium, which is of far greater significance. The body deficit of intravascular potassium may be much greater.

Therefore potassium should be added to IV fluids when the serum potassium level nears 4.5 mmol/L. However, potassium should not be added to IV fluids of patients who are anuric. This added potassium could result in dangerously high values that could precipitate ventricular dysrhythmias such as Mr. Wilson's unifocal premature ventricular contractions. Adding one half of the potassium as the chloride salt and the other half as the phosphate salt is recommended since this avoids delivery of excess chloride to the patient and prevents hypocalcemia.

To prevent complications from treatment of DKA, weight and vital signs are obtained at admission and an indwelling catheter is used for tracking fluids. Blood glucose and potassium levels should be monitored at least hourly. Cardiac monitoring throughout the course of treatment is essential. Hemodynamic monitoring (right atrial pressure and pulmonary capillary wedge pressure) may be necessary in patients with preexisting cardiac disease to evaluate fluid resuscitation. Prevention of cerebral edema and pulmonary edema is also important (Bucher & Melander, 1999).

8. Identify Mr. Wilson's abnormal laboratory values and describe the treatment modalities used with a patient with DKA in regard to these values.

Mr. Wilson's sodium level was low at 126 mmol/L, and the potassium level was high at 5.3 mmol/L. Chloride was low at 95 mmol/L. Sodium and chloride were low because of the vomiting and polyuria. Potassium was high because potassium moves from the intracellular compartment to the extracellular compartment in an exchange for the hydrogen ions (metabolic acidosis). Potassium levels drop as a result of vomiting and polyuria. Once insulin therapy is initiated, potassium returns to the cell.

Mr. Wilson's calcium level was borderline low at 8.8 mmol/L, and his phosphorus level of 6.8 mg/dl was high. It has been shown that high phosphate levels can precipitate hypocalcemia and hypomagnesemia. Therefore close monitoring of calcium, magnesium, and phosphate is strongly recommended as the electrolyte therapy is instituted. However, it is now recommended that phosphate and magnesium levels be allowed to correct themselves, if possible. If phosphorus is required, phosphorus and potassium therapy should begin simultaneously, using potassium phosphate. Excessive phosphate repletion could lead to hypocalcemia; therefore serum phosphate and calcium levels should be observed carefully (Bucher & Melander, 1999).

If patients have severe acidosis (pH <7.0), bicarbonate replacement should be initiated. In severe acidosis, the body uses bicarbonate to buffer the high concentration of ketoacids that results when insulin is unavailable to promote glucose entry into the cell (Porth, 1998). Bicarbonate should be administered with extreme caution because excessive bicarbonate replacement may lead to hypokalemia. If bicarbonate is administered, it should be given slowly and should not be given as a bolus (Bucher & Melander, 1999).

Hypomagnesemia occurs in many persons with diabetes, primarily because of unregulated excessive glucosuria. In general, an inverse relation exists between magnesium levels and glycosuria. In addition, mobilization of fats and protein catabolism are responsible for further magnesium deficits. Therefore patients with DKA often have extreme magnesium deficits. However, the laboratory value for magnesium was unavailable for Mr. Wilson.

9. What are the major complications associated with DKA and its treatment?

Bucher and Melander (1999) state that the major complications associated with DKA primarily are initial hyperkalemia, late or initial hypokalemia, late hypoglycemia, cerebral and pulmonary edema, and acute renal failure. Hypokalemia is potentially lethal and must be avoided. Brain edema is rare in the adult but occurs more often in children. Neurologic signs should be assessed frequently to prevent its effects. Acute renal failure is caused by severe depletion of body fluids and/or necrosis of the renal papillae.

10. Review Mr. Wilson's history and laboratory values to determine the complications of diabetes to which Mr. Wilson is most predisposed?

Mr. Wilson's blood urea nitrogen and creatinine levels were both high, which sometimes occurs in DKA. However, the presence of blood in his urine was undoubtedly associated with the DKA. Mr. Wilson's creatinine level of 4.9 mg/dl could have been caused by ketoacids interfering with the measurement but could also reflect prior damage to the kidneys. If urine output is normal, a creatinine level of 2 to 3 mg/dl should rapidly return to normal. No laboratory measure of albumin was ordered, even though this value would have been helpful. Hypertension and (micro)albuminuria have been described as the most sensitive markers of renal involvement in diabetic patients (Rubin & Farber, 1999). Mr. Wilson's blood pressure during the current DKA episode is 124/80 mm Hg, which, although not in the hypertensive range, is relatively high for a person in the dehydrated state. Current therapy for prevention of nephropathy includes administration of angiotensin-converting enzyme (ACE) inhibitors such as enalapril (Vasotec) or captopril (Capoten).

Annual screening for microalbuminuria and aggressive treatment of hypertension with ACE inhibitors are both recommended in the ADA Position Statement for persons with type I diabetes (Molitch et al, 1998). Persistent levels of albumin in the urine in the range of 30 to 300 mg/24 hr had been identified to be the earliest stage of diabetic nephropathy (American Diabetes Association, 1998b).

11. Mr. Wilson's current insulin regimen is 16 U of 70/30 insulin in the morning and 12 U of 70/30 insulin in the evening. Discuss Mr. Wilson's insulin coverage and its adequacy. Include the essential aspects of intensive insulin therapy.

Adults should receive insulin at 0.5 to 1.5 U/kg/day. Lower ranges are for adults who have hyperglycemia but no ketones, whereas higher dosages are used for patients with DKA. Intensive insulin therapy improves control of diabetes. According to the Diabetes Control and Complications Trial, intensive insulin therapy reduces retinopathy, microalbuminuria, and clinical neuropathy and allows better hemoglobin A_{1c} values to be achieved (Stein, 1998).

Using the aforementioned ranges and calculating Mr. Wilson's probable needs for insulin reveals the following: if the lowest value is used (0.5 U/kg/day), 140 lb must be to kilograms by dividing by 2.2, which yields 63.6 kg × 0.5 U/kg/day = 31.8 U/day of insulin. This is the minimum dose Mr. Wilson should receive according to the intensive insulin therapy guidelines.

Mr. Wilson is receiving only 28 U, so he is not receiving sufficient insulin coverage, even if he did not have the possible acute inflammatory process and was taking his insulin. Mr. Wilson probably should be receiving at least 1 U/kg/day, approximately 64 U. According to the intensive insulin therapy regimen, insulin should initially be administered in four injections with 35% being given before breakfast, 22% before lunch, 28% before supper, and 15% before bedtime. Therefore Mr. Wilson's injections should be 22 U before breakfast, 14 U before lunch, 18 U before supper, and 10 U at bedtime. This regimen should be accompanied by blood glucose monitoring four times a day and compliance with a low-fat, low-sodium, and low-protein diabetic diet. The low-fat diet is suggested because of Mr. Wilson's high cholesterol level. The low-sodium, low-protein diet is beneficial because of Mr. Wilson's predisposition to nephropathy. Mr. Wilson's should also be consuming a high-fiber diet with approximately 40 g of fiber per day. This amount of fiber will reduce his glucose values and cholesterol and triglyceride levels (American Diabetes Association, 1998a).

After Mr. Wilson's blood glucose level has stabilized, his insulin schedule can be altered so that he receives two thirds before breakfast and one third of his injection before supper. His 70/30 premixed insulin will continue to work well for this intensive insulin therapy.

For intensive insulin therapy, multiple injections or continuous subcutaneous pumps and multiple blood glucose monitoring (BGM) tests per day are required. Regimens suggest three to five BGM tests per day for intensive insulin therapy, whereas only three are suggested for conventional therapy (American Diabetes Association, 1998b).

Exercise is another important aspect of intensive insulin therapy. Patients are encouraged to exercise to prevent hypoglycemia and are further advised to use injection sites most distant from the muscles that will be most active.

12. What nursing considerations are important in planning Mr. Wilson's discharge?

With Mr. Wilson's cooperation, future complications from type I diabetes can be reduced by 50% to 70% by intensive insulin therapy (American Diabetes Association, 1998b). The diabetes support team needs Mr. Wilson's cooperation to maintain strict control over his diabetes. The nurse must work with Mr. Wilson to develop a health contract that is realistic and geared toward Mr. Wilson's concept of health. Mr. Wilson must understand the dangers of elevated glucose levels, know the signs and symptoms of hyperglycemia and hypoglycemia, and be able to verbalize interventions for both. The nurse, dietitian, and Mr. Wilson should discuss his present eating habits and decide what changes can be made. An exercise plan should also be discussed. Finally, Mr. Wilson should be informed of local support groups who can help him maintain a regimen of care that will provide an optimum outcome.

The hypoglycemia common to intensive insulin therapy can be handled nutritionally by using the glycemic index of foods. Food are ranked from 0 to 110 based on postprandial glucose responses (Bell & Forse, 1999). Foods with different glycemic indices (GIs) should be eaten together to avoid the pitfalls of hypoglycemia. Foods with the highest GIs (>90) include most breads, corn chips, and most potatoes. Those with intermediate GIs (70 to 90) include oatmeal, sweet potatoes, and most cookies. Most pasta, nuts, barley, and cracked wheat have lower GIs (<70) according to Bell and Forse (1999).

Other considerations to keep in mind during the discharge component are the psychosocial implications of a disease such as diabetes. These patients will have lifelong consequences caused by this illness. Patients who present with DKA are also at times thought to be "noncompliant," when in actuality they have tried to successfully deal with their illness. It must be remembered how difficult it can be for people to accept something that threatens their lives, that requires extensive changes in lifestyle, and that imposes a financial burden. The stresses of diabetes are significant for individuals and their families.

DIABETIC KETOACIDOSIS

References

Alspach, J. G. (Ed.). (1998). *American Association of Critical-Care Nurses: Core curriculum for critical nursing* (5th ed.). Philadelphia: Saunders.

American Diabetes Association (1998a). Nutritional recommendations and principles for people with diabetes mellitus. *Diabetes Care* 21(S1), S32-S39.

American Diabetes Association (1998b). Standards of medical care for patients with diabetes mellitus. *Diabetes Care* 21(S1), S23-S31.

Bell, S. J., & Forse A. (1999). Nutritional management of hypoglycemia. *The Diabetes Educator* 25(1), 41-47.

Bucher, L., & Melander, S. (1999). *Critical care nursing*. Philadelphia: Saunders.

Bullock, B. L. (1996). *Pathophysiology: Adaptations and alterations in function.* (4th ed.). Philadelphia: Lippincott.

Griffin, J. E., & Ojeda, S. R. (1996). *Textbook of endocrine physiology* (3rd Ed.) New York: Oxford University Press.

Hadley, M. (1996). *Endocrinology* (4th ed.). Englewood Cliffs, NJ: Prentice Hall.

Molitch, M. E., DeFronzo, R. A., Franz, M. J., Keane, W. F., Mogenson, C. E., Parving H.-H., and Steffes, M. W. (1998). Diabetic nephropathy. *Diabetes Care* 21(S1), S50-S53.

Porth, C. M. (1998). *Pathophysiology: Concepts of altered health states* (5th ed.). Philadelphia: JB Lippincott.

Rubin, E., & Farber, J. L. (1999). *Pathology* (3rd ed.). Philadelphia: Lippincott-Raven.

Stein, J. (1998). *Internal medicine* (5th ed). St Louis: Mosby.

Thelan, L., Urden, L., Lough, M., & Stacy, K. (1998). *Critical care nursing: Diagnosis and management*. St Louis: Mosby.

CHAPTER 23

MULTIPLE ORGAN DYSFUNCTION SYNDROME

Debra L. Harmon, RN, MSN, CCRN

CASE PRESENTATION

Mrs. Whitman, a 77-year-old white woman, was admitted to the hospital with abdominal pain. History on admission revealed that she had an abrupt onset of severe generalized abdominal pain after eating breakfast this morning. She experienced some nausea but no vomiting. The pain remained unremitting, and she was brought to the emergency department and admitted. She complained of having felt a "band" around her stomach for 5 days with pain radiating to her back, but she felt no pain on the morning of admission. She has a history of chronic back pain with long-term use of nonsteroidal antiinflammatory drugs (NSAIDs). She denies any history of heartburn, gallbladder disease, or pancreatitis.

She has a history of intraabdominal carcinomatosis from carcinoma of the ovaries 6 years previously. Review of systems revealed some dyspnea on exertion caused by her back pain. She complained of dizziness this morning, but she had no complaint of headaches. She denied any chest pain. She has left-sided weakness from a prior cerebrovascular accident (CVA).

BP	100/53 mm Hg	Respirations	28 breaths/min
HR	105 bpm	Temperature	36.3° C (97.3° F)

She appeared to be in acute distress. Breath sounds were decreased throughout her lungs. Heart tones were normal. The abdomen was flat with absent bowel sounds and tender to palpation. There were no palpable masses or abnormal pulsations. Her Glasgow Coma Scale (GCS) score was normal (15).

Laboratory data at admission were the following:

Hgb	12.5 g/dl	BUN	39 mg/dl
Hct	38.6%	Creatinine	1.8 mg/dl
WBCs	$4.34 \times 10^3/mm^3$	Bilirubin	0.4 mg/dl
Platelets	210,000/mm^3	Alkaline	56 U/L
Na$^+$	136 mmol/L	phosphatase	
K$^+$	4.5 mmol/L	AST (SGOT)	31 U/L
Cl$^-$	101 mmol/L	LDH	140 U/L
CO$_2$	25 mmol/L	Albumin	2.3 g/dl
Glucose	189 mg/dl		

The patient was given intravenous fluids and pain medications after admission to the hospital. A computed tomographic scan of the abdomen showed an intraabdominal inflammatory process or a tumor, plus a subdiaphragmatic abscess. A surgical consultation was obtained. On day 2 of the hospitalization, the patient underwent an exploratory laparotomy for an acute condition of the abdomen, which revealed a perforated duodenal ulcer. A pulmonary artery catheter was inserted in the operating room for monitoring her hemodynamic status. After surgery the patient was admitted to the intensive care unit (ICU).

On admission to the ICU, Mrs. Whitman required dopamine and fluid challenges to maintain her blood pressure. Triple antibiotic therapy was started in response to a temperature elevation, noted immediately after surgery. Total parenteral nutrition was started immediately after surgery because she had an endotracheal tube, a nasogastric tube, and a duodenostomy tube that were set at low suction. Diagnostic data immediately after surgery were as follows:

BP	82/60 mm Hg (MAP 68)	PAP	38/18
HR	123 bpm	PCWP	15
Temperature	38.8° C (101.8° F)	CO/CI	4.2/2.6
CVP (RAP)	8		

Ventilator settings were as follows:

Fio_2	50%
SIMV rate	10
V_T	700 ml

Arterial blood gas (ABG) values were as follows:

pH	7.41	Po_2	123 mm Hg
Pco_2	35 mm Hg	HCO_3^-	23 mmol/L

On the second postoperative day, the patient's respiratory status stabilized and the endotracheal tube was removed. Dopamine was continued at 5 μg/kg/min, and as Mrs. Whitman's blood pressure stabilized, the dopamine was titrated and then discontinued.

On the fourth postoperative day, Mrs. Whitman's condition deteriorated, requiring reintubation and mechanical ventilation. Her hemoglobin and hematocrit also dropped significantly, requiring a blood transfusion of 2 units of packed red blood cells. She did not want to be using the ventilator and continuously tried to extubate herself. Her GCS score decreased to 13. On postoperative day 4, diagnostic data after blood transfused were the following:

Hgb	7.1 g/dl	Glucose	90 mg/dl
Hct	21.7%	BUN	32 mg/dl
WBCs	$14.4 \times 10^3/mm^3$	Creatinine	225 mg/dl
Platelets	5000/mm^3	Bilirubin	1.1 mg/dl
Na$^+$	128 mmol/L	Alkaline phosphatase	69 U/L
K$^+$	5.6 mmol/L	AST (SGOT)	120 U/L
Cl$^-$	102 mmol/L	LDH	580 U/L
CO$_2$	32 mmol/L	Albumin	1.8 g/dl

Vital signs and hemodynamic values were the following:

BP	90/64 mm Hg	CVP (RAP)	10
	(MAP 70)	PAP	42/30
HR	130 bpm	PCWP	15
Temperature	38.9° C (102° F)	CO/CI	3.8/2.1

Ventilator settings were as follows:

Fio_2	60%	V_T	700 ml
SIMV rate	10	PEEP	5 cm H_2O

ABG values were as follows:

pH	7.32	Po_2	54 mm Hg
Pco_2	57 mm Hg	HCO_3^-	32 mmol/L

By postoperative day 10, Mrs. Whitman showed worsening signs of respiratory and liver failure. Triple antibiotic therapy continued, yet Mrs. Whitman's temperature continued to spike at 38.9° C (102° F) throughout her hospitalization. Multiple cultures were obtained, yet all showed no growth.

After consultation with Mrs. Whitman's family and in view of the patient's previous wishes regarding ventilatory support, the ventilator was removed. Mrs. Whitman died shortly thereafter.

MULTIPLE ORGAN DYSFUNCTION SYNDROME

Questions

1. Define the evolution of multiple organ dysfunction syndrome (MODS).
2. List etiologic factors for and discuss the incidence of MODS. What are some theories or hypotheses for the cause of MODS?
3. Describe the primary and secondary classifications of MODS. Which classification of MODS has Mrs. Whitman developed? Identify any predictors of mortality or significant manifestations associated with the classifications. Approximate Mrs. Whitman's mortality risk.
4. What pathophysiologic changes occur with MODS?
5. How is the release of oxygen-free radicals and TNF related to the development of MODS?
6. What special considerations are there with children and elderly patients who are predisposed to MODS? What were Mrs. Whitman's predisposing factors?
7. Identify assessment findings and effects of MODS on individual organ systems.
8. Discuss collaborative management measures for MODS.
9. Describe the impact of anemia on MODS. Is intravenous erythropoietin (EPO) an appropriate treatment? Did Mrs. Whitman develop anemia? If so, what treatment was used?
10. What are the nursing diagnoses for the patient with MODS?
11. What ethical considerations play a role in the diagnosis of MODS?
12. What are the future trends for the treatment of MODS?

MULTIPLE ORGAN DYSFUNCTION SYNDROME

Questions and Answers

1. Define the evolution of multiple organ dysfunction syndrome (MODS).

Multiple organ failure (MOF), the precursor to MODS, has been described since the mid-1970s and is a separate entity from single organ failure. *MOF* is the failure of two or more organ systems. MOF is a result of malignant intravascular inflammation, which is often associated with infection or sepsis (Carlson, 1999). In the late 1980s, research on MOF revealed that organ failure can also occur in the absence of infection with disorders such as shock, tissue injury, ischemic conditions, and pancreatitis (Carlson, 1999; Piper & Sibbald, 1997; Thelan, Urden, Lough, & Stacy, 1998).

Subsequently, MOF became a less accepted universal definition for organ failure. The 1991 consensus conference of the Society of Critical Care Medicine and the American College of Chest Physicians suggested that the term *multiple system organ failure (MOF)* be replaced with *multiple organ dysfunction syndrome (MODS)*. The reason for this suggestion was that MOF denotes actual organ failure, which is not actually the case (Piper & Sibbald, 1997). The new term is considered more appropriate because organs such as the heart, lungs, and kidneys show signs of dysfunction but do not actually fail.

MODS is the result of a systemic inflammatory response system (SIRS), which results from the injury and implies an ongoing physiologic phenomenon rather than the presence or absence of organ failure (Carlson, 1999). The SIRS may directly result in MODS or may be a result of sepsis. Although no widely accepted definition of MODS exists, the definition of MODS that was developed at the 1991 consensus conference states that "MODS is the presence of altered organ function in an acutely ill patient such that homeostasis cannot be maintained without intervention" (Carlson, 1999; Sommers, 1998).

2. List etiologic factors for and discuss the incidence of MODS. What are some theories or hypotheses for the cause of MODS?

Etiologic Factors for MODS

According to Sommers (1998), etiologic or predisposing factors for MODS include the following:

- Chronic diseases and preexisting organ dysfunction such as diabetes mellitus, heart failure, and liver failure
- Immunosuppressive therapy
- Extremes of age such as very old or very young
- Malnutrition and alcoholism
- Cancer
- Complications of multiple trauma with prolonged highly invasive surgical procedures, perfusion deficits, hemorrhagic shock
- Burns
- Sepsis

Most etiologic theories favor a common pathway that creates a systemic reaction as the cause, instead of the result, of cardiovascular instability and poor oxygen delivery (Carlson, 1999). The thought is that this systemic response is the result of a prolonged inflammatory response that creates a perfusion deficit. The perfusion deficit is then the trigger for MODS. Examples of triggers of MODS are conditions such as shock and cardiopulmonary arrest (Carlson, 1999).

Incidence of MODS

The incidence of MODS is increasing because patients with chronic illnesses and/or severe trauma are surviving longer. Despite advances in the management of severely traumatized or ill patients, the mortality has been the same for the past 20 years (Carlson, 1999; Sommers, 1998). Depending on the number of organs involved, mortality ranges from 40% to 80%. Mortality approaches 100% when three or more systems are involved (Carlson, 1999; Sommers, 1998). Sommers (1998) stated that MODS develops in 15% of all patients admitted to intensive care units and is responsible for up to 80% of deaths of patients in intensive care units. A study cited by Carlson (1999) described a simple scoring system, based on dysfunctional systems found on the first day of a critical care stay, that could accurately predict mortality approximately 75% of the time.

Theories or Hypotheses for the Cause of MODS

The following are theories regarding the cause of MODS:

1. Activation of interrelated systems such as the compensatory antiinflammatory response syndrome and SIRS that can produce a battle of opposing forces
2. Systemic host defense activation that is overwhelming and chemical mediators that become detrimental rather than beneficial
3. Uncontrolled normal inflammatory response that can further impair organ function
4. Systemic consequences of cardiovascular instability and poor oxygen delivery, which results in possible vascular occlusion
5. Injury, shock, and sepsis that produce ischemia, triggering the four preceding events (Carlson, 1999; Piper & Sibbald, 1997)

3. Describe the primary and secondary classifications of MODS. Which classification of MODS has Mrs. Whitman developed? Identify any predictors of mortality or significant manifestations associated with the classifications. Approximate Mrs. Whitman's mortality risk.

Primary and Secondary Classifications of MODS

Primary MODS is the direct result of a well-defined organ insult in which organ dysfunction occurs early and can be related to an identifiable insult (Carlson, 1999; Piper & Sibbald, 1997; Thelan et al, 1998). *Secondary MODS* is organ dysfunction that develops days after admission. It occurs with a persistent effect of the SIRS-to-sepsis process on the body, rather than with an insult (Carlson, 1999; Piper & Sibbald, 1997). It appears that Mrs. Whitman had developed secondary MODS in response to the persistent SIRS-to-sepsis process over several days postoperatively. The clinical manifestations of SIRS-to-sepsis process associated with MODS are described in Table 23-1 (Carlson, 1999; Piper & Sibbald, 1997).

Predictors of Mortality or Significant Manifestations Associated with MODS

MODS scoring was developed by Marshall and associates in 1995. They identified physiologic descriptors in six organ systems that correlate with the risk of mortality

TABLE **23-1**	Clinical Manifestations of SIRS Associated with MODS
Clinical Manifestation	Description
Temperature	> 38° C (100.4° F) or <36° C (96.8° F)
Heart rate	> 90 bpm
Respiratory rate	> 20 breaths/min
Paco$_2$	< 32 mm Hg (hyperventilation)
White blood cell count	> 12,000/mm^3 or <4000/mm^3 or >10% immature (band) forms

TABLE **23-2**	Organ-Specific Descriptors Correlating with MODS Mortality				
	Score				
System	0	1	2	3	4
Respiratory (Po/Fio$_2$ ratio)	> 300	266-300	151-225	76-150	≤ 75
Renal (serum creatinine)	≤ 100	101-200	201-350	351-500	> 500
Hepatic (serum bilirubin)	≤ 20	21-60	61-120	121-240	> 240
Cardiovascular (PAR = HR × RAP/MAP)	≤ 10	10.1-15.0	15.1-20.0	20.1-30.0	> 30.0
Hematologic (platelet count)	> 120	81-120	51-80	21-50	≤ 20
Neurologic (Glasgow Coma Scale)	15	13-14	10-12	7-9	≤ 6

Reprinted with permission from Alspach, J. G. (Ed.). (1998). *American Association of Critical-Care Nurses: Core curriculum for critical care nursing* (5th ed.). Philadelphia: WB Saunders.

from MODS (Piper & Sibbald, 1997; Sommers, 1998). However, there remains no universal agreement on a uniform way of diagnosing or tracking the progress of MODS in critically ill patients (Piper & Sibbald, 1997).

Organ-specific descriptors correlating with mortality from MODS are described in Table 23-2 (Piper & Sibbald, 1997; Sommers, 1998). The descriptor score in relation to mortality is as follows:

- Score of 9 to 12: mortality 25%
- Score of 13 to 16: mortality 50%
- Score of 17 to 20: mortality 75%

Mrs. Whitman's approximate mortality score was 14 based on her data on postoperative day 4. A score of 14 places her in the 50% mortality category.

4. What pathophysiologic changes occur with MODS?

The pathogenesis of MODS is complex. All of the systems and mediators identified under the interrelated inflammatory system are normally active during any episode of inflammation. However, if the inflammatory state continues over time, the mediators lose control because of the overwhelming inflammatory activation, and normal body responses become unregulated and detrimental (Carlson, 1999). As MODS progresses, three additional levels of pathophysiologic changes occur: a maldistribution of blood flow, an oxygen supply and demand imbalance, and abnormal metabolic control. These pathophysiologic changes occur in the following cascade of events (Carlson, 1999; Thelan et al, 1998):

  I. *Initial insult or injury*
 II. *Simultaneous activation of interrelated inflammatory systems*
    A. Complement system, the first system to be activated
       1. Stimulates neutrophil aggregation and white blood cells to begin phagocytosis
       2. Releases mediators (histamine, oxygen free radicals, interleukins, TNF, B- and T-cell activity, and coagulation factors)
       3. Contains, suppresses, and eliminates infecting organisms and clears damaged tissue of cellular debris and foreign material
    B. Kinin system: second system activated by inflammation
       1. Releases bradykinin, a mediator, that responds much like histamine, causing vasodilation and increased capillary permeability
    C. Renin-angiotensin-aldosterone system, activated by decreased renal perfusion or low volume states
       1. Causes systemic vasoconstriction and increased sodium and water reabsorption
       2. Leads to increased blood pressure
    D. Clotting system
       1. Causes stimulation of the clotting cascade, which can lead to hypercoagulopathy and microemboli formation
       2. Results may play a major role in the development of disseminated intravascular coagulation
    E. Sympathetic nervous system: the fight or flight response
       1. Releases catecholamines (epinephrine and norepinephrine), causing peripheral vasoconstriction
       2. Assists with stimulation of the renin-angiotensin-aldosterone system
    F. Endorphins: "morphinelike substances" in the brain
       1. Cause vasodilation
    G. Myocardial depressant factor: stored in the pancreas
       1. Produces a negative inotropic effect from any hypotensive episode
III. *Maldistribution of blood flow caused by increased capillary permeability results in the following*
    A. Vasoconstriction and vasodilation
       1. Lead to vascular fluid leaks into the interstitium and pooling in the periphery
       2. Give the appearance of edema and decreases vascular volume and blood pressure
    B. Vascular occlusion
       1. Further complicates the maldistribution of blood flow from formation of microemboli (renal system very vulnerable to this)
 IV. *Imbalance between oxygen supply and demand related to the following:*
    A. Decrease in blood pressure
    B. Poor control of tissue perfusion in the microcirculation
    C. Fever
    D. Lung abnormalities such as adult respiratory distress syndrome (ARDS) because of the leaky pulmonary capillary beds
    E. Possible low hemoglobin levels

  V. *Abnormal metabolic control*
    A. Hyperdynamic and hypermetabolic state
        1. Occurs when endocrine activation overcompensates for damage
    B. Protein breakdown from muscle tissue
        1. Leads to rapid wasting and atrophy of muscles
        2. If the underlying condition is not reversed, hypodynamic and decompensated states occur, leading to organ damage and failure
    C. Amino acids converted into glucose
        1. Depletion of glucose stores and inhibition of the synthesis of new glucose may lead to hypoglycemia

5. How is the release of oxygen-free radicals and TNF related to the development of MODS?

Piper and Sibbald (1997) stated that the systems of inflammation release mediators that decrease tissue perfusion and alter cellular oxygen metabolism. This creates byproducts of anaerobic metabolism and mediators such as lactic acid, oxygen-free radicals, and TNF.

Oxygen-Free Radicals

Oxygen-free radicals, produced in excessive amounts, have been implicated as part of the reason for cellular destruction during multisystem organ failure. Normally, antioxidant enzymes are present in sufficient numbers to prevent cellular destruction. However, during conditions such as sepsis and multisystem organ failure, patients have depleted their antioxidant defense system and are especially vulnerable to these destructive effects. Oxygen metabolites cause lipid peroxidation and damage cell membranes like nervous system tissue that is high in lipid content. Oxygen-free radicals can activate the coagulation cascade and cause damage to DNA (Carlson, 1999; Piper & Sibbald, 1997).

Tumor Necrosis Factor

TNF is believed to be the primary mediator of toxic effects of endotoxins released from destroyed bacterial cells. TNF produces many of the signs and symptoms seen in patients with shock: hypotension, tachycardia, tachypnea, hyperglycemia, metabolic acidosis, third spacing, gastrointestinal ischemia, alveolar thickening, acute tubular necrosis, and dramatic changes in body temperature. Therefore TNF plays a major role in the development of MODS and septic shock (Carlson, 1999).

6. What special considerations are there with children and elderly patients who are predisposed to MODS? What were Mrs. Whitman's predisposing factors?

Special Considerations with Children

MODS in children usually develops from a primary, obvious insult as described in the classification of primary and secondary MODS. MODS can be identified in most children within 24 hours of hospital admission via diagnostic criteria. Once MODS is diagnosed, aggressive interventions and treatments must occur for positive outcomes. Mortality is not associated with ongoing sepsis and is less than that for adults with primary MODS. However, the progression of organ failure in children varies from that seen in adults. In children, organ failure usually occurs in the pulmonary, cardiovascular, and neurologic systems, compared with the pulmonary, renal, and hepatic systems in the adult (Piper & Sibbald, 1997).

Special Considerations with Elderly Patients

Management of elderly patients with MODS is more difficult than that of younger adult patients. Physiologic changes occur in elderly patients that cause a decrease in functional reserve and an inability to compensate during periods of stress. To meet the challenge of caring for elderly patients, it is imperative that a complete and detailed physical and psychosocial history and comprehensive physical and laboratory assessments be obtained. Prevention of MODS is the most critical consideration in elderly patients. Aggressive interventions for organ preservation, management of all infectious processes, a balance of oxygen supply and demand, and the provision of nutritional support are essential for successful treatment of MODS (Rauen & Stamatos, 1997).

Mrs. Whitman's Predisposing Factors

Risk factors for MODS include preexisting conditions such as cancer and chronic illnesses, medications (steroids and NSAIDs), and age older than 65 years (Rauen & Stamatos, 1997). Mrs. Whitman's predisposing factors included her age of 77 years, her long-term use of NSAIDs for chronic back pain, and her preexisting conditions—prior intraabdominal carcinoma and CVA. The diagnosis of MODS may be difficult in elderly patients because of the delay in appearance or even absence of symptoms of infection and inflammation. Rauen and Stamatos (1997) state that the first and possibly the only clinical symptom may be a change in mental status or generalized malice. Elderly patients with the aforementioned predisposing factors who display these subtle symptoms should undergo thorough investigation for MODS.

7. Identify assessment findings and effects of MODS on individual organ systems.

Clinical presentation varies from patient to patient depending on the patient's underlying health, degree of organ dysfunction, number of organs involved, and progression of time (Sommers, 1998). According to Carlson (1999) and Sommers (1998), the assessment findings for individual organ systems are the following.

Cardiovascular System

- Tachycardia
- Ventricular arrhythmias refractory to standard intervention
- Mean arterial pressure < 70 mm Hg
- Pulmonary capillary wedge pressure < 12 mm Hg
- Central venous pressure < 8 mm Hg
- Cardiac output > 8 L/min initially; later < 4 L/min
- Cardiac index > 4 L/min initially; later < 2.5 L/min
- Peripheral edema with bounding or diminished pulses
- S_3 heart sound with auscultation
- Skin pale and warm initially; later pale, cool, and clammy

Pulmonary System

- Bradypnea or tachypnea
- Dyspnea with increased work of breathing and cyanosis
- Crackles or wheezes with auscultation

- ABG values: $Pao_2 < 60$ mm Hg, $Paco_2 > 45$ mm Hg, may have metabolic acidosis, respiratory alkalosis, or both
- Decreased pulmonary compliance and ARDS requiring mechanical ventilatory assistance
- Ventilator settings: frequent Fio_2 manipulation and 5 cm H_2O of positive end-expiratory pressure (PEEP)
- Chest x-ray film with diffuse infiltrates (consistent with ARDS)

Renal System
- Oliguria or anuria
- Creatinine clearance < 30 ml/min
- Serum osmolarity > 295 mOsm/kg
- BUN > 20 mg/dl
- Serum creatinine > 2.0 mg/dl or double the serum creatinine level on admission
- Other serum electrolytes
  - Potassium > 5 mEq/L
  - Magnesium < 1.5 mEq/L
  - Sodium < 130 mEq/L
  - Calcium < 8.5 mg/dl
  - Phosphate > 4.5 mg/dl

Hematologic System
- Bleeding tendencies with petechiae or purpura
- Susceptibility to infections
- Laboratory tests
  - WBC > 10,000 mm^3 initially; < 5000 mm^3 later
  - Platelets < 100,000/ml
  - Hematocrit and hemoglobin levels decreased
  - Prothrombin time > 25% above normal
  - Activated partial thromboplastin time > 25% above normal
  - Thrombin time prolonged
  - Fibrin split products > 10 µg/ml

Central Nervous System
- Altered level of consciousness with a GCS score < 6
- Headache with intracranial pressure > 15 mm Hg
- Respiratory depression
- Hypothermia or hyperthermia

Gastrointestinal System
- Anorexia, nausea, vomiting
- Bleeding tendencies with stress ulcers and hematemesis
- Ileus with nasogastric output > 600 ml/24 hr
- Diarrhea or constipation
- Guaiac-positive nasogastric output and stool
- Jaundice
- Laboratory tests
  - Bilirubin > 2.0 mg/dl
  - Albumin < 2.8 g/dl
  - Liver enzymes (lactic acid dehydrogenase, aspartate aminotransferase [serum glutamic-oxaloacetic transferase]) > 50% above normal
  - Hyperglycemia initially and hypoglycemia later

8. Discuss collaborative management measures for MODS.

No definitive therapy exists for MODS. The goal of most treatments is supporting each dysfunctional organ system. However, treatment must be individualized for the whole patient because interventions for one system may cause harm to another system (Carlson, 1999). Carlson (1999) identifies the following three overall goals for the medical treatment of MODS:

1. Treat the underlying cause.
2. Eliminate or control the source or initial insult.
3. Support dysfunctional systems aggressively.

Carlson (1999) also identifies five primary goals of nursing care of MODS as the following:

1. Prevent or control infection.
2. Provide adequate oxygenation.
3. Support appropriate circulating volume.
4. Maximize the effectiveness of heart pumping.
5. Support the patient and family.

Prevent and Control Infection

Prevention and control of infection must be given a high priority in the medical treatment and nursing care of patients with MODS. Prophylactic antibiotics should be considered once cultures are done on blood, sputum, urine, and invasive catheter tips. If fever continues with antibiotic therapy, antipyretics and a hypothermia blanket may be necessary. Other measures to prevent infection include maintenance of skin integrity, impeccable oral hygiene, and screening of visitors with active infections (Carlson, 1999).

An area that has been researched extensively in regard to the prevention and control of infection is the gastrointestinal (GI) tract. Sommers (1998) and Stechmiller, Treloar, and Allen (1997) stated that the gut acts as a bacteria and endotoxin reservoir that exacerbates the development of MODS. However, current studies cited by Carlson (1999) on the efficacy of gut decontamination showed no impact on reducing mortality. Current literature does support aggressive nutritional interventions to minimize catabolism in patients with MODS (Carlson, 1999; Rauen & Stamatos, 1997; Sommers, 1998; Stechmiller et al, 1997). Nutritional support should begin as early as 12 hours after surgery or traumatic injury for the best results (Rauen & Stamatos, 1997). Recommendations for nutritional support include a combination of a slow-drip enteral feeding (5 to 10 ml/hr) for maintenance of GI integrity along with total parenteral nutrition to balance individual needs (Carlson, 1999; Klein, Stanek, & Wiles, 1998; Klein & Wiles, 1997; Rauen & Stamatos, 1997). The goal is to maintain a positive nitrogen balance without overfeeding. Monitoring gastric output for color and amount as well as gastric alkalization with H_2-blockers and antacids is essential for complete GI stabilization.

Provide Adequate Oxygenation

Adequate oxygenation of tissues is another difficult task in patients with MODS. Carlson (1999) and Rinaldo and Clark (1998) support "early, aggressive ventilation, often with PEEP, that is aimed at keeping the Pao_2 greater than 80 mm Hg." Collaboration among nurses and respiratory therapists to institute aggressive pulmonary toilet for maximum air exchange is important. Close monitoring of oxygenation with ABG values, oximetry, or oximetric pulmonary artery catheters is required in patients with MODS. The use of paralytic agents such as vecuronium (Norcuron) with sedation may be necessary when an acceptable Pao$_2$ value cannot be reached. Propofol (Diprivan) is another agent that may be ideal for patients with MODS who are undergoing mechanical ventilation (Carlson, 1999; Rinaldo & Clark, 1998).

Support Appropriate Circulating Volume to Maximize Heart Pumping Effectiveness

Cardiovascular support, continuous cardiac monitoring, and antiarrhythmic therapy are other important areas of collaborative treatment of MODS. These interventions go hand in hand with hemodynamic monitoring and maintenance of fluid balance. Establishing an appropriate balance of circulating volume is challenging in patients with MODS. The use of aggressive invasive monitoring of hemodynamic values is the foundation for restoration of function and stabilization of both cardiovascular and renal systems. Using pulmonary artery monitoring to evaluate and adjust preload, afterload, inotropic agents, and blood oxygen content is vital to successfully maintaining cardiopulmonary status. Fluid resuscitation with crystalloid or colloid remains a debate; it should be administered with caution to avoid fluid overload. The use of diuretics and low-dose dopamine may be necessary to support renal function. Consideration must be given to adequately balancing fluids and supporting renal function. It may be necessary to initiate hemodialysis and/or slow continuous ultrafiltration to allow administration of additional fluid or parenteral nutrition. If blood loss is significant, administration of blood products should be considered. The main complication from fluid resuscitation is pulmonary and peripheral edema. Edema is an expected consequence and is not necessarily considered a sign of intravascular volume overload (Carlson, 1999).

Support the Patient and Family

Support of the patient with MODS and the family dealing with MODS is a final and important medical and nursing collaborative measure. Because of the high mortality and use of costly available medical resources, the patient with MODS presents many ethical dilemmas. Patients and families need frequent and clear information related to progress and plan of care (Carlson, 1999). An aggressive versus a conservative approach to treatment has been shown to influence mortality (Rauen & Stamatos, 1997). Because many of these patients are unable to articulate their wishes, the decision to discontinue treatment falls to the family. Advanced directives and living wills play an important role and can be used to convey the patient's wishes.

9. **Describe the impact of anemia on MODS. Is intravenous erythropoietin (EPO) an appropriate treatment? Did Mrs. Whitman develop anemia? If so, what treatment was used?**

Impact of Anemia on MODS

Anemia is often seen in sepsis (Gabriel et al, 1998). In MODS, anemia reduces the oxygen-carrying capacity and oxygen delivery of blood cells, worsening already impaired oxygen-extraction capacity of tissues. Although MODS may be irritated by an episode of hemorrhagic shock, the anemia of sepsis is caused by cytokine action. Cytokines impair stored iron release into the reticuloendothelial system, causing a functional iron deficit. In addition, increased cytokine levels cause erythropoietic bone marrow suppression, thus inhibiting EPO production and action. Other causes of reduced EPO production in MODS include renal or hepatic failure and repeated blood transfusions. Therefore the vicious cycle of MODS continues with increased cytokines leading to an iron deficit and EPO suppression, which causes or worsens anemia.

Treatment with Intravenous EPO

In a 1998 study on high-dose human EPO administration in patients with MODS, Gabriel et al. concluded that patients receiving 600 IU/kg of EPO intravenously three times a week were able to overcome the impairments of EPO production and iron utilization. The erythropoietic system remained responsive to the high dosages of human EPO during MODS and aided in reducing or correcting anemia. The investigators recommended further study to confirm their results.

Mrs. Whitman developed anemia several days after surgery. She received 2 units of packed red blood cells, which did not improve her hemoglobin and hematocrit values. Her respiratory, renal, and hepatic systems continued to fail, which did not help with her anemia. She did not receive any EPO, and it is uncertain whether the EPO would have helped her outcome.

10.   What are the nursing diagnoses for the patient with MODS?

Nursing diagnoses for MODS are numerous and may cover an entire list of problems with a high rate of occurrence or actual problems depending on the organ systems involved. Carlson (1999) and Sommers (1998) provided an extensive list of nursing diagnoses for the patient with MODS, which includes but may not be limited to the following:

- Alteration in tissue perfusion
- Fluid volume deficit or excess
- Impaired gas exchange
- Ineffective airway clearance
- High risk for infection
- Alteration in nutrition
- Alteration in skin integrity
- Impaired mobility
- Decreased cardiac output
- Anxiety and/or fear
- Pain
- Ineffective thermoregulation
- Impaired communication
- Ineffective family coping

11.   What ethical considerations play a role in the diagnosis of MODS?

Early in the course of the illness, Mrs. Whitman expressed a desire not to be intubated and to "let me just die." Despite Mrs. Whitman's wishes, she received many life support interventions. The question arises whether treatment was aggressive enough. The all or nothing philosophy applies to MODS. Conservative, middle-of-the-road treatment of MODS increases mortality (Rauen & Stamatos, 1997). The issue of advanced directives, such as living wills and durable power of attorney, will continue to play an important role in today's health care environment. It is important that nurses be prepared to inform patients of the existence of advance directives and to assist them in developing their own before becoming critically ill and facing the possibility of not having their wishes carried out. Other future ethical considerations for these patients are the rationing of health care dollars and the futility of care. Families and health care workers will face the fact that rehabilitation after recovery of the patient with MODS is costly, involving months of care before the patient achieves a functional level. Quality versus quantity of life issues may need to be addressed.

12. What are the future trends for the treatment of MODS?

The future for the treatment of MODS is ever changing as research and technology advance. Carlson (1999) cited several current studies for the treatment of MODS but only two with any promise. One study suggested the use of human recombinant interleukin-1 receptor antagonist and another the use of anti-TNF antibodies. Progress in treatment of MODS increases ethical and economic dilemmas faced by patients, families, and health care providers.

MULTIPLE ORGAN DYSFUNCTION SYNDROME

References

Carlson, K. (1999). Multiple organ dysfunction syndrome. In L. Bucher & S. Melander (Eds.), *Critical care nursing* (pp. 1070-1087). Philadelphia: WB Saunders.

Gabriel, A., Kozek, S., Chiari, A., Fitzgerald, R., Grabner, C., Geissler, K., Zimpfer, M., Stockenhuber, F., & Bircher, N. (1998). High-dose recombinant human erythropoietin stimulates reticulocyte production in patients with multiple organ dysfunction syndrome. *The Journal of Trauma, Injury, Infections, and Critical Care, 44*, 361-366.

Klein, C., Stanek, G., & Wiles, C. (1998). Overfeeding macronutrients to critically ill adults: Metabolic complications. *Journal of the American Dietetic Association, 98*, 795-804.

Klein, C., & Wiles, C. (1997). Evaluation of nutrition care provided to patients with traumatic injuries at risk for multiple organ dysfunction syndrome. *Journal of the American Dietetic Association, 97*, 1422-1424.

Piper, R., & Sibbald, W. (1997). Multiple organ dysfunction syndrome; the relevance of persistent infection and inflammation. In A. Fein, E. Abraham, R. Balk, G. Bernard, R. Bone, D. Dantzker, & M, Fink (Eds.), *Sepsis and multiorgan failure* (pp. 189-207). Baltimore: Williams & Wilkins.

Rauen, C., & Stamatos, C. (1997). Caring for geriatric patients with MODS. *American Journal of Nursing, 97*(5), 16bb-16ii.

Rinaldo, J., & Clark, M. (1998). Multiple organ dysfunction in the context of ARDS. In Stein, J. (Ed.), *Internal medicine* (5th ed., pp. 421-423). St Louis: Mosby.

Sommers, M. (1998). Multisystem. In Alspach, J. (Ed.), *American Association of Critical-Care Nurses: Core curriculum for critical care nurses* (5th ed., pp. 715-798). Philadelphia: WB Saunders.

Stechmiller, J., Treloar, D., & Allen, N. (1997). Gut dysfunction in critically ill patients: A review of the literature. *American Journal of Critical Care, 6*, 204-209.

Thelan, L., Urden, L., Lough, M., & Stacy, K. (1998). Systemic inflammatory response syndrome and multiple organ dysfunction syndrome. In L. Thelan, L. Urden, M. Lough, & K. Stacy (Eds.), *Critical care nursing: Diagnosis and management* (3rd ed., pp. 1121-1140). St Louis: Mosby.

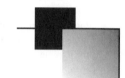

CHAPTER **24**

SEPSIS/SEPTIC SHOCK

Lynn Rodgers, RNC, MSN, CCRN, CNRN, ACNP

CASE PRESENTATION

Emergency Department

John Roberts, a 72-year-old man, arrived in the emergency department unconscious, with stab wounds to the upper-right abdomen and lower-right chest that were sustained in his home while fighting off a burglar. The paramedics secured two large-bore intravenous (IV) catheters in his right and left antecubital spaces and infused lactated Ringer's solution wide open in both sites. An endotracheal tube was inserted, and ventilation with a resuscitation bag with 100% oxygen was begun. Medical antishock trousers (MAST) were in place. Pressure dressings to both wounds were secured.

A 5-cm (2-inch) stab wound to his right lower chest and a 7.5-cm (3-inch) stab wound to his upper-right abdomen were inspected. Chest tubes were inserted into the upper-right and lower-right midaxillary regions. Immediately, 500 ml of red drainage returned via the lower chest tube. His heart rate (HR) was 125 bpm, and the monitor showed sinus tachycardia without ectopy. His blood pressure (BP) was 70/50 mm Hg. Inserting a Foley catheter resulted in drainage 400 ml of clear dark yellow urine. After infusion of more than 2000 ml of lactated Ringer's solution, Mr. Roberts was sent to surgery, still in a hypotensive state. Preoperative body weight was 74 kg (165 lb).

Surgical Intervention

During surgery, a right thoracotomy and right abdominal laparotomy were performed. The right chest wound was explored, and a lacerated intercostal artery was ligated. Exploration of his upper-right abdominal wound revealed more extensive damage. The liver and the duodenum were lacerated. Extensive hemorrhage and leaking of intestinal contents were apparent after opening the peritoneum. Mr. Roberts' injuries were repaired, the peritoneal cavity was irrigated with antibiotic solution, and incisional sump drains were placed in the duodenum.

During the 4-hour surgery, Mr. Roberts received 6 units of blood and an additional 3 L of lactated Ringer's solution. A pulmonary artery catheter (PAC) and right radial arterial line were inserted.

Intensive Care Unit: Immediately after Surgery

When Mr. Roberts arrived in the surgical intensive care unit (ICU), he was receiving ventilatory support. Ventilator settings were as follows:

Assist mode	
Rate	12
Fio_2	60%
V_T	800 ml

Vital signs and hemodynamic parameters immediately after surgery were the following:

BP	92/52 mm Hg	PCWP	6 mm Hg
HR	114 bpm	CVP	4 mm Hg
Respirations	12 breaths/min	CO	5 L/min
Temperature	36.2° C (97.2° F)	CI	2.9 L/min/m^2
PAP	20/8 mm Hg	SVR	1040 dynes/s/cm^{-5}

Arterial blood gas values were normal. Except for a white blood cell (WBC) count of 13.6×10^3/mm^3 and a hemoglobin level of 10 g/dl, Mr. Roberts' other laboratory values were within normal limits.

Intensive Care Unit: Postoperative Day 1

Mr. Roberts remained drowsy but received ventilatory support for 24 hours. His pain was controlled by IV morphine sulfate. The nasogastric tube (NGT) continued to drain large amounts of green fluid, and an incisional duodenal sump tube drained large amounts of greenish brown fluid. His chest and abdominal dressings remained dry. Breath sounds were diminished on the right side but clear on the left. His chest tubes continued to drain small amounts of bloody fluid. Urine output was 40 to 60 ml/hr. His abdomen was slightly firm and distended, and he had no bowel sounds.

Intensive Care Unit: Postoperative Day 2

Mr. Roberts' condition remained stable until his second postoperative day. At this time, he became difficult to arouse but did respond to commands. His respirations were 28 breaths/min, shallow, and labored. His urine output dropped to 20 ml/hr. His skin became warm, dry, and flushed. Other clinical data included the following:

BP	80/50 mm hg	CO	8 L/min
HR	132 bpm	CI	4.7 L/min/m^2
Temperature	36.2° C (97.2° F)	SVR	560 dynes/s/cm^{-5}
PAP	14/7 mm Hg	WBCs	22,000/mm^3
PCWP	4 mm Hg	Glucose	270 mg/dl
CVP	2 mm Hg		

Culture and sensitivity reports from wound drainage indicated gram-negative bacilli. Appropriate IV antibiotics were administered, as well as IV hydrocortisone and naloxone (Narcan). A pharmacy consultation to formulate and calculate nutritional needs was done, and total parenteral nutrition was started. To prepare for the suspected hyperdynamic phase of septic shock, infusion of lactated Ringer's solution was increased to 150 ml/hr, and dopamine at 5 µg/kg/min was started with a concentration of 200 mg/250 ml of 5% dextrose in water (D5W).

Intensive Care Unit: Postoperative Day 6

By the sixth postoperative day, Mr. Roberts' condition had deteriorated dramatically. His skin was cool, mottled, and moist. His sclerae were yellow tinged. He no longer responded to stimuli. A norepinephrine (Levophed) drip infused at 6 µg/min with a concentration of 4 mg/250 ml of D5W, along with a dopamine drip at 2 µg/kg/min was begun. His monitor showed sinus tachycardia with short runs of ventricular tachycardia. ST-segment elevation, T-wave inversion, and the development of Q waves over most of the anterior V leads on his electrocardiogram (ECG). A 75-mg bolus of lidocaine was given followed by a continuous infusion at 2 mg/min with a concentration of 2 g/500 ml of D5W. His breath sounds revealed crackles throughout his chest. Urinary output was only 3 to 5 ml/hr and was grossly bloody. His abdomen was enlarged and firm. His abdominal suture lines had dehisced, and the peritoneum could be seen. The duodenal sump and NGT drainage started to turn red. All arterial and venous puncture sites began oozing blood. Further clinical data included the following:

BP	70/52 mm hg	PCWP	24 mm Hg
HR	140 bpm	CVP	8 mm Hg
Respirations	14 breaths/min	CO	2 L/min
Temperature	35.8° C (96.4° F)	CI	1.1 L/min/m^2
PAP	44/26 mm Hg	SVR	2000 dynes/s/cm^{-5}

Other abnormal laboratory results included the following:

pH	7.14	Lipase	3.9 U/L
P$_{CO_2}$	49 mm Hg	ALT (SGOT)	100 U/L
P$_{O_2}$	46 mm Hg	AST (SGPT)	82 U/L
Sa$_{O_2}$	85%	FDP	39
HCO$_3$$^-$	12 mmol/L	Platelets	75,000/mm^3
Lactic acid	3.0 mEq/l	PT	22 sec
Na$^+$	152 mmol/L	PTT	98.5 sec
K$^+$	5.9 mmol/L	Fibrinogen	130 mg/dl
Creatinine	3.4 mg/dl	CK	640 U/L
Amylase	290 U/L	Troponin I	>50

Final Developments

Despite attempts to reduce afterload with sodium nitroprusside (Nipride) and increase contractility with dobutamine (Dobutrex), Mr. Roberts' hemodynamic status failed even further. When his cardiac rhythm deteriorated into ventricular fibrillation, resuscitation efforts were unsuccessful. An autopsy revealed several small abscessed areas in the lung, acute hepatic failure, multiple hemorrhagic areas, and an acute myocardial infarction (MI).

SEPSIS/SEPTIC SHOCK

Questions

1. Discuss the magnitude of bacteremia and sepsis in hospitalized patients and the relationship between these two diagnoses.
2. What are the risk factors for infection and development of septic shock? Identify those that applied to Mr. Roberts.
3. Discuss the rationale for use of a PAC in monitoring septic shock.
4. What organisms most commonly cause septic shock and in which sites is infection most often seen?
5. What pathophysiologic processes occur with septic shock? What are the effects of these processes on the patient's vascular tank, volume, and pump?
6. Discuss clinical and laboratory changes that occurred on Mr. Roberts' second postoperative day.
7. What is the rationale for each of the following therapeutic modalities ordered for Mr. Roberts on the second postoperative day?

   - IV rate increased to 150 ml/hr
   - Dopamine 5 µg/kg/min
   - Hydrocortisone IV
   - Naloxone (Narcan) IV infusion
   - Total parenteral nutrition

8. Discuss the clinical changes that occurred during Mr. Roberts' sixth postoperative day.
9. What is the rationale for each of the following therapeutic modalities ordered on the sixth postoperative day? Calculate how many milliliters per hour should be infused for each drug listed.

   - Norepinephrine 6 µg/min
   - Dopamine 2 µg/kg/min
   - Lidocaine 2 mg/min

10. What are the reasons for the changes in the following hemodynamic parameters noted on the sixth postoperative day?

    - SVR
    - CO and CI
    - PCWP

11. Interpret Mr. Roberts' blood gas levels on the sixth postoperative day.
12. Why are the renal, liver, and pancreatic laboratory values reported on the sixth postoperative day abnormal?
13. What complications do the hematologic laboratory values suggest?
14. What would account for the ECG changes described?
15. Mr. Roberts' liver was lacerated during the stabbing. What effect, if any, did this have on his eventual outcome?

16. Describe the differences in the parameters below between hyperdynamic or warm septic shock and hypodynamic or cold septic shock.

	Hyperdynamic	**Hypodynamic**
LOC		
BP		
HR		
Respirations		
Pulse pressure		
Skin		
SVR		
CO and CI		
Urine output		

17. How do elderly patients manifest symptoms of sepsis?
18. What does the future hold for therapy in septic shock?

SEPSIS/SEPTIC SHOCK

Questions and Answers

1. **Discuss the magnitude of bacteremia and sepsis in hospitalized patients and the relationship between these two diagnoses.**

The American College of Chest Physicians and the Society of Critical Care Medicine have developed standardized definitions for sepsis and related conditions with the continuum extending from bacteremia, sepsis, and severe sepsis to finally septic shock. These organizations define bacteremia as the presence of live bacteria in the bloodstream. Bacteremia does not always create systemic complications nor lead to sepsis. *Systemic inflammatory response syndrome (SIRS)* is a systemic reaction to infection as evidenced by two or more of the following:

> Temperature > 100.4° F (38° C) or < 96.8° F (36° C)
> HR > 90 bpm
> Respiratory rate > 20/min or $Paco_2$ < 32 mm Hg
> WBC count > 12,000/mm^3 or < 4000/mm^3 or > 10% band forms

When a confirmed infection is associated with SIRS, sepsis has developed. Sepsis can be caused by pathogens other than bacteria, such as fungi, viruses, and protozoa (Astiz & Rackow, 1998). Mortality is highest, however, when sepsis is associated with confirmed bacteremia (Cohen, 1998). Regardless of the causative organism, sepsis can result in systemic complications that occur when circulating chemical mediators released by the inflammatory response compromise the patient's cardiovascular system.

Severe sepsis also occurs when hypoperfusion, hypotension, and organ dysfunction develop. If hypotension and perfusion abnormalities occur despite aggressive fluid resuscitation and inotropic therapy, septic shock is present (Zimmerman, 1997).

Septic shock is the most common cause of deaths in the ICU and the 13th leading cause of death in the United States. Each year sepsis develops in 400,000 to 800,000 patients, resulting in septic shock in 200,000 patients (Jones & Bucher, 1999; Talan, 1997). Mortality from sepsis is reported to be 20% to 50%, and death from septic shock is estimated to be 40% to 70% or higher (Astiz & Rackow, 1998; Porter, 1997).

The incidence of death from sepsis has actually increased over the past 15 years despite the development of advanced treatments and new antibiotics. Increased virulence of organisms, mutated antibiotic-resistant organisms, weakened host resistance, and the aging of our population are all factors in the losing battle against sepsis (Pinner, Teutsch, & Simonsen, 1996). Unfortunately 60% to 79% of all deaths from sepsis occur in the geriatric population (Stanley, 1996).

2. What are the risk factors for infection and development of septic shock? Identify those that applied to Mr. Roberts.

Risk factors for infection and development of septic shock are patient and/or treatment related. Patient-related risk factors include burns, trauma, malnutrition, leukemia, age older than 70 years or newborn, debilitating diseases (especially chronic lung disease, cardiovascular disease, diabetes mellitus, or renal or liver failure), pregnancy, sleep deprivation, immunocompromised states, and response to physiologic and psychologic stressors.

Treatment-related risk factors include foreign body insertion, drugs (especially immunosuppressives, cytotoxins, and antibiotics), artificial airways, surgery, immobility, and hospital understaffing.

Mr. Roberts had the following risk factors: IV infusion, endotracheal tube, chest tube, Foley catheter, PAC and right radial arterial line, abdominal trauma, age older than 70 years, and leaking of gastrointestinal contents into the peritoneum.

3. Discuss the rationale for use of a PAC in monitoring septic shock.

A PAC is often used for monitoring patients with severe septic shock and is helpful for differentiating the type of shock. Cohen (1998) postulated that invasive interventions such as a PAC may actually contribute to increased morbidity and mortality in patients with septic shock and should not be used routinely. Cardiovascular and metabolic abnormalities can be readily determined from the hemodynamic profile obtained from the PAC. Appropriate pharmacologic, medical, and nursing treatments can be determined by careful analysis of this information. Monitoring the patient's response further assists in adjusting treatment for maximal response.

Rice (1997) and Tangredi (1998) described septic shock as having two distinct phases: hyperdynamic and hypodynamic. Initially, a hyperdynamic response occurs. During this phase, systemic vascular resistance (SVR) is decreased. An increase in cardiac muscle contractility also develops as a compensatory mechanism. The decrease in SVR and increase in cardiac contractility result in abnormally high cardiac output (CO) and cardiac index (CI). In addition, pulmonary artery and capillary wedge pressures (PAWP and PCWP, respectively) can be below normal because of the venous vasodilation and decreased venous return.

During the hypodynamic phase of septic shock, compensatory mechanisms begin to fail. Fluid escapes the vascular tree into the tissues because of an increase in capillary permeability. Sympathetic nervous system stimulation causes profound vasoconstriction. The heart muscle itself is depressed, and contractility decreases. Hypotension then results from decreased intravascular volume, increased SVR, and decreased cardiac contractility. CO and CI are decreased; however, PAWP and PCWP are increased. Treatment is guided by the hemodynamic information that a PAC provides. With this information, the patient's chances of survival are increased.

4. What organisms most commonly cause septic shock and in which sites is infection most often seen?

Bacteria are the most common causes of septic shock. In the past, gram-negative bacteria were overwhelmingly the organisms most likely to cause septic shock, specifically *Escherichia coli, Klebsiella, Enterobacter, Serratia, Pseudomonas aeruginosa, Bacteroides,* and *Proteus.* However, the incidence of sepsis caused by gram-positive bacteria such as *Staphylococcus aureus, Staphylococcus epidermidis, Streptococcus pyrogenes, Listeria,* and pneumococcal pathogens has risen to almost equal that of gram-negative bacteria (Talan, 1997).

In 1998, a 40-year review of the literature by Friedman, Silva, and Vincent revealed interesting historical information concerning septic shock. Before 1990, the primary source of infection in sepsis was the abdomen. From 1991 through 1997, this source had changed to the chest, with the abdomen becoming the second most common site. The urogenital system has remained the third most common site of infection in sepsis.

5. What pathophysiologic processes occur with septic shock? What are the effects of these processes on the patient's vascular tank, volume, and pump?

Once a microbial infection develops, a general but complex inflammatory response develops, resulting in increased capillary permeability and blood flow. These responses allow immunologic cells to migrate toward the site of infection, begin phagocytic actions, and activate the complement system. Once the complement system is activated, more WBCs come to the site of the infection and as many as 40 inflammatory mediators are released. Cytokines are one of the primary mediators that signal other cells to release additional mediators such as tumor necrosis factor-α (TNF-α) and interleukin (IL)-1 and IL-6, interferon, leukotrienes, histamine, bradykinin, prostaglandins, thromboxane A_2, serotonin, nitric oxide, arachidonic acid, platelet-activating factor (PAF), oxygen-free radicals, and myocardial depressant factor. If the invading organism is a gram-negative bacterium, endotoxins are also released, which further stimulate the production of these inflammatory mediators (Jones & Bucher, 1999).

The three major effects of septic shock within the cardiovascular system are (1) vasodilation, (2) maldistribution of blood volume, and (3) myocardial depression. Two interacting factors result in vasodilation in septic shock (Carpati, Astiz, & Rackow, 1999). First, a loss of vascular reaction to sympathetic nervous system stimulation occurs and, second, production of substances from the endothelial lining relax the vascular smooth muscle layer of the vessels. Profound dilation in the arterial and venous circulation results and decreases in SVR and preload develop. Initially, compensation occurs by an increase in CO. However, tissue perfusion continues to decrease because of the maldistribution of blood flow and impaired cardiac function.

Maldistribution of blood flow develops as a consequence of blood volume displacement from intravascular areas to extracellular spaces. Although septic shock is usually associated with vasodilation, pulmonary, renal, hepatic, splenic, and pancreatic vasoconstriction occurs with associated organ dysfunction. Increased capillary permeability allows serum to migrate into the interstitial spaces. Parenchymal edema in the pulmonary, cardiac, and renal vascular beds results in functional failure of these organs. The interstitial fluid shift also depletes the circulating volume and increases blood viscosity. Blood flow becomes sluggish, WBCs and platelets accumulate, and microemboli develop. Vascular occlusion and inadequate tissue perfusion progress (Crowley, 1996). Anaerobic metabolism with elevations in lactic acid levels leads to metabolic acidosis. Hotchkiss et al. (1999) postulated that cellular stress response during septic shock results in downregulation or hibernation of the cell with a shift to fetal gene expression. Through these actions, the cell reverts to a lower energy–using state and avoids death. Unfortunately, only enough energy is produced to keep the individual cells alive but not enough to continue whole organ function. Multiorgan failure eventually results.

Although the exact mechanism of the septic inflammatory response is unclear, various mediators are thought to depress the function of the myocardium. Some findings suggest that microvascular and myocyte damage depresses the myocardial function and affects the responsiveness of the myofilament to calcium. Other studies found evidence that the myocardium is hyporesponsive to catecholamines because of impaired β-adrenergic receptor stimulation of cyclic adenosine monophosphate. Still other researchers found indirect evidence of specific myocardial depressant substances (Carpati et al, 1999). Regardless of the mechanism, the depressed myocardium meets no resistance in the profoundly vasodilated systemic vascular bed. Thus CO and CI initially are maintained and often are increased.

In summary, the common cardiovascular patterns demonstrated initially in septic shock consist of high CO, low SVR, decreased left ventricular ejection fraction, a dilated left ventricle, and a normal or increased stroke volume. Death is usually a result of hypotension, which results from a progressively increasing SVR, a perpetual decrease in CO, and eventual multiple organ system failure.

6. **Discuss clinical and laboratory changes that occurred on Mr. Roberts' second postoperative day.**

Difficult to Arouse

Difficult to arouse is an early cardinal sign of systemic infection and inflammatory response to circulating endotoxins. In a patient with sepsis, the level of consciousness continues to deteriorate with impending shock as a result of decreased cerebral perfusion.

Respiration 28 breaths/min, Shallow and Labored

The lungs become a target organ as septic shock progresses. Circulating endotoxins cause deterioration of the patient's pulmonary status. The initial pulmonary response to endotoxins creates bronchoconstriction. Pulmonary edema as a result of increased capillary permeability occurs. Tachypnea is also an early cardinal sign of systemic infection, hypoxemia, and physiologic stress.

Urine Output Decreased to 20 ml/hr

As renal blood flow in the patient in septic shock is reduced, urine output decreases. Antidiuretic hormone and aldosterone are released to increase intravascular water and sodium in an attempt to maintain CO and renal blood flow, often with no success. In addition, aminoglycoside antibiotics, frequently effective in sepsis, are nephrotoxic.

Warm, Dry, Flushed Skin

In the early stages of septic shock, vasoactive mediators create a flushed appearance because of peripheral vasodilation. This early stage is known as *hyperdynamic* or *warm septic shock.*

BP 80/50 mm Hg

Hypotension commonly is caused by the vasodilation when cardiac compensation fails.

HR 132 bpm

Tachycardia is another early cardinal sign of a systemic infection and inflammatory response. An increase in heart rate is also a compensatory mechanism to maintain perfusion and CO.

Temperature 40° C (104° F)

The hypothalamus responds to bacteremia with an increase in temperature. As blood is shunted away from the skin during shock, the normal ability of the skin to disperse heat is decreased. Fever also is one of the cardinal signs of infection and inflammation.

CI 4.7 L/min/m^2; SVR 560 dynes/sec/cm^{-5}

The initial hyperdynamic pattern of septic shock consists of high CI as a result of low SVR. Toxic bacterial endotoxins are thought to decrease the vasomotor tone of the blood vessels by activating the release of endorphins and histamine and the complement system.

WBCs 22,000/mm^3

Leukopenia is an early finding in an immunocompromised patient with sepsis. However, as sepsis progresses, the inflammatory response signals the bone marrow to accelerate leukocyte synthesis and release. Consequently, the WBC count will increase to more than 10,000/mm^3.

Glucose Level 270 mg/dl

The reaction of the adrenal cortex to shock is to release glucocorticoids. The glucocorticoids release glucagon. Glucagon stimulates the conversion of glycogen to glucose (glycolysis) and gluconeogenesis in the liver. Therefore, the serum glucose level may be elevated.

Culture and Sensitivity Reports Indicate Gram-Negative Bacilli

Gram-negative bacteria are the organisms that account for 60% of sepsis in adults. Gram-positive bacteria are the causative organisms 35% of the time, with fungi and other organisms at 5% (Talan, 1997).

7. **What is the rationale for each of the following therapeutic modalities ordered for Mr. Roberts on the second postoperative day?**

IV Rate Increased to 150 ml/hr

Restoration of adequate intravascular volume is an important aspect of patient care during episodes of hypotension. Vasodilation during sepsis dramatically decreases preload and afterload. The vascular tree is too large for the circulating volume. The circulating volume is also further decreased because increased capillary permeability allows fluid to escape into interstitial spaces (Astiz & Rackow, 1998).

Dopamine 5 μg/kg/min

Low-dose dopamine increases renal blood flow, creates a moderate pressor effect, and improves cardiac performance.

Steroids

Use of corticosteroids is controversial and should be reserved for patients in septic shock who have a suspected or documented adrenal insufficiency. According to Briegel et al. (1999) infusion of steroids reduced the length of vasopressor therapy and resulted in earlier resolution of organ dysfunction related to sepsis. Mortality of patients with sepsis or septic shock who receive corticosteroids may not be significantly reduced and in some cases may be higher owing to development of secondary infections.

Naloxone (Narcan) IV Infusion

Naloxone is a narcotic antagonist generally used to reverse the respiratory depression caused by narcotics. As described by Jones and Bucher (1998), naloxone is now given to patients with severe septic shock before compensatory mechanisms cease. Its primary action is to block opioid receptors and other receptors that mediate vasodilation. Levels of endogenous endorphins and myocardial depressant factor are reduced, thereby combating vasodilation and decreased contractility.

Total Parenteral Nutrition

Because of the disruption of Mr. Roberts' gastrointestinal system, tube feedings were not feasible. Nutrition via parenteral means was required. Uehara, Plank, and Hill (1999) studied resting energy expenditure during the first week after onset of severe sepsis and found it drastically increased to 40% greater than normal. Further findings indicated that activity energy expenditure increased by three to four times normal requirements. Finally, overall total energy expenditure can increase to 50 to 60 kcal/kg/day with severe sepsis.

8. **Discuss the clinical changes that occurred during Mr. Roberts' sixth postoperative day.**

As described by Rice (1997), the following clinical changes occur as septic shock progresses.

Cool, Mottled, Moist Skin

The skin indicates the change from hyperdynamic (warm) to hypodynamic (cold) septic shock. This is a poor prognostic sign for the patient, as it indicates failure of the compensatory mechanisms.

Yellow Sclerae

As chemical mediators continue to shunt blood to various organs, the patient's liver and kidneys become hypoperfused. Hyperbilirubinemia and jaundice are common clinical indicators that the liver is adversely affected. In addition, Mr. Roberts' liver was lacerated during his injury.

ECG Changes—Sinus Tachycardia with Short Runs of Ventricular Tachycardia

Sinus and ventricular tachycardia indicate further myocardial damage from the circulating endotoxins and the decreased CO. Because the kidneys are hypoperfused, the patient may be experiencing acute renal failure. The K^+ level of 5.9 mmol/L could suggest acute renal failure and is probably responsible for the ventricular tachycardia. The 12-lead ECG indicated a massive anterior wall MI.

BP 70/52 mm Hg, CO 2 L/min, CI 1.1 L/min/m², PAP 44/26 mm Hg, PCWP 24 mm Hg, SVR 2000 dynes/sec/cm⁻⁵, CVP 8 mm Hg

Mr. Roberts' hemodynamic changes are classic indications of the hypodynamic phase of septic shock. Afterload is drastically increased, and contractility is decreased. Multisystem failure is imminent.

Respirations 14/min, Congested Breath Sounds

Mr. Roberts' respiratory assessment indicates further deterioration of respiratory status caused by circulating endotoxins, pulmonary edema, and left ventricular failure.

Temperature 35.8° C (96.4° F)

The low temperature is another indication that septic shock has progressed from hyperdynamic to hypodynamic.

Abdomen Large and Firm, Wound Dehiscence

Because of increased capillary permeability, accumulation of inflammatory fluids, and cardiac failure, ascites is present. The increased intraabdominal pressure and poor healing produced wound dehiscence.

9. **What is the rationale for each of the following therapeutic modalities ordered on the sixth postoperative day? Calculate how many milliliters per hour should be infused for each drug listed.**

Norepinephrine 6 μg/min = 22.5 ml/hr

Norepinephrine is indicated for hemodynamically significant hypotension unresponsive to other vasopressors.

Dopamine 2 μg/kg/min = 11.25 ml/hr

Dopamine at 1 to 3 μg/kg/min dilates the renal and mesenteric vessels. Norepinephrine constricts the renal and mesenteric vessels, and adding low dosages of dopamine counteracts some of this effect.

Lidocaine 2 mg/min = 30 ml/hr

Lidocaine was started to decrease the ventricular irritability, which is evidenced by the ventricular tachycardia and most likely is caused in part by the K^+ level of 5.9 mmol/L.

10. **What are the reasons for the changes in the following hemodynamic parameters noted on the sixth postoperative day?**

SVR

The SVR increased from 560 to 2000 dynes/sec/cm⁻⁵. Clinically, the SVR represents the resistance against which the left ventricle must pump to eject its volume. This elevation indicates a change from hyperdynamic to hypodynamic septic shock.

CO and CI

The CO decreased from 8 to 4.7 L/min, and the CI decreased from 2 to 1.1 L/min/m^2 on the sixth postoperative day. Because CO represents the amount of blood pumped by the ventricle in 1 minute, it can be concluded that an increase in SVR will decrease the CO and CI. A drop in CO and CI indicates that hypodynamic septic shock has developed.

PCWP

The PCWP increased from 4 to 24 mm Hg, indicating an increase in the pressure in the left side of the heart. This could be from the ventricular dilation and decreased ejection fraction that occur in late septic shock and from the release of various chemical and hormonal mediators that depress myocardial function.

11. Interpret Mr. Roberts' blood gas levels on the sixth postoperative day.

Mr. Roberts' blood gas levels indicate metabolic and respiratory acidosis. Lactic acidosis caused by increased oxygen debt from abnormal cellular metabolism is a common finding in patients with septic shock. During the progression of septic shock, a ventilation-perfusion mismatch also develops as chemical mediators create pulmonary interstitial edema and a maldistribution in pulmonic blood flow. In addition, localization of activated neutrophils in the microvasculature of the pulmonary system is thought to contribute to the sepsis-induced pathologic lung damage (Protopapas & McLuckie, 1996).

12. Why are the renal, liver, and pancreatic laboratory values reported on the sixth postoperative day abnormal?

As described by Talan (1997), the kidneys, liver, brain, and lungs are the organs most frequently affected by septic shock. As renal blood flow is reduced, urine output decreases, and the body is unable to eliminate waste products. Acute renal failure ensues. As chemical mediators continue to shunt blood to various organs, the liver and pancreas become hypoperfused. Shock liver and acute cholestatic jaundice are common. Disseminated intravascular coagulation (DIC) is an ominous complication that occurs most often in sepsis caused by gram-negative organisms. Sepsis increases procoagulant effects, early fibrinolysis, and plasminogen activator inhibitor 1 protein and decreases antithrombin III anticoagulation activity (Jones & Bucher, 1999). Laboratory results of liver function and clotting factors reflect development of DIC. The increased lactic acid level is also significant as this indicates the severity of perfusion failure and oxygen debt and is associated with impending death.

13. What complications do the hematologic laboratory values suggest?

Possible complications based on the hematologic laboratory values include acute renal and hepatic failure, DIC, adult respiratory distress syndrome, and acute MI (Gawlinski, McCloy, Caswell, & Quinones-Baldrich, 1999).

14. What would account for the ECG changes described?

Mr. Roberts' ECG changes could indicate an acute anterior wall MI. This diagnosis can be made by the ST-segment elevation, T-wave inversion, and diagnostic Q waves evident in the V anterior chest leads. His elevated creatinine kinase, troponin I, and aspartate aminotransferase levels verified the diagnosis.

15. Mr. Roberts' liver was lacerated during the stabbing. What effect, if any, did this have on his eventual outcome?

Patients at greatest risk for development of septic shock are those who have sustained open wounds, open fractures, massive tissue injury, or significant head injury. The lacerated liver was directly related to the acute hepatic failure noted on the autopsy.

16. Describe the differences in the parameters below between hyperdynamic or warm septic shock and hypodynamic or cold septic shock.

Jones and Bucher (1999) summarized the differences in the hyperdynamic and hypodynamic stages of septic shock as follows:

	Hyperdynamic	Hypodynamic
LOC	Mental cloudiness	Continued deterioration
BP	Normal to just below baseline	Profound hypotension
HR	Bounding pulses, tachycardia	Thready pulsed, tachycardia
Respiration	Decreased rate or mild respiratory distress	Decreased rate with severe respiratory complications
Pulse pressure	Normal to wide	Narrow
Skin	Warm, dry	Cool, moist, mottled
SVR	Decreased	Increased
CO and CI	Increased	Decreased
Urine output	Normal	Decreased

17. How do elderly patients manifest symptoms of sepsis?

Many elderly patients demonstrate blunted responses to sepsis. Temperature elevations may only be primary to secondary or hypothermia may develop. Elevations in WBC counts may not occur; however, a shift to the left may be seen, indicating an increase in the number of immature cells. Cell-mediated immunity is also decreased as evidenced by a decrease in T-cell production. Elderly patients also demonstrate a decrease in physiologic reserve. Cardiovascular compensatory mechanisms are decreased because the usual response to catecholamine release with tachycardia and vasoconstriction does not readily occur in elderly patients. Colonization of the lungs with infective organisms with resulting pneumonia is more common and occurs more quickly in elderly patients with sepsis. Nonspecific signs and symptoms such as delirium, decreased functional status, anorexia, vomiting, incontinence, urinary frequency or oliguria, or hypotension may be present. The most common presenting symptom of sepsis in elderly patients, although nonspecific and elusive, is a sudden mental status change (Stanley, 1996). This vague picture of sepsis in elderly patients accounts for delayed treatment, increased severity of sepsis, and resulting high mortality.

18. What does the future hold for therapy in septic shock?

Most research on therapy of septic shock is targeted to neutralizing or preventing damage from the many inflammatory mediators. Development and testing of several endotoxin antibodies such as IL-1 receptor agonists, anti-TNF antibodies or binders, and PAF receptor antagonists are presently in progress. Wardle (1996) discussed experimental and futuristic approaches in the treatment of septic shock. Medications that decrease stimulation of the complement pathway such as C1 esterase inhibitor and heparin are used. Coagulation control using such substances as heparin, antithrombin III, hirudin, protein C, or thrombomodulin demonstrates some effectiveness against DIC, which is a prevalent complication of severe septic shock. The use of pentoxifylline and monoclonal antibodies to decrease leukocyte adherence has produced mixed clinical outcome results. Defense boosting with antiproteases, antioxidants, growth hormone, and vaccines is being explored.

Because of the complex nature of the body's inflammatory response, the ability of researchers to influence the course of sepsis and septic shock remains disappointing (Vincent, 1997). The dose and timing of various interventions may be crucial. Many researchers too narrowly focus their approach on only single-agent therapies when multiple agents may need to be considered for an optimal outcome. In addition, much has been written on the medical-ethical consequences of the specific therapies for sepsis (Sbarbaro, 1997). Several of the potential treatments are extremely costly, and insurance plans may refuse payment. At what price do we treat the patient with sepsis? How can we as a society get the best value for our health care dollars?

Withholding proven medical treatment on the basis of financial reimbursement presents several ethical issues. Some interventions may actually increase morbidity and mortality in some patients (Cohen, 1998). Much is yet to be learned about the treatment of this devastating disease process. Truly, treatment of sepsis and septic shock will remain a medical research priority and an ethical dilemma in the 21st century.

SEPSIS/SEPTIC SHOCK

References

Astiz, M. E., & Rackow, E. C. (1998). Septic shock. *The Lancet, 351*(9114), 1501-1505.

Briegel, J., Forst, H., Haller, M., Schelling, G., Killer, E., Kuprat, G., Hemmer, B., Lenhart, A., Heyduck, M., Stoll, C., & Peter, K. (1999). Stress doses of hydrocortisone reverse hyperdynamic septic shock: A prospective, randomized, double-blind, single-center study. *Critical Care Medicine, 27*(4), 723-732.

Carpati, C. M., Astiz, M. E., & Rackow, E. C. (1999). Mechanisms and management of myocardial dysfunction in septic shock. *Critical Care Medicine, 27*(2), 231-232.

Cohen, N. H. (1998). Reduced mortality from septic shock-lessons for the future. *Critical Care Medicine, 26*(12), 1956-1958.

Crowley, S. R. (1996). The pathogenesis of septic shock. *Heart & Lung, 25*(2), 124-136.

Friedman, G., Silva, E., & Vincent, J. (1998). Has the mortality of septic shock changed with time? *Critical Care Medicine, 26*(12), 2078-2086.

Gawlinski, A., McCloy, K., Caswell, D., & Quinones-Baldrich, W. J. (1999). Cardiovascular disorders. In A. Gawlinski and D. Hamwi (Eds.), *Acute care nurse practitioner clinical curriculum and certification review* (pp. 136-294). Philadelphia: WB Saunders.

Hotchkiss, R. S., Swanson, P. E., Freeman, B. D., Tinsley, K. W., Cobb, J. P., Matuschak, G. M., Buchman, T. G., & Karl, I. E. (1999). Apoptotic cell death in patients, with sepsis, shock, and multiple organ dysfunction. *Critical Care Medicine, 27*(7), 1230-1251.

Jones, K. M., & Bucher, L. (1999). Shock. In L. Bucher & S. Melander (Eds.), *Critical care nursing* (pp. 1010-1035). Philadelphia: WB Saunders.

Pinner, R., Teutsch, S., & Simonsen, L. (1996). Trends in infectious diseases mortality in the United States. *Journal of the American Medical Association, 275*(3), 189-193.

Porter, S. B. (1997). Current status of clinical trials with anti-TNF. *Chest, 112*(6), 339S-341S.

Protopapas, M., & McLuckie, A. (1996). Sepsis in the intensive care unit. *Care of the Critically Ill, 12*(1), 21-24.

Rice, V. (1997). *Shock: A clinical syndrome.* Aliso Viejo, CA: American Association of Critical-Care Nurses.

Sbarbaro, J. A. (1997). Ethical considerations on the use of monoclonals in the managed care environment. *Chest, 112*(6), 342S-344S.

Stanley, M. (1996). Sepsis in the elderly. *Critical Care Nursing Clinics of North America, 8*(1), 1-6.

Talan, D. A. (1997). Sepsis and septic shock. *Emergency Medicine, 29*(3), 54-68.

Tangredi, M. (1998). Septic shock. *American Journal of Nursing, 98*(3), 46-47.

Uehara, M., Plank, L. D., & Hill, G. L. (1999). Components of energy expenditure in patients with severe sepsis and major trauma: a basis for clinical care. *Critical Care Medicine, 27*(7), 1295-1302.

Vincent, J. (1997). New therapies in sepsis. *Chest, (112)*6, 330S-338S.

Wardle, E. N. (1996). Experimental and futuristic approaches to treatment of septic shock. *Care of the Critically Ill, 12*(6), 217-220.

Zimmerman, J. L. (1997). Sepsis. *Emergency Medicine, 29*(1), 73-82.

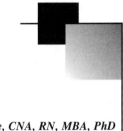

CHAPTER *25*

BURNS

Ann H. White, CNA, RN, MBA, PhD

CASE PRESENTATION

Tony Knight, a 21-year-old man, was involved in an industrial fire. Mr. Knight was welding a steel structure when a spark from his torch ignited a barrel of flammable material that was inadvertently placed in his work area. Mr. Knight sustained full-thickness burns over the upper half of his chest and circumferential burns to both arms. He also sustained superficial partial-thickness burns to his face, neck, and both hands. His entire abdomen, upper half of his back, and front of his upper legs sustained deep partial-thickness burns.

He was transported to a small community hospital where two intravenous (IV) lines were started, a Foley catheter and nasogastric tube were inserted, and humidified oxygen at 3 L/min was started through a nasal cannula. He was given mannitol 12.5 g IV before being transported to a major burn center. Vital signs immediately before transport were as follows:

BP	136/84 mm Hg	Respirations	24 breaths/min
HR	96 bpm	Temperature	37.2° C (99° F) (oral)

Mr. Knight's preburn weight was 72 kg (160 lb). Mr. Knight was received in the burn unit 4 hours after sustaining the burn injury.

At admission to the burn unit, Mr. Knight was alert and oriented, and his vital signs were as follows:

BP	140/90 mm Hg	Respirations	24 breaths/min
HR	110 bpm	Temperature	36.1° C (97° F)

Mr. Knight's lungs were clear in all fields on auscultation, and he had an occasional productive cough of a small amount of carbon-tinged sputum. His voice was becoming hoarse. No bowel sounds were heard, and the nasogastric tube was draining dark yellow-green liquid. Peripheral pulses were obtained with a Doppler stethoscope because they could not be palpated manually. The Foley catheter was draining burgundy-colored urine. Urine output totaled 280 ml since the insertion of the Foley catheter 4 hours before. Fluid resuscitation efforts since the burn injury included 4 L of lactated Ringer's solution through the

IV lines. The following laboratory results were determined after Mr. Knight's arrival in the burn unit:

WBCs	$12 \times 10^3/mm^3$	SMAC	20
RBCs	$34.8 \times 10^6/mm^3$	Na^+	151 mmol/L
Hgb	12.8 g/dl	K^+	5.2 mmol/L
Hct	52%	Cl^-	112 mmol/L
pH	7.37 (with 3 L oxygen)	BUN	22 mg/dl
P_{CO_2}	35 mm Hg	Creatinine	1.6 mg/dl
P_{O_2}	105 mm Hg	Myoglobin (RIA)	90 ng/ml
HCO_3^-	18 mmol/L	Carboxyhemoglobin	6%
Sao_2	99%		

Urinalysis revealed the following:

Specific gravity	1.040	Blood	Trace
Glucose	+1	Protein	Trace
Ketones	Trace		

The burn unit physician performed a fiberoptic bronchoscopy, which showed minimal redness of the glottis and no edema. Escharotomies were performed on Mr. Knight's arms immediately after admission to the burn unit. Mr. Knight was bathed, his scalp was shaved, and his burns were dressed in occlusive silver sulfadiazine (Silvadene) dressings. Mr. Knight's burns were then dressed twice a day with silver sulfadiazine. The following regimen was prescribed: ranitidine (Zantac) 150 mg IV push every 12 hours; antacid 30 ml every hour instilled through a nasogastric tube and clamped for 15 minutes for the first 48 hours after the burn; and morphine sulfate 3 mg IV push every hour as needed for pain.

Bowel sounds returned on day 3, the nasogastric tube was removed, and a high-calorie, high-protein diet was begun. On day 5 of the hospital stay, Mr. Knight was taken to surgery for the first of a series of surgical procedures to excise and graft the areas of full-thickness injury with split-thickness autografts. The donor sites included his buttocks and the backs of his legs. Mr. Knight was discharged from the hospital after a 65-day hospital stay with follow-up and rehabilitation scheduled.

BURNS

Questions

1. Discuss the pathophysiology of burns, including the classification of burn depth and severity of burn injury.
2. Using the rule of nines and the Lund and Browder chart, calculate the percentage of TBSA burned.
3. Describe the initial assessment and stabilization of a burn victim at the scene of the injury and in the emergency department.
4. Describe the three phases of burn physiology, including a discussion of the effects on the following systems during the emergent and acute phases:

   - Cardiovascular
   - Respiratory

- Immunologic
- Gastrohepatic
- Genitourinary

5. Based on Mr. Knight's preburn weight, use the Parkland formula to calculate the fluid requirement for adequate resuscitation.
6. What significance, if any, would the administration of mannitol have on fluid resuscitation?
7. What assessment findings would indicate myoglobinuria?
8. Describe the treatment protocol for myoglobinuria.
9. What assessment findings are critical to establishing the presence of an inhalation injury? Which of Mr. Knight's assessment findings warrant concern?
10. Describe the treatment protocol of a burn patient with an inhalation injury or a suspected inhalation injury.
11. What is the purpose of escharotomies?
12. Discuss pain management in the treatment protocol for the patient with a burn injury.
13. Using the Curreri formula for nutrition, calculate Mr. Knight's nutritional needs. Discuss the need for a high-calorie, high-protein diet.
14. Discuss burn wound care and dressing techniques. Include the types of topical antimicrobial agents commonly used in wound care, listing advantages and disadvantages of each.
15. Describe the types of biologic and synthetic dressings currently being used in wound care.
16. Discuss the use of autografts and the nursing care required.
17. Describe the appropriate care for donor sites.
18. Discuss the splinting and positioning required for Mr. Knight to maintain use of his extremities and upper body.
19. List the nursing diagnoses, outcomes, and interventions appropriate for the care of the patient with a burn injury during the emergent and acute phases of burn physiology.
20. Discuss the psychosocial aspects of caring for the patient with a burn injury and the impact on the patient's support system.

BURNS

Questions and Answers

Introduction

The skin is the largest organ of the human body and consists of two layers: the epidermis and dermis (Thelan, Urden, Lough, & Stacy, 1998). The epidermis is composed of avascular cells that act to protect the body from the environment. The dermis contains the structures of the skin, including blood vessels, glands, hair follicles, nerves, and capillaries that bring nourishment to the epidermis and sensory fibers.

The skin serves to maintain body temperature, control evaporation and fluid loss, produce vitamin D, and protect the body against the environment (Jordan & Harrington, 1997). A burn injury results in the loss of all or portions of the epidermis and dermis and the associated functions.

Experts estimate that 1.4 million people in the United States sustain a burn injury each year (Jones & Bucher, 1999). Approximately one third of the burn victims are children (Gordon & Goodwin, 1997). An estimated 100,000 people are hospitalized for a burn injury each year, with 12,000 of these dying during their hospitalization (Thelan et al, 1998). A burn injury, while directly affecting the skin, also has dramatic effects on every system in the body.

1. Discuss the pathophysiology of burns, including the classification of burn depth and severity of burn injury.

A burn injury results in the coagulation of cellular proteins in the cells of the skin. The denaturation of protein is produced by the heat or actual contact from a thermal, chemical, electrical, or radiation exposure (Alspach, 1998).

The coagulation of the cellular proteins leads to irreversible cell injury with local production of histamine and oxygen-free radicals. The release of these substances leads to increased capillary permeability, alteration of the cell membrane, and possible alteration of the DNA structure, leading to cell death (Alspach, 1998).

Thermal Burn

A thermal burn is a heat-related injury produced through exposure to hot liquids, steam, flames from a fire, or direct contact with some heat source. This exposure disrupts the function of the skin and its appendages. The extent or severity of this disruption depends on the length of contact time with the heat source, extent of tissue exposed to the heat source, and ability of the heat source and tissue to dissipate the heat (Jones & Bucher, 1999).

Chemical Burn

A chemical burn causes denaturation of the protein through actual contact of the chemical with the skin. The extent of the damage depends on the chemical, the chemical's action, the concentration of the chemical, and the length of contact of the chemical with the skin (Jones & Bucher, 1999). The chemical will continue to burn the skin until totally removed from the body.

Electrical Burn

Although electrical burns account for only about 5% of all of the burns sustained, these burns have a much higher mortality rate than the other types of burns because of the severity of the tissue damage (Jones & Bucher, 1999). There may be minimal damage to the skin, but the structures under the skin, including muscle, nerves, blood vessels, and bones, may sustain extensive damage because of the amount of heat produced as the electrical current passes through the body.

Radiation Burns

Radiation burns may result from exposure to radiation therapy as a treatment modality for certain types of cancer or industrial exposure to certain types of equipment (Thelan et al, 1998). These burns are typically localized, and damage depends on the amount of radiation exposure.

Classification of Burn Depth

Traditionally, burns have been classified as first, second, and third degree. Today, burns are described as superficial, partial thickness, and full thickness. Table 25-1 describes each type of burn and the common characteristics of each.

Severity of Burn Injury

The American Burn Association (ABA) established guidelines to determine the severity of the burn injury. These guidelines rate a burn as minor, moderate, or major, depending on the areas of the body involved in the burn injury and the total body surface area (TBSA) burned (Gordon & Goodwin, 1997). A minor burn for adults usually has a small surface area (less than 15% of the TBSA), with no involvement of the face, hands, feet, or perineum, and can be treated in the home environment. A moderate burn injury has a larger surface area (usually 15% to 25% of the TBSA), including partial- and full-thickness burns. A major burn has a TBSA of more than

TABLE 25-1	Classification of Burn Depth			
		Partial Thickness		
	Superficial	**Superficial**	**Deep**	**Full Thickness**
Morphology	Destruction of epidermis (no other layers involved)	Destruction of epidermis and minimal dermis	Destruction of epidermis and dermis; skin appendages (e.g., hair follicles) intact	Destruction of epidermis and dermis; loss of skin appendages and possible loss of subcutaneous tissue
Skin function	Intact	Intact	Absent	Absent
Tactile and pain sensors	Intact	Intact	Diminished	Absent
Blisters	May be present after 24 hr	Fluid-filled blisters appear immediately after injury	Usually not present, eschar formation	Not present, eschar formation
Appearance of wound	Redness of area with local edema	Moist, pink, or mottled red	Mottled with areas of waxy white, dry surface; absence of blanching	Thick, leathery eschar; white, cherry red, or brown-black; blood vessels may be thrombosed
Healing time	3-5 days	10-14 days	21+ days	Will not heal
Scarring	None	Low incidence; may be influenced by genetic predisposition	High incidence due to slow healing; may be influenced by genetic predisposition	High incidence; depends on time of grafting and surgical techniques used

Modified from Solotkin, K., & Knipe, C. (2000). Patients with burns. In S. Lewis, M. Heitkemper, & S. Dirksen (Eds.), *Medical-surgical nursing* (pp. 523-550). St Louis: Mosby.

25% of the TBSA, including partial- and full-thickness burns. Any burns involving parts of the face, hands, feet, or perineum are included in this category. Moderate and major burn injuries should be treated in a burn center or a critical care area with expertise in the care of patients with burns.

Three concentric zones of injury and their impact on the severity of the burn injury have been described (Alspach, 1998; Jones & Bucher, 1999):

1. *Zone of hyperemia:* the least damaged area; it typically heals in 3 to 5 days.
2. *Zone of stasis:* area in which tissue perfusion is compromised. If resuscitative methods are effective in returning tissue perfusion, the tissue may survive.
3. *Zone of coagulation:* area of permanent burn injury; it is characterized by cellular death.

Fig. 25-1 depicts the three concentric zones of a burn injury.

2. Using the rule of nines and the Lund and Browder chart, calculate the percentage of TBSA burned.

Based on the percentage of TBSA and depth of burn, how would you classify Mr. Knight's burn?

The two methods most commonly used to determine the TBSA of the burn injury are the rule of nines and the Lund and Browder chart (Jones & Bucher, 1999). To ensure adequate fluid resuscitation, an accurate estimate of the TBSA must be obtained. Only partial- and full-thickness burns are calculated as part of the burn injury.

The rule of nines is most commonly used at the site of the burn injury by emergency medical technicians or paramedics and in the emergency department. This method quickly provides an estimate of the TBSA so that fluid resuscitative efforts can begin. It should be noted here that because of differences in proportion of body surface areas, two forms of the rule of nines are available. One form should be used for adults and a second form for children. The form used in this case presentation is for adults only.

The Lund and Browder method is a more accurate estimate of the burn injury, but it takes longer to complete. This method is used in most burn centers because a more accurate determination of the burn injury is needed.

Figs. 25-2 and 25-3 depict the rule of nines and the Lund and Browder charts. Based on the information provided in the case presentation, Mr. Knight sustained a 65% TBSA burn. According to the ABA classification of burn injuries, Mr. Knight sustained a major burn injury because of the amount of TBSA involved in the burn and the location of the burns around the neck and face.

3. Describe the initial assessment and stabilization of a burn victim at the scene of the injury and in the emergency department.

The care received at the site of the burn injury is critical. The basic concern at the scene of a burn injury is to stop the burning process. With a thermal burn, the flames must be extinguished and the clothing removed. Articles of clothing should be removed if there is concern that the clothing may be smoldering and continuing to burn the injured person. If the clothing is embedded in the burn, trying to remove the

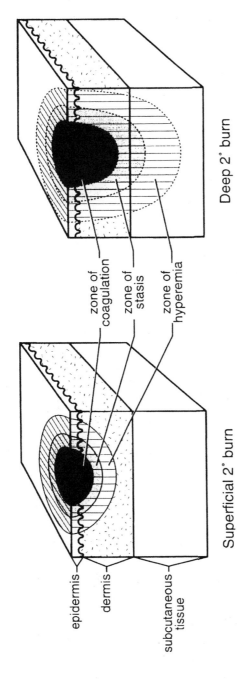

FIGURE 25-1 A diagrammatic rendition of Jackson's three zones of burn injury. If the zone of stasis progresses to necrosis, the potential for conversion of partial-thickness injury to full-thickness injury exists. (From Williams G, Phillips L: Pathophysiology of the burn wound. In: Herndon DN (ed): Total Burn Care. London, W.B. Saunders, 1996.)

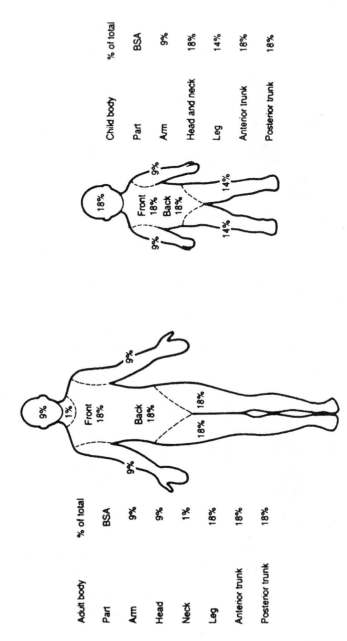

FIGURE 25-2   The "rule of nines" is useful in estimating the extent of burn injury. Note the differences between adults and children. BSA, body surface area. (From Micak RP, et al: Prehospital management, transportation, and emergency care. In: Herndon DN (ed): Total Burn Care. London, W.B. Saunders, 1996.)

Adult body		
Part	BSA	% of total
Arm	9%	
Head	9%	
Neck	1%	
Leg	18%	
Anterior trunk	18%	
Posterior trunk	18%	

Child body		
Part	BSA	% of total
Arm	9%	
Head and neck	18%	
Leg	14%	
Anterior trunk	18%	
Posterior trunk	18%	

AGE vs AREA

Area	Birth 1 yr	1-4 yr	5-9 yr	10-14 yr	15 yr	Adult	2°	3°	Total	Donor Areas
Head	19	17	13	11	9	7				
Neck	2	2	2	2	2	2				
Ant Trunk	13	13	13	13	13	13				
Post Trunk	13	13	13	13	13	13				
R Buttock	2½	2½	2½	2½	2½	2½				
L. Buttock	2½	2½	2½	2½	2½	2½				
Genitalia	1	1	1	1	1	1				
R U Arm	4	4	4	4	4	4				
L.U. Arm	4	4	4	4	4	4				
R L Arm	3	3	3	3	3	3				
L L Arm	3	3	3	3	3	3				
R Hand	2½	2½	2½	2½	2½	2½				
L Hand	2½	2½	2½	2½	2½	2½				
R Thigh	5½	6½	8	8½	9	9½				
L. Thigh	5½	6½	8	8½	9	9½				
R Leg	5	5	5½	6	6½	7				
L Leg	5	5	5½	6	6½	7				
R. Foot	3½	3½	3½	3½	3½	3½				
L Foot	3½	3½	3½	3½	3½	3½				

TOTAL

BURN DIAGRAM

AGE_____

SEX_____

WEIGHT_____

COLOR CODE

Red — 3°

Blue — 2°

BAMC Form 290 NS
1 May 74

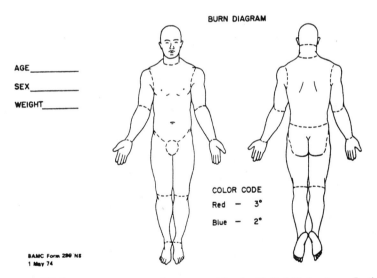

FIGURE 25-3 This is the burn diagram used by the United States Army Institute of Surgical Research. It is based on the Lund and Browder chart using the Berkow formula to take into account the anatomic and age differences in body size. This diagram is also used to map the patient's extent of injury and color code depth of injury for partial-thickness and full-thickness burns.

clothing may not be warranted (Jones & Bucher, 1999). With a chemical burn, the victim must be removed from the source of the chemical. Once that is accomplished, copious amounts of water should be used to flush the chemical from the skin. In most cases, trying to find an antidote for the chemical is not advised (Gordon & Goodwin, 1997). While the antidote is being sought, the chemical continues to burn the skin

TABLE *25-2*	ABCDEF Assessment	
Letter	Assessment	Findings and Care
A	Airway	Patency of airway, oxygen
B	Breathing	Support ventilation
C	Circulation	Check pulses, may need cardiopulmonary resuscitation
D	Disability	Should be alert and oriented
E	Exposure	Cover with clean sheet
F	Fluid	Begin fluid resuscitation

and valuable time is lost. The victim of an electrical injury should be removed from the source of the electricity as soon as possible. A major concern during this effort is to keep the rescuer from becoming a part of the circuit and sustaining an electrical injury as well.

Gordon and Goodwin (1997) cited the Guidelines for Advanced Burn Life Support as the most appropriate method for conducting a primary survey once the victim has been removed from the source of the burn injury. These guidelines use an ABCDEF assessment to ensure adequate care of the burn victim at the site. Table 25-2 depicts the assessments and emergency care required based on each letter.

A burn victim should receive the same management as any other trauma victim. Maintaining the airway and circulation is paramount, followed by an assessment of any other types of injury. Evaluation of circulatory status includes checking the peripheral pulses to ensure adequate perfusion to all the extremities. A burn victim is alert and oriented. If there is a change in the person's mental status or if the person is disoriented or confused, other types of injury must be investigated.

Once the burn victim's condition is stabilized, he or she should be transported to the closest facility. If the burn injury is moderate or major, the preference is to transport the person to a burn center. When the burn victim reaches the emergency department or burn center, a thorough head-to-toe assessment should be conducted (Gordon & Goodwin, 1997). A complete history, including allergies, current medications, immunizations (current tetanus), and drug and tobacco use, should be completed. The emergency department of a hospital without a burn center should be in immediate contact with a burn center to coordinate transporting the burn victim to the center and to provide effective treatment of the burn injury.

4. **Describe the three phases of burn physiology, including a discussion of the effects on the following systems during the emergent and acute phases:**

    - Cardiovascular
    - Respiratory
    - Immunologic
    - Gastrohepatic
    - Genitourinary

The first phase of burn physiology is the emergent or shock phase. This phase typically lasts 48 hours and is a crucial period for the patient. The second phase begins when diuresis is noted and lasts until wound closure. This phase is referred to as the *acute* or *fluid resuscitation phase*. The third and last phase is the rehabilitation phase. This phase should begin immediately after the burn injury to help maintain or restore function and cosmetic appearance so the patient can function in society.

Emergent or Shock Phase

During the emergent phase, the patient experiences a type of hypovolemic shock. This shock is the result of increased capillary permeability, which permits the shift of fluid from the plasma to the interstitial spaces. Direct cell damage increases capillary permeability, permitting the escape of large amounts of fluid, electrolytes, protein, and debris (Alspach, 1998). Changes in capillary permeability begin within 30 minutes of the thermal injury, and fluid and electrolyte losses peak within 6 to 8 hours of the burn injury (Jones & Bucher, 1999). In addition, the fluid regulators, including the osmotic and hydrostatic pressures and the sodium pump, are lost. Again, these changes are caused by direct cellular damage from the thermal injury. The cumulative effect of the loss of these regulatory mechanisms is hypovolemic shock, also referred to as *burn shock*. Rapid fluid shifts result in multisystem changes.

Cardiovascular System

The cardiovascular system responds to the hypovolemic shock by attempting to compensate for the massive loss of fluid. Catecholamines are released, decreasing cardiac output and increasing peripheral resistance in an attempt to increase the fluid volume in the vascular system. Ultimately, if fluid resuscitation efforts are not initiated, cardiac output is further decreased and there is hemoconcentration of blood cells with diminished perfusion to major organs (Jones & Bucher, 1999).

Respiratory System

The respiratory system may sustain an inhalation injury (see questions 7 and 8). Even if an inhalation injury is not sustained, lung compliance may decrease as a result of the extensive injury, and pulmonary care similar to that required for an inhalation injury may be necessary (Alspach, 1998)

Immunologic System

In the immunologic system, the mechanical barrier response and the cellular immune response are lost. Loss of the mechanical barrier means a loss of the body's ability to protect itself from invading organisms. Immediately after the injury, the arachidonic acid cascade and the inflammatory cytokine cascade are activated (Jones & Bucher, 1999). After the first 3 to 4 days, changes in the leukocytes, neutrophils, and macrophages are noted (Jones & Bucher, 1999). The final result is that the body loses powerful mechanisms to protect itself from invading organisms. Infection is one of the greatest concerns in a patient with a burn injury. Because of colonization of bacteria on the burn wound itself and loss of the defense mechanisms to fight against this colonization, a massive infection can develop in a patient with a burn injury.

Gastrohepatic System

The gastrohepatic system responds to a burn injury by shutting down, which results in the development of a paralytic ileus. This response probably is a result of the decrease in perfusion of this system and the endocrine response to the trauma (Jones & Bucher, 1999).

Genitourinary System

The genitourinary system responds by decreasing kidney function through secretion of antidiuretic hormone and renal vasoconstriction. The body attempts to use compensatory mechanisms to offset the hypovolemia. In this case, the kidneys may be compromised because of the extensive loss of fluid volume in the vascular system. Adequate fluid resuscitation to maintain effective kidney function is vital.

Acute or Fluid Resuscitation Phase

The second phase of burn physiology is the acute or fluid resuscitation phase. This phase begins when the return of fluid control mechanisms effects diuresis. The eschar begins to separate, and the focus of care turns to the preparation of the wound for healing or grafting. The cardiovascular system begins to stabilize because capillary permeability decreases, and fluid shifts are less severe. Cardiac output and lymphatic system functions return to normal. The respiratory system may be prone to development of pulmonary edema or pneumonia because of the massive fluid shifts and hospitalization. Patients with previous cardiovascular or pulmonary disease are more likely to develop respiratory problems. The patient remains immunosuppressed, and all efforts to prevent any type of infection should continue.

The gastrohepatic system begins to function, which leads to the concern for adequate nutritional intake. An additional concern is the development of stress ulcers. Careful monitoring of the gastric contents, stool, and any emesis for blood is imperative. The use of antacids and histamine-receptor antagonists to prevent the occurrence of stress ulcers is critical. Renal function should return. However, careful monitoring of kidney function is imperative as the body attempts to excrete waste products and debris from the burn injury. Renal failure is a possibility at this stage as well.

Rehabilitation Phase

The rehabilitation phase focuses on the return of the patient to his or her previous roles and responsibilities in society. With adequate fluid resuscitation efforts and care in the first two stages, the systems will have stabilized by the time the patient enters the third phase.

5. **Based on Mr. Knight's preburn weight, use the Parkland formula to calculate the fluid requirement for adequate resuscitation.**

The Parkland formula permits the calculation of fluid needs for the first 24 hours immediately after the burn injury (Hudak, Gallo, & Morton, 1997). However, this formula calculates the fluid need of crystalloids only:

4 ml of lactated Ringer's solution × kg of body weight × %TBSA burned

Mr. Knight's fluid need based on 65% TBSA burned is 4 ml × 72 kg × 65% TBSA = 18,720 ml of fluid in the first 24 hours. Half the fluid (9360 ml) should be infused during the first 8 hours after the burn. This time is calculated from the *time of the actual burn injury,* not from the time the patient is first seen by medical personnel. Therefore it is essential that the critical care nurse know the actual time of the injury and the amount of fluid that has been infused before the patient arrives in the unit. (Note: 4 L had been infused thus far, and a total of 9.36 L must be infused. The nurse has 4 hours to infuse the remaining 5.36 L.) The remaining half of the fluid requirement is then infused over the next 16 hours.

Some experts use the modified Brooke formula, which is similar to the Parkland formula (Hudak et al, 1997). The modified Brooke formula calculates the fluid needs as follows:

2 ml of lactated Ringer's solution × kg of body weight × %TBSA burned

With this formula, Mr. Knight's fluid needs for the first 24 hours would be 9360 ml.

Lactated Ringer's solution without dextrose is the crystalloid solution most often used to provide a balanced salt solution. Because a burn injury affects the fluid and electrolyte balance of the body, the amount and type of IV fluid is important. In the first 24 hours after a burn injury, the capillary permeability is increased and the selectivity is decreased (Jones & Bucher, 1999). Because of these physiologic changes in the capillary seal, large amounts of fluid shift from the intravascular space, leading to the loss of osmotic pressure and with it the body's ability to pull fluid back into the intravascular space. These changes lead to hypovolemic shock and massive edema. Additional fluid is lost through the burn injury itself in the form of wound drainage and evaporation.

The destruction of the cells in a burn injury also leads to a loss of electrolytes during the first 24 hours. The loss of sodium and potassium is of greatest concern. The sodium loss is the result of the fluid shifts and the cellular destruction. Potassium is lost into the extracellular fluid because of the cellular destruction.

Replacement therapy focuses on maintenance of the patient's condition until the capillary permeability and selectivity are restored. As stated earlier, lactated Ringer's solution is the IV solution of choice because the composition of this solution closely resembles the composition of the fluid being lost. Table 25-3 compares the composition of lactated Ringer's solution and the extracellular fluid.

The use of colloids (albumin or fresh frozen plasma) during the first 24 hours continues to be controversial. As capillary integrity is restored, colloids may be infused to aid in the reestablishment of the fluid regulators, including osmotic and hydrostatic pressures. However, most burn units do not begin to infuse colloids until after the first 24 hours (Jones & Bucher, 1999). Each burn unit will have an accepted fluid resuscitation protocol to maintain the cardiovascular status.

An important consideration when calculating fluid requirements for the patient with a burn injury is to understand that these formulas are guidelines. The patient's urine output and vital signs must be monitored carefully, and age and response of the patient must be taken into consideration. The rate of fluid administration must be adjusted according to the patient's needs.

Hourly urine output is the most valuable parameter to assess the adequacy of fluid resuscitation and renal perfusion. Hourly outputs should range from 0.5 to 1 ml/kg of body weight for adults (Thelan et al, 1998). Typically, this results in an hourly output of 30 to 50 ml of urine. If no prior renal disorder is present, hourly outputs less than 0.5 ml/kg may indicate hypovolemia.

TABLE 25-3	Comparison of Ringer's Lactated Solution and Extracellular Fluid	
Electrolyte	Lactated Ringer's Solution (mmol/L)*	Extracellular Fluid (mmol/L)†
Na^+ (mmol/L)	130	135-145
K^+ (mmol/L)	4	3.5-5.5
Cl^- (mmol/L)	109	96-106
HCO_3^- (mmol/L)	28	20-30

Modified from Lewis, S., Heitkemper, M., & Dirksen, S. (Eds.). (2000). *Medical-surgical nursing*, St Louis: Mosby.
*Normal value ranges may differ slightly between clinical laboratories.
†Plus 80 to 100 ml of free water per liter.

6. What significance, if any, would the administration of mannitol have on fluid resuscitation?

Mannitol functions as an osmotic diuretic to increase water excretion by osmotic action (Horne & Bond, 2000). Mannitol is administered to maintain urinary output adequate to prevent acute renal failure during trauma such as a burn injury. Also, osmotic diuretics are sometimes recommended when there is evidence of myoglobinuria, which necessitates the flushing of the kidneys to prevent sludging and possible acute tubular necrosis (Jones & Bucher, 1999). The major problem with this treatment approach is the absolute need for accurate measurement of hourly urine output. As presented in question 3, careful monitoring of the patient with a burn injury is required to ascertain fluid resuscitation needs. Hourly urine outputs are the major parameter in this monitoring. If an osmotic diuretic is administered, the burn unit staff treating the patient has no way of knowing if the urine output is a result of adequate fluid resuscitation or infusion of the osmotic diuretic.

Typically, osmotic diuretics should be used only as a last resort in an attempt to protect the kidneys. Adequate fluid resuscitation should maintain kidney functioning. If assessment findings support the presence of myoglobinuria, the amount of IV fluids administered should be increased first to flush out the kidneys and prevent sludging of the myoglobin. If forced diuresis is attempted, the patient must be monitored carefully for fluid overload, especially elderly patients and those with previous cardiac or renal diseases.

7. What assessment findings would indicate myoglobinuria?

Myoglobin is a pigment released when muscle tissue is damaged and may be evident with large thermal or electrical burn injuries. Myoglobin is a fairly large molecule that the body attempts to excrete through the kidneys. However, myoglobin has a tendency to sludge in the kidneys. If inadequate amounts of urine are produced, sludging may occur. Acute tubular necrosis may result from the kidneys' inability to remove the myoglobin.

Assessment findings that would indicate the presence of myoglobin in the urine include the TBSA of the burn, the type of burn injury, and the color of the urine produced. Urine that contains myoglobin is usually a burgundy-to-rust color.

Mr. Knight sustained a large (65%) TBSA thermal burn. Also when Mr. Knight arrived at the burn unit, the color of his urine was burgundy. Both assessment findings indicate a high possibility for the presence of myoglobin in the urine.

8. Describe the treatment protocol for myoglobinuria.

Two treatment protocols are available to ensure adequate urine output to flush the myoglobin from the kidneys. The first option is adequate fluid resuscitation. With a possibility of myoglobin in the urine the hourly output should be greater than 30 ml to ensure the flushing of the kidneys. The urine output may need to be increased to between 40 and 50 ml/hr to protect the kidneys. Patient response to the fluid resuscitation must also be monitored. The patient's cardiovascular, respiratory, and renal systems must be able to withstand the amount of fluids required to sustain the target hourly urine output.

A second option is the use of osmotic diuretics. Mannitol, administered intravenously with the dosage based on body weight, is usually the drug of choice. The decision to administer an osmotic diuretic must be made cautiously because it destroys the validity of the hourly urine output measurement.

9. **What assessment findings are critical to establishing the presence of an inhalation injury? Which of Mr. Knight's assessment findings warrant concern?**

The extent of pulmonary injury depends on the anatomic location of the insult, the agent inhaled such as steam or smoke, the toxic substances in the agent inhaled, and the length of exposure to the agent (Alspach, 1998). Inhalation injuries are typically observed within the first 12 hours after the burn injury (Lentz & Peterson, 1997).

Inhalation injuries can be classified according to the location of the injury relative to the glottis (Jones & Bucher, 1999). Upper airway inhalation injuries (above the glottis) should be suspected if there are obvious burns to the face, neck, or upper chest. The potential for an inhalation injury is increased if the burn injury is sustained in an enclosed space.

A lower airway inhalation injury is a direct burn below the glottis and usually results from inhaling heated air or steam. An inhalation injury below the glottis is rare because of the ability of the trachea to dissipate heat and the reflex action of the vocal cords to close off the lower airway when they are exposed to toxic air.

Smoke inhalation, which is often the cause of death in burn-related injuries, typically results in carbon monoxide or cyanide toxicity. The fire also consumes the oxygen, and hypoxia may occur if the burn victim is in an enclosed space and/or trapped.

Edema formation may also lead to airway obstruction and respiratory distress. The edema may be the result of an actual burn to the tissues in the airway or may result from fluid resuscitation efforts, especially if the face, neck, and chest are involved in the burn.

The following clinical indicators increase the risk of a possible inhalation injury (Lentz & Peterson, 1997):

- A burn injury sustained in an enclosed space
- Burns to the face, neck, and chest*
- Singed nasal hair or eyebrows
- Carboniferous material in mouth
- Carboniferous sputum*
- Carboxyhemoglobin level more than 10%
- Wheezing
- Hoarseness of the voice*
- Deep, labored respirations
- Altered level of consciousness
- Cough
- Tachypnea

---

*Documented findings in case study.

10. **Describe the treatment protocol for a burn patient with an inhalation injury or a suspected inhalation injury.**

Monitoring of the respiratory status of a patient with a burn injury is critical and should take priority over all other concerns. The basic ABCs of survival (airway, breathing, and circulation) must be met first, as with any trauma patient. Monitoring of the respiratory system and the treatment protocols include the following:

- Assess the respiratory rate, rhythm, and quality frequently.
- Monitor arterial blood gas (ABG) and carboxyhemoglobin values periodically.
- Deliver humidified oxygen. The type of delivery system used depends on the extent of the inhalation injury. It can vary from a nasal cannula to intubation and ventilator support if the inhalation injury is severe. Delivery of 100% humidified oxygen through a nonrebreather mask or ventilator promotes oxygenation and excretion of carbon monoxide.
- Perform pulmonary hygiene efforts including positioning, coughing and deep breathing, incentive spirometry, or ultrasound nebulizers.
- Elevate the head of the bed at least 30 to 40 degrees unless contraindicated by another condition.
- Obtain chest x-ray films.
- Use fiberoptic bronchoscopy to directly visualize the airway.
- Obtain a xenon-133 ventilation-perfusion lung scan: xenon-133 is injected intravenously with serial scans done to monitor the clearance of the xenon by the lungs. Xenon is usually washed out of the alveoli within 90 seconds (Jones & Bucher, 1999).
- Perform escharotomies if chest expansion is compromised.

Initially, the chest x-ray film, ABG values, and carboxyhemoglobin findings may appear normal. The initial results become baseline data for comparison with subsequent laboratory results. Serial studies can identify deterioration of the pulmonary function. A xenon-133 lung scan and fiberoptic bronchoscopy can accurately diagnose 93% of inhalation injuries (Jones & Bucher, 1999).

11. **What is the purpose of escharotomies?**

Escharotomies are incisions made through the eschar to allow for swelling without compromising tissue perfusion. An eschar is typically thick and leathery, allowing little expansion if there is swelling under it. If the burn is circumferential, the swelling from the burn injury itself and the swelling associated with fluid resuscitation can compromise the arterial blood flow to the area. Escharotomies may be necessary if there is extensive burn injury to the anterior or posterior trunk. If eschar is present, the respiratory effort and therefore ventilation may be compromised. Escharotomies on both sides of the chest through the midaxillary line may aid in decreasing the respiratory effort (Jordan & Harrington, 1997).

The incisions should extend through the eschar down to the subcutaneous fat to allow adequate separation of the edges of the incision and to relieve the pressure from the swelling. Incisions are made in the midlateral or midmedial line, moving from the proximal to the distal end of the involved extremities. The locations of the incisions are critical to prevent causing trauma to nerves, tendons, and the vascular structure. The incisions may be performed at the bedside because there is no pain sensation in these types of burn injuries. Antimicrobial agents should be applied after the incisions are made to delay colonization of bacteria (Jordan & Harrington, 1997).

12. Discuss pain management in the treatment protocol for the patient with a burn injury.

Pain management is a major concern in the care of the patient with a burn injury. Continual monitoring of both the physical and emotional pain experienced by these patients during all phases of the burn injury is important. Many believe that anyone experiencing a full-thickness burn does not have pain because of the loss of pain sensors in the burned tissue. However, total full-thickness burns are rare. There is usually a mixture of partial- and full-thickness burns. Because the pain sensors are intact with partial-thickness burns, the patient may experience severe pain. Initially, because of the massive edema resulting from the burn and fluid resuscitation efforts, only IV pain medication such as morphine should be administered. Massive edema compromises the absorption of the pain medication if it is given intramuscularly or subcutaneously. Once the patient enters the acute and rehabilitation phases, other routes of administration of pain medication can be considered. Alternative methods of pain management should also be considered. For example, guided imagery has been used very successfully for some patients with burn injuries.

Initial interventions for pain should include small doses of IV narcotic medications such as morphine by IV push or patient-controlled anesthesia pump. After the first 24 to 48 hours, other forms of pain medication may be used, including oral doses of morphine or meperidine and transcutaneous doses of fentanyl (Jones & Bucher, 1999).

Medication other than narcotics may aid in pain control after the initial 48 hours. Anxiolytics such as diazepam (Valium) and lorazepam (Librium) may decrease the anxiety associated with the anticipation of painful dressing changes. Diphenhydramine (Benadryl) and hydroxyzine (Atarax) may also be used to decrease the itching associated with wound healing (Jones & Bucher, 1999)

13. Using the Curreri formula for nutrition, calculate Mr. Knight's nutritional needs. Discuss the need for a high-calorie, high-protein diet.

Many formulas have been developed to calculate caloric requirements (Jones & Bucher, 1999). The Curreri formula is used to establish the number of calories required by the patient with a burn injury. The formula estimates only the number of calories and does not address the percentage of proteins, fats, and carbohydrates the patient requires.

$$(25 \text{ kcal} \times \text{weight [kg]}) + (40 \times \text{TBSA}) = \text{total calories}$$

Mr. Knight's caloric need per day would be calculated as follows:

$$(25 \text{ kcal} \times 72 \text{ kg}) + (40 \times 65\%) = 4400 \text{ kcal}$$

Some experts advocate the use of several parameters such as indirect calorimetry, daily weight, and nitrogen balance to estimate nutritional needs (Jones & Bucher, 1999).

Nutritional support becomes paramount once the condition of the patient with a burn injury has stabilized. Hypermetabolism that is directly proportional to the extent of the burn injury results. The basal metabolic rate may double in a patient with a 40% or greater TBSA burn injury (Hudak et al, 1997).

Because of the high metabolic rate and the need for a positive nitrogen balance to promote healing, a diet high in calories and protein is essential. Once the patient's condition is stabilized, nutritional intake must begin. If the patient cannot consume enough calories orally, enteral feedings may be required to meet the extensive nutritional needs. These includes oral supplements or continuous feedings through a nasoenteric (intestinal) tube. Specific types of feedings and tubes used for enteral therapy depend on the condition of the patient, the anticipated time of nutritional support required to meet the metabolic needs, and the risk of aspiration.

The protein intake per day for the patient with a burn injury can range from 1.6 to 3.2 g/kg of body weight (Thelan et al, 1998). For Mr. Knight, this would result in an intake of 115 to 230 g of protein per day.

Pharmacologic nutrition, including the use of glutamine, arginine, and (n-3) fatty acids, is currently being investigated. Studies have shown that with the use of these pharmacologic nutrients, immunologic function is improved, occurrence of infections is reduced, and the nitrogen balance is maintained (De-Souza & Greene, 1998). Further research is necessary in the use of these nutrients (Le Boucher & Cynober, 1997).

14. **Discuss burn wound care and dressing techniques. Include the types of topical antimicrobial agents commonly used in wound care, listing advantages and disadvantages of each.**

With the loss of integrity of the skin and the colonization of bacteria in the burn wound and under eschar, management of the burn wound becomes imperative (Greenfield & McManus, 1997). If a wound becomes infected, consequences such as conversion of a partial-thickness to full-thickness wound may occur, healing may be delayed, and the wound infection can lead to septic shock and death.

Five goals of burn wound care include closing the wound as soon as possible, supporting the development of granulation tissue, cleaning the wound for grafting, reducing scar formation and contractures, and providing patient comfort (Hudak et al, 1997).

The first step in the process of burn wound care is wound cleansing. Hydrotherapy is begun as soon as possible to promote meticulous cleansing and wound debridement. The type of hydrotherapy depends on the infection control policies of the unit and the condition of the patient. Some patients are placed in a Hubbard tank or are given a shower. Typically, hydrotherapy is completed at least daily but may be performed more often if ordered by the burn unit team. The goal is to wash all areas carefully, being sure to thoroughly remove all antimicrobial agents previously placed on the burn wound. Also, any eschar that is beginning to separate may be removed with forceps and scissors. All hair should be shaved around the burn wound to decrease the chance of infection.

Hydrotherapy can be a painful ordeal for the patient. Adequate premedication is required. The actual time of the hydrotherapy (usually 20 minutes) should be monitored carefully to prevent hypothermia. Heat lamps may be used to decrease the amount of heat lost by the patient.

During hydrotherapy, the wound must be assessed continually for color and appearance: the presence of eschar and healing as seen by budding of the skin; presence of drainage, including odor, color, and amount; and any exposed deep tissue such as tendons and bone (Greenfield & McManus, 1997).

Once the wound is cleansed, an antimicrobial agent is applied. These agents are the best method to control burn wound sepsis and to reduce the number of bacteria colonizing in the wound. The agents ideally will also restrain colonization of bacteria to a level that the body can control through its internal defense mechanisms (Hudak et al, 1997). Four of the most commonly used antimicrobial agents are listed in Table 25-4. Selection of an antimicrobial agent depends on the wound depth, location, condition, and specific organism isolated, which is established by wound culture (Greenfield and McManus, 1997).

There are two methods of dressing a burn wound. The first method is the open method. An antimicrobial cream is applied with a sterile glove with no dressing applied. This approach allows direct visualization of the wound, less discomfort for the patient during wound care, and simplicity in wound care. However, the patient

TABLE 25-4	Commonly Used Antimicrobial Agents	
Agent	Indications	Nursing Considerations
Clotrimazole cream	Fungal colonization of wounds	Apply thin coat of agent to wound and wait 20 min before applying any dressings; make use of an antibacterial agent in addition to the antifungal agent; painless; may cause skin irritation and blistering.
Mafenide acetate (Sulfamylon)	Active against most gram-positive and gram-negative wound pathogens; drug of choice for electrical and ear burns	Apply once or twice daily with sterile glove; do not use dressings that reduce effectiveness and cause maceration; monitor respiratory rate, electrolyte values, and arterial pH for evidence of metabolic acidosis; painful on application to partial-thickness burns for about 30 min.
Silver nitrate	Effective against a wide spectrum of common wound pathogens and fungal infections; used in patients with sulfa allergy or toxic epidermal neurolysis; poor penetration of eschar	Apply 0.5% solution wet dressings two or three times a day; ensure that dressings remain moist by wetting every 2 hr; preserve solution in a light-resistant container; protect walls, floors, and so son, with plastic to prevent black staining that occurs; monitor for hyponatremia and hypochloremia.
Silver sulfadiazine (Silvadene)	Active against a wide spectrum of microbial pathogens; use with caution in patients with impaired renal or hepatic function	Apply once or twice a day with sterile gloved hand; leave wounds exposed or wrap lightly with gauze dressing; painless.

may experience hypothermia, may further traumatize the wound, or may have psychologic difficulty looking at the wound.

A second method is the closed method in which dressings are applied to the wound. Antimicrobial cream is applied to the wound using a sterile glove or is coated on a gauze pad and laid on the wound, which is then covered with an additional dressing. If a solution is used, the dressing is saturated and placed on the wound and covered with additional dressings. These dressings should be wrapped distal to proximal with no two burn surfaces touching each other. The advantages of this type of dressing are limitation of fluid loss through evaporation, debridement of the wound when the dressings are removed, absorption of the exudate from the wound, and patient comfort. Disadvantages of this type of dressing are the discomfort experienced by the patient during dressing changes and the warm moist environment created under the dressings.

15. Describe the types of biologic and synthetic dressings currently being used in wound care.

Biologic dressings are used as temporary wound coverings until autografts are available. Reasons why biologic dressings aid in the management of burn wounds include the following:

- Decreasing bacterial proliferation on the wound
- Preventing necrosis of viable elements in the dermis
- Preventing wound desiccation
- Assisting in control of evaporation of fluid and heat loss through the open wound
- Decreasing protein loss in fluid exudate
- Decreasing pain experienced by patients
- Protecting exposed structures such as blood vessels, tendons, and nerves
- Stimulating healing and preparing the wound bed for autograft skin
- Facilitating joint motion

The most commonly used biologic and synthetic dressings are described in Table 25-5.

New forms of dressings and debridement material are now on the market. Each of these new products has properties that aid in the debridement and healing of burn injuries. Burn centers will continue to investigate and develop wound management care that will promote healing, decrease scarring, and decrease the threat of infection.

16. Discuss the use of autografts and the nursing care required.

With a full-thickness burn, healing and reepithelialization are not possible. As a result, an autograft using viable skin from the patient is the only option for covering the wound.

For the autograft to "take," the wound itself must be pink, firm, and free of exudate or eschar, which is accomplished through wound cleansing and debridement. Once the wound is ready for the graft, the patient is taken to surgery, where the autograft is obtained. Autografts may be split thickness, full thickness, pedicle flaps, or free flaps, depending on the area of the body requiring the autograft. Most

TABLE 25-5	Common Biologic and Synthetic Dressings
Type of Dressing	**Definition**
Biologic dressing	Temporary wound cover of human or animal species tissue
Allograft (homograft)	Temporary wound cover composed of a graft of skin transplanted from another human, living or dead
Xenograft (heterograft) skin	Used as a temporary wound cover to promote healing; a graft of skin, usually pigskin, transplanted between animals of different species
Biosynthetic dressing	A wound covering composed of both biologic and synthetic materials
Temporary skin substitute (Biobrane)	A bilaminar wound dressing composed of nylon mesh enclosed in a collagen derivative with a silicone rubber outer membrane; permeable to some antibiotic ointments
"Artificial skin" (Integra)	A wound dressing composed of two layers: (1) a "dermal" layer made of animal collagen that interfaces with an open wound surface; (2) an "epidermal" layer made of polymeric silicone (Silastic) that controls water loss from the dermis and acts as a bacterial barrier; the dermal layer biodegrades within several months and is reabsorbed; the epidermal layer may be removed and replaced with autograft skin when appropriate

autografts are split-thickness grafts to cover the wound early. If the area requiring coverage is large, the autograft is meshed so that it can cover a larger surface area. The autograft can be meshed by a ratio of 1:1.5 to 1:4. This means that the autograft can cover 1.5 to 4 times its own surface area. Meshed grafts have a tendency to adhere better to the wound and allow exudate and debris to ooze through the open meshed areas. A ratio of 1:4 is typically the largest ratio used to prevent longer healing time and scarring (Jordan & Harrington, 1997). The graft is laid on the wound and stapled or sutured in place. Some burn units use fibrin glue to hold the autograft in place. Further investigation of this approach is needed. Once the autograph is secured to the wound, a dressing is applied and the patient is returned to the burn unit.

The nurse must take special care not to disrupt the autograft. The patient may be confined to bed rest or the extremity may be immobilized with splints to promote proper positioning and to prevent disruption of the graft. The nurse must ensure proper positioning while being fully aware of the potential for other complications, such as respiratory infection and skin breakdown as a result of the immobility.

An autograft "takes" when it becomes a permanent part of the wound. Blood flow through capillaries growing into the autograft is established by the third to fifth day after the graft. Wound closure is anticipated within 7 to 10 days after graft placement.

17. Describe the appropriate care for donor sites.

Selection of autograft skin donor sites is based on the location and the extent of the burn. Once the autograft skin is obtained, the donor site must be monitored because of the creation of a partial-thickness injury. In surgery, fine mesh gauze (either dry or impregnated with a substance such as scarlet red or a synthetic material) is placed over the donor site to promote healing and prevent further injury. On the patient's return to the burn unit, the donor site should be exposed to air. Some burn units apply a radiant heat source to the area to increase drying. Once the donor site begins to heal, usually 7 to 14 days after the graft is obtained, the gauze or synthetic material will begin to separate from the wound (Solotkin & Knipe, 2000). As this separation occurs, the material can be trimmed from the wound with scissors.

The nurse must be careful to keep the donor site clean, dry, and trimmed. A donor site can be used more than once if there are no complications such as an infection. If the donor site becomes infected, it should be treated as the burn wound.

18. Discuss the splinting and positioning required for Mr. Knight to maintain use of his extremities and upper body.

Most burn units have physical therapists and occupational therapists available to assist patients with burn injuries. In collaboration with the nursing staff, their goal is to maintain as much function as possible so that the patient can return to society. All joints should be placed in a neutral position if possible. Splints must be applied correctly. If necessary, the therapist should apply the splints or provide in-service training for nurses on the application of splints (Pessina & Ellis, 1997). Footboards or shoes are used to prevent foot drop. Early ambulation requires coordination of the nursing staff and physical therapist to provide the optimal environment for the patient to accomplish this goal. Pain management that allows the patient to ambulate and participate in exercises becomes an important issue.

19. List the nursing diagnoses, outcomes, and interventions appropriate for the care of the patient with a burn injury during the emergent and acute phases of burn physiology.

Solotkin and Knipe (2000) created a nursing care plan identifying the most common nursing diagnoses for a patient with a burn injury. Although many nursing diagnoses may be important for this type of patient, this care plan presents the most common interventions (Table 25-6).

20. Discuss the psychosocial aspects of caring for the patient with a burn injury and the impact on the patient's support system.

Burn injuries are some of the most devastating injuries to sustain. An individual's identity and self-image are directly related to his or her appearance. Disfigurement from burns to the face can be especially difficult for the patient.

The nurse must constantly assess the patient and the support system available through family or friends. This assessment includes identifying feelings of guilt, abandonment, pain, loss, and fear. In addition, the patient may experience anxiety, sleep deprivation, and disorientation (Davis & Sheely-Adolphson, 1997). The nurse can encourage the patient, family, and friends to verbalize their concerns and provide them with appropriate information. Also, a referral to a social worker, psychologist, or chaplain may be necessary to provide additional psychosocial or spiritual support.

TABLE 25-6	Nursing Care Plan for Resuscitative and Acute Care Phase of the Patient with a Major Burn Injury		
Nursing Diagnosis	Outcome	Interventions	
Ineffective airway clearance or impaired gas exchange related to tracheal edema or interstitial edema secondary to inhalation injury and manifested by hypoxemia and hypercapnia	Po_2 >90 mm Hg, Pco_2 <40 mm Hg, O_2 saturation >95% Respirations 16-20 min Clear mentations Ability to mobilize secretions Clear to white secretions Absence of dyspnea and increased work of breathing with appropriate positioning	Assess respiratory rate and character qh, breath sounds q4h, and level of consciousness qh. Evaluate need for chest escharotomy during fluid resuscitation. If patient is not intubated, assess for stridor, hoarseness q1hr. Monitor oxygen saturation q1hr; obtain and evaluate ABG values prn. Administer humidified oxygen as ordered. Cough and deep breathe qh while awake. Suction q1-2h or prn; monitor sputum characteristics and amount. Schedule activities to avoid fatigue and dyspnea. Turn q2h to mobilize secretions. Assist with obtaining chest x-ray film as ordered.	
Fluid volume deficit secondary to fluid shifts and evaporate loss of fluids from the injured skin	Hourly urine output: 30-50 ml; 1 ml/kg—children <30 kg body weight; 75-100 ml—electrical injury Stable vital signs Clear sensorium	Titrate calculated fluid requirements in first 48 hr to maintain acceptable urinary output. Obtain and evaluate urine specific gravity and sugar and acetone q2h. Monitor vital signs qh until hemodynamically stable. Monitor mental status qh for at least 48 hr. Obtain and record daily weights. Record hourly intake and output measurements and evaluate trends. Monitor laboratory values for first 48 hr and then as required by patient status.	

Continued

TABLE 25-6	Nursing Care Plan for Resuscitative and Acute Care Phase of the Patient with a Major Burn Injury— cont'd	
Nursing Diagnosis	**Outcome**	**Interventions**
High risk for impaired vascular perfusion in extremities with circumferential burns manifested by decreased or absence peripheral pulses	Absence of tissue injury in extremities secondary to inadequate perfusion related to vascular compression from edema	Check peripheral pulses qh for 72 hr by palpation or ultrasonic flowmeter; evaluate sensation of pain and capillary refill in extremities. Notify physician of changes in pulses, capillary refill, or pain sensation; be prepared to assist with escharotomy or fasciotomy. Evaluate upper extremities.
Alteration in comfort: acute pain related to burn trauma	Able to identify factors that contribute to pain Verbalizes improved comfort level Physiologic parameters return to normal Adequate respirations and hemodynamic stability after administration of narcotic analgesia	Medicate before bathing, dressing changes, major procedures, prn. Reduce anxiety; explain all activities before initiating them; talk to patient while performing activities; assess need for analgesic or anxiolytic medication; use nonpharmacologic pain-reducing methods as appropriate. Monitor and document response to analgesics or other interventions
High risk for infection related to loss of skin, impaired immune response, invasive therapies	Absence of infected burn wounds Vital signs stable Laboratory values within normal limits Negative results from sputum, blood, and urine cultures	Assess burn wound and invasive catheter sites. Assess and document characteristics of urine and sputum q8h. Obtain wound, sputum, urine, and blood cultures as ordered. Assess and record temperature and vital signs q1-4h as appropriate. Provide protective isolation appropriate to method of wound care. Provide wound care with antimicrobial topical agents as ordered.

TABLE 25-6	Nursing Care Plan for Resuscitative and Acute Care Phase of the Patient with a Major Burn Injury— cont'd	
Nursing Diagnosis	**Outcome**	**Interventions**
Impaired skin integrity related to burn wound, or consequences of immobility	No evidence of progressive burn wound or donor site injury Burn wound or donor site healing and skin graft adherence within appropriate time frames	Assess and document: skin over pressure areas, burn wounds, donor sites, pressure points under splints, dependent area of unburned skin. Pad pressure areas: heels, elbows, sacrum, scapulas, and burned ears. Check circulation distally and digits in splinted extremities. Promote drying of donor sites as appropriate; keep heat lamps at a safe distance to prevent injury. Immobilize skin graft sites for 5-7 days after grafting to promote graft adherence.
High risk for aspiration *R/T; hypoactivity of gastrointestinal tract	No aspiration of gastric contents No respiratory complications from aspirations	Insert and maintain nasogastric tube to low suction until bowel sounds return. Auscultate for bowel sounds q4h. Test stools and gastric contents for pressure of blood. Administer histamine blockers and antacids as ordered.
High risk for nutritional deficit related to increased metabolic demands due to wound healing	Consumption of daily requirement of nutrients, based on formulas for appropriate calorie calculation Positive nitrogen balance Progressive wound healing	Monitor weights every day or biweekly. Assess abdomen, bowel sounds q8h. Record all oral intake. Activate enteral, parenteral feeding protocol as appropriate prn. Provide adaptive devices to facilitate self-feeding.

Continued

TABLE 25-6	Nursing Care Plan for Resuscitative and Acute Care Phase of the Patient with a Major Burn Injury— cont'd	
Nursing Diagnosis	**Outcome**	**Interventions**
High risk for hemorrhage related to presence of a stress ulcer	No occurrence of stress ulcer while in hospital	Assess all stools, emesis, and residual of the tube feedings for blood. Monitor hemoglobin and hematocrit levels. Administer histamine blockers and antacids as ordered. Auscultate abdomen and monitor for bowel sounds and pain. Encourage oral diet as soon as possible.
High risk for hypothermia related to loss of skin or external cooling	Rectal and core temperature is 37.2-37.8° C (99-100° F)	Monitor and document rectal and core temperature q1-2h.
High risk for ineffective patient and family coping related to acute stress of critical injury and potential life-threatening crisis; alteration in family processes related to critical injury	Patient or family verbalize goals of treatment regimen Patient or family demonstrate knowledge of support systems that are available Patient or family able to express concerns and fears Patient or family coping functional and realistic for phase of hospitalization, family processes at precrisis level	Support adaptive and functional coping mechanisms. Use interventions to reduce patient fatigue and pain. Promote use of group support session for patients and families. Orient patient and family to unit and support services and reinforce information frequently. Involve patient and family in treatment goals and plan of care.

BURNS

References

Alspach, J. (Ed.). (1998). *American Association of Critical-Care Nurses: Core curriculum for critical care nursing* (5th ed.). Philadelphia: Saunders.

Davis, S. T., & Sheely-Adolphson, P. (1997). Burn management. Psychosocial interventions: Pharmacologic and psychologic modalities. *Nursing Clinics of North America, 32*(2), 331-342.

De-Souza, D., & Greene, L. (1998). Pharmacological nutrition after burn injury. *The Journal of Nutrition, 128*(5), 797-803.

Gordon, M., & Goodwin, C. (1997). Initial assessment, management, and stabilization. *Nursing Clinics of North America, 32*(2), 237-249.

Greenfield, E., & McManus, A. (1997). Infectious complications. *Nursing Clinics of North America, 32*(2), 297-309.

Horne, M., & Bond, E. (2000). Fluid, electrolyte, and acid-base imbalances. In S. Lewis, M. Heitkemper, & S. Dirksen (Eds.), *Medical-surgical nursing* (5th ed., pp. 323-351). St Louis: Mosby.

Hudak, C., Gallo, B., & Morton, P. (1997). *Critical care nursing: A holistic approach* (7th ed.). Philadelphia: Lippincott.

Jones, K., & Bucher, L. (1999) Burns. In L. Bucher & S. Melander (Eds.). *Critical care nursing* (pp. 1036-1069). Philadelphia: Saunders.

Jordan, B., & Harrington, D. (1997). Management of the burn wound. *Nursing Clinics of North America, 32*(2), 251-273.

Le Boucher, J., & Cynober, L. (1997). Protein metabolism and therapy in burn injury. *Annals of Nutrition and Metabolism, 41*, 69-82.

Lentz, C., & Peterson, H. (1997). Smoke inhalation is a multilevel insult to the pulmonary system. *Current Opinion in Pulmonary Medicine, 3*(3), 221-226.

Pessina, M., & Ellis, S. (1997). Burn management. Rehabilitation. *Nursing Clinics of North America, 32*(2), 365-374.

Solotkin, K., & Knipe, C. (2000). Patients with burns. In S. Lewis, M. Heitkemper, & S. Dirksen (Eds.), *Medical-surgical nursing* (5th ed., pp.523-550). St Louis: Mosby.

Thelan, L., Urden, L., Lough, M., & Stacy, K. (1998). *Critical care nursing*. St Louis: Mosby.

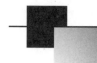

CHAPTER *26*

ACQUIRED IMMUNODEFICIENCY SYNDROME

Connie Cooper, RN, MSN

CASE PRESENTATION

John Michael, a 35-year-old white man, came to the local mental health hospital complaining of impaired concentration, withdrawal from family and friends, mood swings, difficulty with his memory, fatigue, and suicidal ideation. Two months before coming to the hospital, he had moved to the area from San Francisco to be with his family.

On admission, Mr. Michael's assessment revealed he had lost 4.5 to 7 kg (10 to 15 lb) since coming to his parent's home. He has not been able to read or concentrate. His suicidal ideas involve harming himself but no specific plan. Mr. Michael's psychosocial history revealed that he was homosexual and in the mid-1980s had visited several bath houses in San Francisco before settling down with his one close friend. Mr. Michael stated he had returned home to tell his family that his test for human immunodeficiency virus (HIV) was positive. His family told him they would stand by him. He denied the use of intravenous (IV) drugs but has used marijuana on occasion. His medical history included having had diarrhea for the past 3 weeks, night sweats, and enlarged glands in his neck and under his arms. Two of his friends recently had been told that they were HIV positive, and two other friends died from acquired immuno-deficiency syndrome (AIDS). He fears he has become depressed, believes he is losing his mind, and is becoming more confused. He told the nurse he was having difficulty with tremors in his legs, which occasionally have given him problems with walking.

His admitting diagnosis was major depression—single episode; rule out AIDS dementia complex (ADC).

After Mr. Michael's psychiatrist was informed of his history, medication orders were given for fluoxetine (Prozac) and nortriptyline (Pamelor).

Current vital signs and laboratory results are as follows:

BP	134/88 mm Hg	Chest x-ray film	Within normal limits
HR	90 bpm	RBCs	$3.5 \times 10^6/mm^3$
Respirations	20 breaths/min	WBCs	$6.6 \times 10^3/mm^3$
Temperature	37.2° C (98.9° F) (oral)	Hgb	12.9 g/dl
ELISA	positive for HIV antigens	Hct	36.8%
	(confirmed by Western	Lymphocytes	13%
	blot test)		

After 1 week of psychotherapy and medication therapy, Mr. Michael did not show any improvement in mood, affect, or neurologic deficits. He began falling when attempting to walk, had difficulty with the Mini-Mental State Examination, and became more confused. The psychiatrist made a medical referral. Two physicians refused to accept the referral. Finally an oncologist accepted Mr. Michael's case. Two days later, Mr. Michael was transferred to the oncology unit. More tests were ordered.

Results for a complete blood count with differential were the following:

RBCs	$5.5 \times 10^6/mm^3$	Hct	38.9%
WBCs	$4.4 \times 10^3/mm^3$	Lymphocytes	11%
Hgb	12.7 g/dl	Monocytes	3%

The lymphocyte subset results were the following:

Total lymphocyte count	$411/mm^3$	Helper:suppressor	0.07
Absolute B-cell count	$99/mm^3$	ratio (CD4+:	
Absolute T-cell count	$206/mm^3$	CD8+)	

Routine chemistry results were the following:

Na^+	137 mmol/L	Total protein	6.3 g/dl
Glucose	120 mg/dl	K^+	3.7mmol/L
Creatinine	0.8 mg/dl	Cl^-	100 mmol/L
Albumin	2.6 g/dl	CO_2	26 mmol/L
BUN	9 mg/dl		

Results of other tests were the following:

VDRL	Negative	Stool culture	*Salmonella*
Hepatitis B serology	Negative	CT scan	Mild brain atrophy and
Viral load	230,000 copies/ml		white matter changes

Once Mr. Michael was transferred to a medical floor, treatment with zidovudine (Retrovir), lamivudine (Epivir, 3TC), and indinavir (Crixivan) and ampicillin (Ampicin) for *Salmonella* infection was begun. During Mr. Michael's hospitalization, his assessment revealed no previous opportunistic diseases. He reported that his first symptoms were night sweats, diarrhea, and difficulty with his memory. Difficulty walking began shortly thereafter. His respiratory status began to change. On day 9, he developed a nonproductive cough, dyspnea, chills, and a few crackles in the base of his lungs. The physician was informed of changes, and orders included oxygen via mask at 40%, a chest x-ray film, and a second CD4+ count. The chest x-ray examination revealed bilateral infiltrates. A flexible fiberoptic bronchoscopy revealed *Pneumocystis carinii* pneumonia (PCP). Mr. Michael was treated with IV pentamidine. On day 13, his respiratory status worsened. There were indications of respiratory failure, and a decision had to be made about intubation and mechanical ventilation. Mr. Michael had difficulty with decision making and also exhibited some psychomotor slowing. His family was kept informed of his physical condition. Mr. Michael wanted his family to help him make this difficult decision. Considering the quick onset of his symptoms and change in condition, the family chose admission to the intensive care unit (ICU) and mechanical ventilation. He was admitted to the ICU. Treatment with IV ampicillin and IV hydrocortisone was initiated.

Within 2 days, Mr. Michael was afebrile and was weaned from the ventilator. His respiratory rate had fallen from 40 to 25 breaths/min, and his respiratory distress had lessened. Mr. Michael was then transferred back to the medical unit, receiving oxygen via nasal cannula. A third $CD4^+$ cell count was 190/mm^3. Tables 26-1 and 26-2 show diagnostic data at Mr. Michael's return to the medical unit.

After his return to the medical unit, Mr. Michael was treated for oral candidiasis with nystatin (NeoDerm) and ketoconazole (Nizoral). His skin tests indicated

TABLE *26-1*	Vital Signs					
	Day					
	4	7	9	13	14	15
BP (mm Hg)	112/72	154/82	132/84	132/62	112/72	130/84
HR (bpm)	112	112	112	120	112	90
Respirations (breaths/min)	20	22	26	36	40	35
Temperature						
°C	36.7-37.2	36.7-37.2	37.2-37.8	37.8-38.9	38.9-39.4	36.7-37.2
°F	98-99	98-99	99-100	100-102	102-103	98-99

BP, Blood pressure; *HR*, heart rate.

TABLE *26-2*	Laboratory Results				
	Day				
	7 (room air)	9 (40% O_2)	13 (100% O_2)	14 (40% O_2)	15 (room air)
pH	7.48	7.49	7.45	7.48	7.46
P_{CO_2} (mm Hg)	36	32	35	28	32
Pa_{O_2} (mm Hg)	49	44	104	93	85
Sa_{O_2} (%)	89	83	97	97	96
HCO_3^- (mm Hg)	27	25	24	20	23
Mode			A/C	A/C	
Ventilation rate			17	17	
V_T			900	900	
PEEP (cm H_2O)			14	12	

PEEP, Positive end-expiratory pressure.

complete failure of delayed hypersensitivity reactions, and AIDS was diagnosed. After $1^1/_2$ weeks of IV trimethoprim-sulfamethoxazole (TMP-SMX; Bactrim), Mr. Michael was weaned from oxygen and discharged.

After discharge from the hospital, Mr. Michael was treated with zidovudine (formerly azidothymidine [AZT]), lamivudine, indinavir (Crixivan), and oral TMP-SMX.

ACQUIRED IMMUNODEFICIENCY SYNDROME

Questions

1. What factors put Mr. Michael at risk for HIV infection/AIDS?
2. What tests are used to screen for HIV infection?
3. What laboratory tests are done to help determine treatment for HIV infection/AIDS?
4. What clinical indicators would be used to determine whether Mr. Michael has major depression or ADC?
5. What is the difference between HIV infection and AIDS?
6. What clinical indicators confirmed that Mr. Michael's HIV infection had progressed to AIDS?
7. Describe the symptoms of PCP.
8. What symptoms and pulmonary diagnostic findings in Mr. Michael's case indicated the need for transfer to the ICU?
9. Mechanical ventilation and ICU admission for a person with AIDS is controversial. Why was Mr. Michael admitted to the ICU?
10. What treatments did Mr. Michael receive in the ICU to ensure a successful outcome? Include medications for HIV infection such as HAART and PCP prophylaxis.
11. What are some of the nursing interventions that will help Mr. Michael with his psychosocial and physiologic needs?
12. When assigned to an patient with HIV infection, what personal feelings or concerns should be acknowledged?
13. Are the ICU nurses at an increased risk of acquiring AIDS from patients who receive mechanical ventilation?
14. What is the recommended protocol for occupational exposure to HIV?

ACQUIRED IMMUNODEFICIENCY SYNDROME

Questions and Answers

1. What factors put Mr. Michael at risk for HIV infection/AIDS?

Mr. Michael's history revealed that he was homosexual and had had many sexual partners. Researchers have agreed that the greatest risk of exposure to HIV in the homosexual man comes from anal sexual intercourse and sexual practices with multiple sexual partners (Flaskerud & Ungvarski, 1999). Such sexual practices cause trauma to the rectal mucosa, which increases the chances of transmission of the HIV virus and other sexually transmitted diseases.

2. What tests are used to screen for HIV infection?

It is important to do a health history and physical assessment along with gathering diagnostic data (Douglas, 1999). Two tests are used to screen for HIV infection: enzyme-linked immunosorbent assay (ELISA) and Western blot. Exposure to HIV elicits an antigen-antibody reaction and creates antibodies. These antibodies are then detected by the screening tests. The Western blot is a confirmatory test after a positive ELISA (Flaskerud & Ungvarski, 1999). The presence of the antibody indicates that the person is infected and is infectious. The incubation period for AIDS is wide.

The ELISA was first developed to screen the blood supply before transfusion. The Western blot is more specific than the ELISA. It confirms that the antibody in question is specifically reactive with HIV by detecting antibody reactivity to individual components of the virus (Flaskerud & Ungvarski, 1999).

Other tests available to detect HIV infection include p24 antigen, viral isolation, salivary tests (OraSure), and urine tests. Rapid tests for HIV are also available and are licensed by the U.S. Food and Drug Administration. The rapid test can provide results in 30 minutes. This test is important in the situation of occupational exposure when immediate treatment decisions need to be made (Flaskerud & Ungvarski, 1999).

3. What laboratory tests are done to help determine treatment for HIV infection/AIDS?

Lymphocytes are mononuclear white blood cells (WBCs) that are critical in immune defense. Two major classes of lymphocytes are B cells and T cells. Humoral immunity is the B-cell response to harmful antigens. Humoral immunity protects the body by circulating antibodies that are produced by the B cells. The creation of antibodies helps a person's system to fight infections. When the B cells are activated, they release large amounts of immunoglobulins (antibodies). Cellular immunity is immune protection resulting from the direct action of cells of the immune system (Stine, 1998). Key cell types are phagocytes and lymphocytes.

CD4$^+$ T-lymphocyte counts are used to stage the client's immune system in response to infection and provide an indication for antiretroviral therapy and prophylaxis (Douglas, 1999). CD4$^+$ counts are a key in initiating and amplifying both humoral and cell-mediated immune mechanisms (Zeller, McCain, & Swanson, 1996).

Viral load or viral burden is a more direct method of measuring HIV activity. Viral load or HIV RNA in plasma will allow the clinician to more accurately assess the amount of HIV activity that is taking place in the body. Viral load tests help the clinician determine prognosis, the need for antiretroviral treatment, and the patient's response to antiretroviral treatment (Flaskerud & Ungvarski, 1999; Melroe, Stawarz, Simpson, & Henry, 1997).

4. What clinical indicators would be used to determine whether Mr. Michael has major depression or ADC?

A patient with major depression usually complains of depressed mood, diminished interest or pleasure in activities, appetite changes with weight changes (up or down), insomnia or hypersomnia, fatigue or loss of energy, inability to concentrate, feelings of worthlessness or guilt, psychomotor agitation or retardation, and thoughts of death or suicide. The presence of any five of these symptoms, lasting for at least 2 weeks, is a clinical indication of a major affective disorder that requires intervention. Major depression is one of the most common and treatable psychiatric disorders among HIV-infected people in the United States (Valente & Saunders, 1997). It is important to take a careful history to determine symptoms and situational crises that could precipitate the symptoms. Assessment of suicidal ideation is important at the time of the initial interview. Any precipitating factors such as bereavement, reactions to medication, or thyroid problems should be ruled out. Nurses in acute-care or mental health settings must be aware of the psychosocial and neuropsychiatric aspects of HIV disease. It may be necessary to manage the case of a patient who has anxiety or depression associated with a new diagnosis of HIV infection or AIDS or a patient who may be manifesting dementia associated with AIDS (Flaskerud & Ungvarski, 1999).

HIV is capable of invading brain tissue. Neurologic symptoms have been reported in approximately 40% to 70% of all patients with AIDS, with 10% having manifestations of neurologic involvement at the time of diagnosis (Flaskerud & Ungvarski, 1999). According to Douglas (1999), the early manifestations of ADC are decreased memory, inability to concentrate, apathy, slowness in thinking, depressed mood, agitation, unsteady gait, tremor, clumsiness, motor weakness, and psychotic features. HIV-positive patients are often aware of the changes in their neurologic well-being, which may lead to an adjustment disorder with fear, anxiety, or depression.

Mr. Michael had with symptoms that fit both categories. The most significant symptom that precipitated the transfer to a medical unit was the change in his ambulation status. It is important to avoid medications that have anticholinergic side effects because these can cause delirium, including hallucinations, confusion, and sometimes agitation. The medications of choice include zidovudine, lamivudine, psychostimulants, and antidepressants (Douglas, 1999).

5. What is the difference between HIV infection and AIDS?

The terms *HIV infection* and *AIDS* are not synonymous. *AIDS* is used to indicate only the most severe diseases or clinical conditions observed in the continuum of illness related to infection with the retrovirus HIV type 1 (HIV-1) (Flaskerud & Ungvarski, 1999).

The definition and classification system for HIV infection was revised and published in December 18, 1992, by the Centers for Disease Control and Prevention (CDC). The CDC classifies HIV infection according to CD4$^+$ T-lymphocyte counts and clinical conditions associated with HIV infection (CDC, 1992). The CD4$^+$ T-lymphocyte cell is affected by the HIV virus. The CD4$^+$ cell count is a rough measurement of damage already done to the immune system by HIV (Ress, 1998) "Decreases in CD4 cells often precede overt morbidity and mortality; the numbers do not provide a picture of day to day activity of the virus in the blood" (Ress, 1998, p. 59). The compromised immune system allows opportunistic organisms to invade the body, which normally would be able to defend itself from these invaders.

The HIV/AIDS classification system emphasizes the clinical importance of the $CD4^+$ lymphocyte count in the categorization of HIV-related clinical conditions (CDC, 1992). The definition includes all infected persons with $CD4^+$ counts of less than $200/mm^3$ and patients with three additional opportunistic infections: pulmonary tuberculosis, invasive cervical cancer, and recurrent bacterial pneumonia (Douglas, 1999).

According to the CDC (1992) revised classification system, counts of $CD4^+$ T lymphocytes are placed in the following three categories:

1. Category 1: $\geq 500/\mu l$
2. Category 2: 200-$499/\mu l$
3. Category 3: $\leq 200/\mu l$

These categories guide clinical and therapeutic management of adolescents and adults with HIV infections. The $CD4^+$ T-cell count classification presents a continuum for HIV disease. The continuum ranges from an asymptomatic stage to advanced HIV disease.

The asymptomatic stage is manifested by an acute primary HIV infection, an asymptomatic condition, or persistent generalized lymphadenopathy (CDC, 1992). As many as 90% of persons with HIV infections have severe flulike symptoms 1 to 3 weeks after infection. These symptoms may last for 1 to 2 weeks. During this time, their HIV antibody test results are usually negative, although they do have a steady decline in their $CD4^+$ T-lymphocyte count and an increase in viral RNA (Flaskerud & Ungvarski, 1999). The HIV antibody test results usually become positive 2 to 18 weeks after infection.

The early symptomatic stage develops when $CD4^+$ T-cell counts drop to around $500/\mu l$ (Flaskerud & Ungvarski, 1999). Clinical conditions that could occur at this stage include candidiasis, herpes zoster, pelvic inflammatory disease, and peripheral neuropathy (CDC, 1992).

The late symptomatic stage begins when a patient's $CD4^+$ T-lymphocyte cell count drops below $200/\mu l$ (Flaskerud & Ungvarski, 1999). A patient may develop life-threatening infections and cancers. The infections usually are treatable. At this point, the stage of infection reflects the CDC criteria for AIDS. The last stage of HIV infection is the advanced HIV disease stage. The patient's $CD4^+$ T-cell count has dropped to less than $50/\mu l$ (Flaskerud & Ungvarski, 1999). Once this level has been reached, death is likely within 1 year.

6. What clinical indicators confirmed that Mr. Michael's HIV infection had progressed to AIDS?

Laboratory findings in the diagnosis of AIDS include a positive HIV antibody test, decreased WBC and lymphocyte counts, depressed $CD4^+$ T-cell count, an abnormal CD4:CD8 ratio, and an RNA viral load (Douglas, 1999; Flaskerud & Ungvarski, 1999; McCain et al, 1998). According to the CDC's definition and classification of the disease, Mr. Michael's disease progressed from HIV infection to AIDS when his $CD4^+$ count dropped below $200/\mu l$. Mr. Michael also had three opportunistic diseases: PCP, *Candida* infection of the oral mucosa, and *Salmonella* infection of the gastrointestinal tract.

7. Describe the symptoms of PCP.

Persons infected with HIV eventually have at least one episode of PCP. The Pulmonary Complications of HIV Infection Study (1998) indicated that respiratory symptoms are a common complaint of persons with HIV infections, and they increase in frequency as the $CD4^+$ cell count declines below 200/µl (Huang, 1998). Statistics indicate that as many as 75% to 80% of patients with AIDS will have PCP. *P. carinii* was originally classified as a protozoan, but today new data suggest that *P. carinii* is more closely related to fungi. *P. carinii* is a simple fungus that is found in the lungs of humans, rats, cats, dogs, and several other animals. Most children develop antibodies to *P. carinii* at an early age. *P. carinii* is not considered a serious pathogenic organism unless a person is severely immunocompromised. In PCP, the alveoli fill with proteinaceous material that contains cysts and trophozoites. Air distribution into alveoli filled with *P. carinii* is impaired (Flaskerud & Ungvarski, 1999).

Symptoms associated with PCP include fever; high respiratory rate (>30 breaths/min); dyspnea on exertion then at rest; normal or abnormal chest examination results; normal breath sounds or minimal rales; cyanosis around the mouth, nailbeds, and mucous membranes; dry, nonproductive cough (unless the patient is a smoker); and thrush, which indicates immunosuppression (Flaskerud & Ungvarski, 1999; Huang, 1998).

8. What symptoms and pulmonary diagnostic findings in Mr. Michael's case indicated the need for transfer to the ICU?

Mr. Michael's symptoms after his transfer to the medical unit included dyspnea, fever, and nonproductive cough. His chest x-ray examination showed minimal infiltrates in both lobes. Oxygen was necessary for his hypoxia. His vital signs were within normal limits except for his temperature. Mr. Michael required admission to the ICU when his worsening respiratory status became life threatening. Because of his diminished respiratory function, he required intubation and mechanical ventilation.

9. Mechanical ventilation and ICU admission for a person with AIDS is controversial. Why was Mr. Michael admitted to the ICU?

The primary reason for patients with PCP to be admitted to the ICU is for mechanical ventilation related to respiratory failure. Infection with *P. carinii* destroys lung tissue, and repeated infections decrease functioning lung surface area and cause mechanical problems in mobilizing secretions (Flaskerud & Ungvarski, 1999). In the terminal stages of AIDS, mechanical ventilation and endotracheal tube placement are associated with mortality of 85% (Flum & Steinberg, 1998). Endotracheal tube placement allows for better oral hygiene and ventilation. Studies indicate that survival rate is higher for patients with a first episode of PCP than for those with subsequent episodes. PCP is being diagnosed sooner and is being treated more effectively (Flaskerud & Ungvarski, 1999). With early treatment, most patients with AIDS survive their first bout with PCP.

This was Mr. Michael's first episode of PCP. His CD4$^+$ count was below 200/μl but not significantly. There is a wide range of indications for critical care for patients with HIV infections. PCP accounts for approximately 16% of ICU admissions. The use of mechanical ventilation for PCP is associated with high mortality (Flum, & Steinberg, 1998; Rosen et al, 1997). This mortality can be drastically reduced when patients' antiretroviral treatment is not interrupted. An example can be found in Ress's 1998 article in *Critical Care Nurse*. In 1989, a patient with PCP was hospitalized in the ICU, and AZT was discontinued while the patient received TMP-SMX intravenously. The patient died 10 weeks later from complications of HIV infection. Patient 2 in 1998 was admitted to the ICU for PCP and received the same treatment, but the patient's antiretroviral medications were not stopped. Six months later, the patient was in good health with an undetectable "viral load" and no further acute illness (Ress, 1998).

10. What treatments did Mr. Michael receive in the ICU to ensure a successful outcome? Include medications for HIV infection such as highly active antiretroviral therapy (HAART) and PCP prophylaxis.

The results from the flexible fiberoptic bronchoscopic examination indicated PCP. This in turn alerted the physician to begin IV pentamidine. Pentamidine was chosen because Mr. Michael was receiving AZT and high-dose IV TMP-SMX, which could potentially cause bone marrow depression (Ress, 1998). Bone marrow depression is also a side effect of AZT. When Mr. Michael's status did not improve, ampicillin and hydrocortisone were added. His oral candidiasis was treated with ketoconazole.

For his HIV status, Mr. Michael is being treated with AZT, 3TC, and indinavir. AZT and 3TC are nucleoside analog reverse transcriptase inhibitors (NRTIs). When NRTIs are incorporated into the DNA of HIV during its replication phase, the NRTI terminates the replication (Flaskerud & Ungvarski, 1999). Indinavir is a protease inhibitor that inhibits protease in the chronically infected cells, resulting in noninfectious viral particles (Flaskerud & Ungvarski, 1999). The terminology used to describe combination therapy today is highly active antiretroviral therapy (HAART). Monotherapy is no longer recommended. HAART has been considered a great breakthrough for treatment of HIV infection. Some consider it a miracle therapy. Others have called HAART treatment the *Lazarus effect:* patients who were at death's door are now active and productive (Boyle, 1998). Unfortunately, not everyone has the Lazarus effect from HAART. For some patients, the therapy has failed. With successful use of HAART, discontinuation of PCP prophylaxis (primary and secondary) has been possible. The criterion that must be met before the prophylaxis can be discontinued is a CD4$^+$ cell count greater than 200 cells/μl documented twice in a 1-month interval. The study by Schneider, Borleffs, Stolk, Jaspers, and Hoepelman (1999) found that patients whose CD4$^+$ cell count was greater than 200/μl could discontinue their PCP prophylaxis. (See Table 26-3 for medications for HIV infection and Table 26-4 for medications for opportunistic infections.)

Text continued on p. 354

TABLE 26-3	HIV Antiviral Drug Guide			
Common Name	Brand Name	Side Effects*	Common Drug Interactions†	Cost
NUCLEOSIDE ANALOGS				
AZT, zidovudine, ZDV	Retrovir	Bone marrow suppression, myopathy, headaches, fever, chills, muscle soreness, fatigue, nausea, fingernail discoloration	Clarithromycin (Biaxin), rifabutin, and rifampin may decrease AZT levels. Methadone and ganciclovir increase AZT levels. Probenecid increases AZT levels.	$3.98/300 mg tablet $2905/yr
ddl, didanosine	Videx	Avoid if history of heavy alcohol consumption or peripheral neuropathy; visual impairment in children; headache, increased uric acid levels, insomnia, diarrhea, pancreatitis	Indinavir. Take on an empty stomach. Take 2 hr apart from cimetidine (Tagamet), ketoconazole (Nizoral), and dapsone. Antitumor medications may increase neuropathy.	$1.53/100 mg tablet $1675/yr
ddC, dideoxycytidine	Hivid	Headache and fever, peripheral neuropathy, pancreatitis	Amphotericin B, antineoplastics, disulfiram (Antabuse), foscarnet, isoniazid, pentamidine, phenytoin (Dilantin), and probenecid may increase risk of peripheral neuropathy. Antacids decrease ddC levels. Foscarnet and probenecid may increase ddC levels.	$2.29/0.75 mg tablet $2607/yr

Adapted from Gallant, J. E. (1998, January-February). When to switch your drug combo. *Positively Aware*, pp. 29-42; and Ress, B. C. (1998). AIDS/HIV antiretroviral therapy for human immunodeficiency virus disease: Implications for critical care nursing. *Critical Care Nurse 18*(6), 54-62.
*These are common side effects. Some clients may experience others not described.
†These are common drug interactions; they are not all-inclusive.   *Continued*

TABLE 26-3	HIV Antiviral Drug Guide— cont'd			
Common Name	Brand Name	Side Effects*	Common Drug Interactions†	Cost
d4T, stavudine	Zerit	Headache and fever, peripheral neuropathy, pancreatitis	Amphotericin B, foscarnet, and dapsone may increase risk of peripheral neuropathy. Ganciclovir and IV pentamidine (Pentam) may increase the risk of pancreatitis.	$3.88/40 mg tablet $2832/yr
3TC, lamivudine	Epivir	Headache, nausea and fatigue	TMP-SMX (Bactrim) increases 3TC levels.	$3.68/150 mg tablet $2688/yr
AZT/3TC, zidovudine/ lamivudine	Combivir	Bone marrow suppression, headache, fever, chills, muscle soreness, nausea, malaise, fatigue, anemia, fingernail discoloration, runny nose	See AZT and 3TC.	$7.18/tablet $5240/yr
NONNUCLEOSIDE ANALOGS				
Nevirapine, NVP	Viramune	Rash, Stevens-Johnson syndrome, headache, nausea	Reduces levels of saquinavir. May react adversely with rifampin, rifabutin, and oral contraceptives.	$4.13/200 mg tablet $3015/yr
DMP 266, Efavirenz	Sustiva	Rash, confusion, insomnia	Decreases the concentration of clarithromycin; can increase metabolism of various drugs.	$1.75/50 mg tablet

Adapted from Gallant, J. E. (1998, January-February). When to switch your drug combo. *Positively Aware*, pp. 29-42; and Ress, B. C. (1998). AIDS/HIV antiretroviral therapy for human immunodeficiency virus disease: Implications for critical care nursing. *Critical Care Nurse* *18*(6), 54-62.

Table 26-3	HIV Antiviral Drug Guide— cont'd			
Common Name	Brand Name	Side Effects*	Common Drug Interactions†	Cost
Delavirdine	Rescriptor	Rash, headache, nausea	Terfenadine (Seldane), astemizole (Hismanal), cisapride (Propulsid), midazolam, and alprazolam should not be used concurrently. Potential toxicity when given with clarithromycin, dapsone, rifabutin, ergot derivatives, nifedipine, quinidine, and warfarin. Absorption is decreased with antacids.	$0.51/100 mg tablet $2234/yr
Protease inhibitors Saquinavir mesylate, RO31-8959	Invirase	Fewer side effects seen because of low absorption level about 4%-6%	Nevirapine and rifabutin decrease saquinavir levels. Saquinavir may increase dapsone levels.	$2.12/200 mg tablet $6964/yr
Indinavir, MK-639	Crixivan	Headache, nausea, kidney stones	Alcohol consumption may increase risk of kidney stones. Do not be use with rifampin or terfenadine. Ketoconazole may increase indinavir levels by 60%.	$2.50/400 mg tablet $5475/yr

Continued

Table 26-3	HIV Antiviral Drug Guide— cont'd			
Common Name	Brand Name	Side Effects*	Common Drug Interactions†	Cost
Ritonavir, ABT-538	Norvir	Asthenia (weakness), nausea, diarrhea, vomiting, tingling/ numbness around mouth, increased levels of triglycerides and cholesterol	Tobacco and alcohol may lower blood levels of ritonavir. Do not take with select painkillers, select cardiovascular drugs, specific antihistamines, and sedative and sleep drugs. Clarithromycin increases ritonavir levels by 80%. Rifampin decreases ritonavir levels by 35%.	$1.55/100 mg tablet $6789/yr
Saquinavir, RO 31-8959	Fortovase	Diarrhea, nausea, increased levels of triglycerides and cholesterol, abdominal discomfort, flatulence, headaches, insomnia, taste alteration, dyspepsia (compare with Invirase)	Drugs that reduce saquinavir blood levels are rifampin, rifabutin, Phenytoin, dexamethasone (Decadron), and carbamazepine (Tegretol). Potential interactions may occur with terfenadine, astemizole, and cisapride.	$0.84/200 mg tablet $5700/yr
Nelfinavir, AG-1343	Viracept	Diarrhea, increased levels of triglycerides and cholesterol	Many drug interactions are seen.	$4.13/200 mg tablet $3015/yr

Adapted from Gallant, J. E. (1998, January-February). When to switch your drug combo. *Positively Aware*, pp. 29-42; and Ress, B. C. (1998). AIDS/HIV antiretroviral therapy for human immunodeficiency virus disease: Implications for critical care nursing. *Critical Care Nurse* 18(6), 54-62.

Table 26-4   HIV-Related Illnesses — Opportunistic Infections

	Symptoms	Treatment
Bacterial Infections (Causes)		
Mycobacterium avium complex	Persistent fever, night sweats, fatigue, weight loss, chronic diarrhea, low blood platelets, nausea, dizziness, abdominal pain; swollen lymph glands, kidney, or spleen; soft tissue masses	Clarithromycin or azithromycin and ethambutol; ciprofloxacin; rifabutin; amikacin (IV) or sparfloxacin
Tuberculosis (TB)	Night sweats, cough, fever, weight loss, swollen lymph glands, fatigue, organ specific symptoms	Three-drug combination to avoid multidrug-resistant TB using isoniazid, pyrazinamide, and rifampin; Rifater, a combination pill, is available; alternatives: ethambutol, streptomycin, amikacin, l-ofloxacin, sparfloxacin; first-line therapy for resistant TB is combination cycloserine-capreomycin with other anti-TB drugs
Syphilis	Initial signs: chancres or sores on body, especially genitals, caused by treponema spirochete Secondary syphilis: 10-12 wk after infection, a rash on hands and feet that spreads, fever, swollen lymph glands, diarrhea Tertiary syphilis: severe neurologic disorders	Aggressive treatment with penicillins, or other antibiotics if allergic; monitor syphilis for recurrence
Salmonella	Persistent diarrhea, cramping, fever, weakness, loss of appetite	Standard antibiotics

Adapted from HIV related illnesses: On the alert for opportunistic infections (1998, Winter). *OUT Extra: A consumer guide to HIV care*, pp. 22-23; and Casey, K. M., Cohen, F., & Hughes, A.

Continued

TABLE *26-4*	HIV-Related Illnesses — Opportunistic Infections — cont'd	
	Symptoms	Treatment
FUNGAL INFECTIONS		
Candidiasis (thrush) (common to body and inhabits the alimentary tract)	White patches on gums, tongue; pain and difficulty swallowing; loss of appetite; vaginal itching, burning, discharge	Fluconazole, nystatin, clotrimazole, ketoconazole, oral solution itraconazole, amphotericin B lipid complex; natural agents for vaginal infection: yogurt, vinegar douche, garlic
Cryptococcal disease	Meningitis: mild headaches, intermittent fevers, malaise, nausea, fatigue, loss of appetite, altered mental status, seizures (rare); skin ulcers, pneumonia (concurrent with PCP)	Fluconazole, amphotericin B, 5-flucytosine, liposomal amphotericin B, itraconazole, dexamethasone; for meningitis, lowering cranial pressure is vital
Histoplasmosis	Skin infections, fever, swollen lymph glands, weight loss, anemia, difficulty breathing; also pneumonia	Itraconazole, amphotericin B, fluconazole, liposomal ampho-tericin B
PCP (lies dormant in lungs, everyone exposed)	Fever, dry cough, weight loss, night sweats, difficulty breathing, elevated liver enzymes	Systemic treatment recommended: TMP-SMX (Bactrim, Septra), cotrimoxazole, pentamidine, dapsone, trimethoprim, atovaquone, trimetrexate, primaquine or clindamycin
PROTOZOAL INFECTIONS		
Cryptosporidiosis	Diarrhea with watery stool, abdominal cramping, nausea, vomiting, fatigue, flatulence (gas), weight loss, poor appetite, dehydration, electrolyte imbalances	Azithromycin, atovaquone, bovine colostrum, nitroglycerin (NTG), octreotide
Toxoplasmosis	Encephalitis (brain disease); also fever, severe headaches, confusion, lethargy, altered mental state, dementia, sei-zures, coma	Pyrimethamine combined with one of sulfadiazine, clindamycin, azithromycin: plus recombinant interferon-γ, atovaquone, ddI

Adapted from HIV related illnesses: On the alert for opportunistic infections (1998, Winter). *OUT Extra: A consumer guide to HIV care,* pp. 22-23; and Casey, K. M., Cohen, F., & Hughes, A.

TABLE 26-4	HIV-Related Illnesses — Opportunistic Infections — cont'd	
	Symptoms	**Treatment**
Microsporidiosis; isosporiasis	Watery diarrhea, abdominal pain, cramping, nausea, vomiting, weight loss, fever	Experimental: albendazole, metronidazole
VIRAL INFECTIONS Cytomegalovirus (CMV)	Affects different parts of the body, fever is common; in eyes: blurry vision; in esophagus: pain, ulcers, difficulty swallowing; in colon and gut: diarrhea, abdominal pain, wasting; in lungs: pneumonia	Approved: ganciclovir (dihydroxypropoxy-methylguanine) IV or intraocular implants; foscarnet, cidofovir, ganciclovir-foscarnet combination; experimental: intravitreal cidofovir or gel, MSL-109, Lobucavir, GW1263, GEM 132, ISIS 2922, valacyclovir
CMV neurologic disorders	Infections of the central nervous system, encephalitis (brain disease), dementia, apathy, delirium, confusion, lethargy	Standard CMV retinitis treatment seen as suboptimal; promising: aggressive ganciclovir-foscarnet combination
Progressive multifocal leukoencephalopathy	Neurologic problems: gross dementia, paralysis, loss of all senses in late-stage disease	No proven treatments. Experimental: vidarabine, acyclovir, foscarnet, and antiretrovirals
Hairy leukoplakia (caused by the Epstein-Barr virus; white hairy patches cannot be removed)	White, raised patches in mouth and on tongue; also skin rash, thirst, lightheadedness, nausea; may be confused with thrush	Acyclovir (Zovirax), ganciclovir
Herpes simplex virus (HSV) 1 and 2; herpes zoster (transmission is person to person with contact with lesions either orally or sexually; herpes zoster is usually reactivation of previous infection, chickenpox)	Ulcers, painful blister and/or itching on lips (caused by HSV1), anus and/or genitals (caused by HSV2); "shingles" on body caused by herpes zoster	Acyclovir, valacyclovir, famciclovir, foscarnet, trifluridine, cidofovir

Continued

TABLE 26-4 HIV-Related Illnesses — Opportunistic Infections — cont'd		
	Symptoms	Treatment
Hepatitis A, B, C (HAV: transmitted by fecal-oral route, contaminated shellfish; HBV: transmission via contaminated needles, transfusion of blood or products, sexual contacts or transplants; HCV: transmission via percutaneous exposure to contaminated blood, blood products and sexual contacts)	Liver infections, fever; chronic progressive disease is seen for B and C; coinfection with C has been linked to higher HIV viral loads	Vaccine for A and B; no treatment for A; penciclovir and adefovir for B; experimental use of short-term 3TC for B, α-interferon, riba-virin for C
CANCERS		
Kaposi's sarcoma (KS) (KS in healthy homosexual men may support theories of: sexually transmitted KS virus; role of CMV unclear, homosexual men who used/use "poppers" have increased incidence of KS)	Cancer of skin and organs associated with a new herpes virus: HHV-8; small purplish lesions visible on skin; bronchoscopy for diagnosis in lungs	Vinblastine, vincristine, etoposide, bleomycin, doxorubicin, α-interferon (also in combination); surgical excision, radiation, cryotherapy, drugs injected into lesions; experimental: human chorionic gonado-tropin; light therapy; oral all-trans-retinoic acid (Atra) HAART, 9-cis-retinoic acid (Pancreatin)
Non-Hodgkin's lymphoma or B-cell lymphomas (suspected viral etiology, Epstein-Barr virus is passenger virus, coincidentally found)	Cancer of lymphocytes; may also affect bone marrow and central nervous system; B-cell lymphomas linked to Epstein-Barr virus	Combination of anti-cancer drugs; first-line therapy is CHOP (cyclophosphamide, doxorubicin, vin-cristine, and prednisone); experimental: CDE (cyclophosphamide, doxorubicin, etoposide) with ddI, granulocyte-colony-stimulating factor

Adapted from HIV related illnesses: On the alert for opportunistic infections (1998, Winter). *OUT Extra: A consumer guide to HIV care*, pp. 22-23; and Casey, K. M., Cohen, F., & Hughes, A.

TABLE 26-4	HIV-Related Illnesses — Opportunistic Infections — cont'd	
	Symptoms	Treatment
OTHER CONDITIONS		
Wasting syndrome (causes include: decreased nutrient intake; avoidance of food because of diarrhea, course of illness, weakness; anorexia, chronic illness, depression, fever, medication side effect)	Rapid severe weight loss, loss of appetite, chronic diarrhea, fever; involuntary weight loss of >10% from usual weight in addition to diarrhea; tumor necrosis factor and glutathione levels linked to wasting	Drugs to increase food absorption and weight (megestrol [Megace], dronabinol [Marinol], growth hormone) nutritional supplements (oral and IV); exercise, vitamins
Neuropathy	Tingling "pins and needles" in feet and legs, hands and fingers, numbness and pain	Nerve damage possibly a side effect of drugs or HIV infection; experimental: peptide T, nerve growth factor and vitamin B
Idiopathic thrombocytopenia purpura	Excessive bleeding from nosebleeds, cuts; easy bruising; small and large red spots on skin (caused by HIV-related low platelet counts)	Prednisone, a steroid; Win-Rho, an immunoglobulin, gamma globulin
GYNECOLOGIC		
Cervical cancer (etiology: HSV2, human papilloma virus [HPV])	Cervical lesions and cellular abnormalities caused by sexually transmitted viruses, including herpes and HPV; detected by abnormal Pap smear; confirmed by colposcopy	Early stage (microinvasive) cancer: cryosurgery (freezing), scraping and cone biopsy of cervix; invasive cancer: hysterectomy, surgical removal of lymph nodes; regular Pap smears to detect onset of infection
HPV; genital warts	Genital warts can be felt if external; internal warts require examination	Cryosurgery, laser then monitor; HPV can recur; Regular Pap smears to detect onset of infection; experimental: fluorouracil, an injectable gel
Pelvic inflammatory disease	Vaginal discharge, pain, internal ulcers, ectopic pregnancy, linked to *Chlamydia*; screening early detection critical	Ceftriaxone plus tetracycline or doxycycline or erythromycin (if pregnant or allergic)

11. What are some of the nursing interventions that will help Mr. Michael with his psychosocial and physiologic needs?

Mr. Michael's initial admission assessment demonstrated several psychosocial needs. It is important to assess his safety both through necessary suicidal precautions and assistance with ambulation. Mr. Michael's safety should be a priority. It is also important to maintain the patient's support systems.

Potential nursing diagnoses for ADC include the following:

- Anxiety related to unknown progression of HIV/AIDS
- Ineffective coping related to depression and AIDS dementia
- ADC related to unknown progression of HIV/AIDS
- Fear related to the unknown progression of HIV/AIDS

It is necessary to design a plan of care according to assessment data and expected outcomes. For example, because Mr. Michael will have perceptual alterations, including diminishing memory, it is important to have him keep a calendar to help him follow treatment regimens. Instructions should be simple and concise.

During the time that Mr. Michael has PCP, it is important to follow care according to developed nursing diagnoses and expected outcomes.

The nursing care of a patient with ADC and PCP in the ICU depends not only on the nurses' knowledge of the physiology of the disease process but also on the psychosocial needs of the critically ill patient (Ress, 1998). Compliance with medication regimens is a very important to stress to a patient with HIV infection/AIDS. Noncompliance with HIV medication can cause viral mutation and drug resistance.

12. When assigned to a patient with HIV infection, what personal feelings or concerns should be acknowledged?

These fears are going to be very individualized. It is important that the nurse addresses his or her fears related to disease transmission, homophobia, and other feelings that arise when caring for patients with HIV infection. Unfortunately, it is still common in hospitals and in community settings to encounter nurses who are "afraid" to care for these patients. Individual needs should be recognized and educational programs that correct misinformation related to this disease should be developed and implemented. The latest revision of American Nurses Association's Nurses Code is a guide for carrying out nursing responsibilities in a manner consistent with quality in nursing care and the ethical obligations of the profession.

13. Are the ICU nurses at an increased risk of acquiring AIDS from patients who receive mechanical ventilation?

The incidence of medical personnel contracting AIDS from patients is quite low. The use of universal precautions by all medical personnel lessens the risk of infection. It is important to handle blood and body fluids properly. It is important to follow the CDC recommendations for prevention of HIV transmission in health care settings and to follow the Occupational Safety and Health Administration's blood and body fluid precautions.

The risk of acquiring HIV infection from needlesticks or cuts exposed to HIV-infected blood is 0.3% (1 in 300) (CDC, 1998). The risk of exposure of the eyes, nose, or mouth to HIV-infected blood is 0.1% or 1 in 1000 (CDC, 1998). Exposure of skin to a small amount of blood has practically no risk. It is important that ICU staff take precautions to avoid contact with blood and body fluids from all patients. "As of December, 1996 CDC has received 52 documented cases and 111 possible cases of occupationally acquired HIV infection among health care workers" (CDC, 1998; Porche, 1997).

14. What is the recommended protocol for occupational exposure to HIV?

CDC has very specific guidelines for the follow-up of potential occupational exposure. These protocols can be found on their Web site at http://www.cdc.gov/ncidod/hip/faq.htm (CDC, 1999) and include the following:

1. If the source client is seronegative for HIV and has no clinical evidence or risk for HIV infection or AIDS, no further follow-up is indicated.

2. If the source patient has AIDS, is seropositive for HIV, or refuses to be tested, as soon as possible after the exposure, the health care worker (HCW) will be referred for baseline serologic testing for evidence of HIV. The HCW may go to the employee health or emergency room health care provider/facility of choice or may be referred to a designated laboratory/agency. This will depend on the employer's infection control policy. The HCW should be referred for postexposure counseling about the risk of infection, prevention of transmission of HIV during the follow-up period, and the need for appropriate follow-up medical care.

3. Those exposed will have follow-up HIV testing at 6 weeks, 3 months, 6 months, and 12 months postexposure at a health care provider/facility of choice (Table 26-5).

Table 26-5	Type of Exposure and Prophylaxis Suggested	
Type of Exposure	Source Material	Antiretroviral Prophylaxis
Percutaneous	Blood	
	Highest risk	Recommend
	Increased risk	Recommend
	No increased risk	Offer
	Fluid containing visible blood, other potentially infectious fluid, or tissue	Offer
	Other body fluid	No offer
Mucous membrane	Blood	Offer
	Fluid containing visible blood, other potentially infectious fluid, or tissue	No offer
Skin	Blood	Offer
	Fluid containing visible blood, other potentially infectious fluid, or tissue	Offer
	Other body fluid	No offer

Adapted from Porche, D. J. (1997) Treatment review: Postexposure prophylaxis after an occupational exposure to HIV. *Journal of the Association of Nurses in AIDS Care, 8*(1), 83-87.

ACQUIRED IMMUNODEFICIENCY SYNDROME

References

Boyle, B. (1998). Can a broken HAART be mended? *The AIDS Reader 8*(3), 114-120.

Centers for Disease Control and Prevention. (1999). Occupational exposure to HIV. Information for health care workers [WWW document]. URL: http://www.cdc.gov/ncidod/hip/faq.htm.

Centers for Disease Control and Prevention. (1998) Public Health Service guidelines for the management of health-care worker exposures to HIV and recommendations for postexposure prophylaxis [WWW document]. URL: http://ftp.cdc.gov/pub/Publications/mmwr/rr/rr4707.pdf. Also in *Morbidity and Mortality Weekly Report, 47*(RR-7), 1-34.

Centers for Disease Control and Prevention. (1992, December, 18). 1993 revised classification system for HIV infection and expanded surveillance case definition for AIDS among adolescents and adults. *Morbidity and Mortality Weekly Report, 41*(RR-17), 1-19.

Douglas, S. (1999). Human immunodeficiency virus disease. In L. Bucher & S. Melander (Eds.), *Critical care nursing.* Philadelphia: Saunders.

Flaskerud, J. H., & Ungvarski, P. J. (1999). *HIV/AIDS: A guide to primary care management* (4th ed.). Philadelphia: Saunders.

Flum, D., & Steinberg, S. (1998). Bedside percutaneous tracheostomy in acquired immunodeficiency syndrome. *American Surgeon 64*(5), 444-447.

Huang, L. (May 1998). The evaluation of respiratory symptoms in HIV-infected patients. *The AIDS knowledge base* [On-line publication]. URL http://hivinsite.ucsf.edu/akb/1997/05pulm/index.html.

McCain, N. L., Lyon, D. E., Higginson, R., Settle, J., Wheeler Robins, J. L., & Fisher, E. J. (1998). Revision of the HIV Center Medical Staging Scale. *Journal of the Association of Nurses in AIDS Care, 9*(5), 19-23.

Melroe, N. H., Stawarz, K. E., Simpson, J., & Henry, W. K. (1997). HIV RNA quantitation: Marker of HIV infection. *Journal of the Association of Nurses in AIDS Care, 8*(5), 31-38.

Porche, D. J. (1997). Treatment review: Postexposure prophylaxis after an occupational exposure to HIV. *Journal of the Association of Nurses in AIDS Care, 8*(1), 83-87.

Ress, B. C. (1998). AIDS/HIV antiretroviral therapy for human immunodeficiency virus disease: Implications for critical care nursing. *Critical Care Nurse, 18*(6), 54-62.

Rosen, M. J., Clayton, K., Schneider, R. F., Fulkerson, W., Rao, A. V., Stansell, J., Kvale P. A., Glassroth, J., Reichman, L. B., Wallace, J. M., & Hopewell, P. C. (1997). Intensive care of patients with HIV infection: Utilization, critical illnesses, and outcomes. Pulmonary complications of HIV Infection Study Group. *American Journal of Respiratory Critical Care Medicine, 155*(1), 67-71.

Schneider, M. M., Borleffs, J. C., Stolk, R. P., Jaspers, C. A., & Hoepelman (1999). Discontinuation of prophylaxis for *Pneumocystis carinii* pneumonia in HIV-1-infected patients treated with highly active antiretroviral therapy. *Lancet, 353*(9148), 201-203.

Stine, G. J. (1998). *Acquired immune deficiency syndrome biological, medical, social, and legal issues* (3rd ed.). Upper Saddle River, NJ: Prentice Hall.

Valente, S. M., & Saunders, J. M. (1997). Managing depression among people with HIV disease. *Journal of the Association of Nurses in AIDS Care, 8*(1), 51-67.

Zeller, J. M., McCain, N. L., & Swanson, B. (1996). Immunological and virological markers of HIV-disease progression. *Journal of the Association of Nurses in AIDS Care, 7*(1), 15-27.

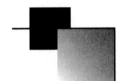

CHAPTER *27*

ABDOMINAL AORTIC ANEURYSM

Brian W. Higgerson, RN, MSN, FNP, CCRN

CASE PRESENTATION

Mr. Stephens, a 54-year-old African-American man, was admitted to the intensive care unit (ICU) after repair of an abdominal aortic aneurysm (AAA). He has a history of coronary artery disease, hypertension, chronic bronchitis, diabetes, and peripheral vascular disease. Before hospitalization, Mr. Stephens was experiencing severe lower back pain accompanied by nausea and vomiting. Mr. Stephens was seen in the emergency department for his progressive symptoms and evaluated for an AAA with possible rupture. A Doppler ultrasound study and computed tomographic (CT) scan confirmed the aneurysm without evidence of a rupture.

Presurgical measures included intubation, arterial catheter placement, and the insertion of an pulmonary arterial catheter. The surgical repair of the aneurysm was without complications. A bifurcated Dacron graft was placed, and the aneurysmal sac was wrapped around the graft and anastomosed. Upon arrival in the ICU, the following data were obtained:

BP	150/40 mm Hg (via arterial line)	Temperature	(96° F [35.5° C]) (core)
HR	120 bpm (sinus tachycardia without ectopy)	PAP	30/10 mm Hg
		PAWP	15 mm Hg
Respirations	12 breaths/min (ventilator with IMV 12)	CO	4.0 L/min
		CI	2.0 L/min

Ventilator settings were the following:

Mode	SIMV	V_T	900 ml
Rate	12	PEEP	5 cm
Fio_2	0.50	Pressure support	12 cm

After the surgery, Mr. Stephens returned to the intensive care unit for recovery and aggressive monitoring. He was nonresponsive upon arrival in the unit. A warming blanket was immediately applied, and his temperature increased to 96° F within a few minutes. Dorsalis pedis and posterior tibial pulses were audible bilaterally via a Doppler. His extremities were cool and pale, and capillary refill was approximately 5 seconds. Arterial blood gas measurements were obtained, and the results were within normal limits.

A midline abdominal dressing was dry and intact. There were no bruits noted over the abdominal dressing. After insertion of nasogastric tube connected to low wall suction, a minimal amount of light green aspirate was seen. His Foley catheter drained large amounts of pale, yellow urine. An as-needed order for sodium nitroprusside (Nipride) was written to maintain arterial blood pressure less than 160/90 mm Hg. A dopamine infusion of 2 µg/kg was initiated on arrival in the unit.

ABDOMINAL AORTIC ANEURYSM

Questions

1. Describe the pathophysiology involved in aortic aneurysms.
2. Describe the pathophysiology involved in aortic dissection.
3. What etiologic or precipitating factors may be associated with AAAs?
4. List the subjective and objective findings that may be associated with an AAA.
5. Discuss the diagnostic studies that contribute to the diagnosis of an AAA.
6. List nursing diagnoses appropriate for care of the patient with an AAA.
7. What are the responsibilities and nursing interventions necessary for postoperative care after repair of an AAA?

ABDOMINAL AORTIC ANEURYSM

Questions and Answers

1. **Describe the pathophysiology involved in aortic aneurysms.**

An *aneurysm* is a defect in the anatomy of an artery resulting in stretching, weakness, and ballooning out of the arterial wall (McCance & Huether, 1998). The artery most commonly affected is the aorta; in 80% of patients, the abdominal area is involved. There are three types of aneurysms: fusiform, saccular, and dissecting. An fusiform aneurysm involves the ballooning of the entire circumference of the artery. A saccular aneurysm involves only one side of the artery ballooning. A dissection occurs from a tear in the intima of the vessel, allowing blood to accumulate between the layers. The most common presentation of an AAA is fusiform in shape, extending below the renal arteries to involve the entire infrarenal aorta and often the common iliac artery. Several factors contribute to the weakening of the aortic medial wall. These include dilation, increased pressures, and thinning of the wall, which lead to the weakening and dilating of the vessel. Complications of an aneurysm include dissection, embolization of thrombus, and end-organ disease.

2. **Describe the pathophysiology involved in aortic dissection.**

A life-threatening complication from an AAA is a dissection or rupture (Urden, 1998). Hypertension is a factor in 80% of dissections. The decreased wall strength, increased turbulence at the bifurcation, and increased systolic pressure may contribute to the progression of the dilation of the aortic wall and increase likelihood of dissection. According to the law of Laplace, tension on the vessel wall is directly proportional to the radius of the wall (McCance & Huether, 1998). As the aneurysm increases in size, the wall is under an increasing amount of tension; thus, the larger the aneurysm and the higher the systemic blood pressure, the more likely the aneurysm is to rupture. Proximal dissections are associated with high mortality (80%).

There are three severe consequences from a dissecting aneurysm. One is downstream ischemia as the blood trapped in the wall forces the inner layer into the lumen (Nowak & Handford, 1999). The second possibility occurs if the aortic wall ruptures near its base, which results in blood that escapes the vessel and becomes trapped in the pericardium. The result of this event is called *cardiac tamponade,* and it is associated with high mortality. The third potential consequence is the disruption of the aortic valve by dissecting of the aortic wall adjacent to it (Nowak & Handford, 1999).

3. What etiologic or precipitating factors may be associated with AAAs?

Several etiologic or precipitating factors may be associated with an AAA. The most prevalent factor seen in 95% of patients is atherosclerosis (Thelan, Urden, Lough, & Stacy, 1998). Other contributing factors include congenital abnormalities, trauma, severe hypertension, arteritis, Raynaud's disease, and a family history of aneurysms (Lessig & Lessig, 1998). Aneurysms are more common in persons older than 50 years of age and are seen in men twice as often as in women (Ferri, 1999).

4. List the subjective and objective findings that may be associated with an AAA.

Subjective Data

Almost 75% of AAAs are asymptotic and are discovered on routine examinations (Phillips, 1998a). Subjective findings may include the following (Lessig & Lessig, 1998):

- Dull abdominal, flank, and/or back pain
- Nausea
- Vomiting
- Complaints of heartburn
- Syncope
- Severe abdominal pain, which may be associate with rupture

Objective Data

Objective findings may include the following (Lessig & Lessig, 1998):

- Pulsating epigastric mass that may or may not be tender
- Bruit over the abdominal aorta
- Hypertension/hypotension
- Wide pulse pressure

5. Discuss the diagnostic studies that contribute to the diagnosis of an AAA.

Because objective and subjective findings can be limited in contributing to the definitive diagnosis of AAA, diagnostic studies are imperative. Abdominal ultrasound is nearly 100% accurate in identifying an aneurysm and estimating the size to within 0.3 to 0.4 cm. However, ultrasound is not as useful for estimating the proximal extension to the renal arteries or involvement of the iliac arteries (Ferri, 1999). A CT scan is recommended for preoperative imaging of the aneurysm and estimating the size to within 0.3 mm. There are no false-negative results, and the CT scan can localize the proximal extent, detect the integrity of the wall, and rule out rupture. An angiogram can provide detailed information about the arterial anatomy, localizing the aneurysm relative to the renal and visceral arteries. According to Ferri (1999), this is the definitive preoperative diagnostic study for surgeons. Magnetic resonance imaging can also be used, but it is more expensive and not readily available.

6. List nursing diagnoses appropriate for care of the patient with an AAA.

- Alteration in tissue perfusion related to arterial occlusive disease
- Anxiety related to critical care environment
- Fluid volume excess related to acute renal failure
- Alteration in skin integrity related to incision site
- Impaired physical mobility related to postsurgical procedure

7. What are the responsibilities and nursing interventions necessary for postoperative care after repair of an AAA?

Aggressive nursing interventions and monitoring are necessary steps in the care of a patients after repair of a AAA. Meticulous assessment is the primary responsibility of the nurse and should focus on blood loss to the organs normally supplied by the aorta, including the stomach, small intestine, ascending and descending colon, rectum, spinal cord, and kidneys (Phillips, 1998b). Postoperative assessment should be performed every 15 minutes for the first 2 hours after the surgery. If the patient's condition is stable, assessments may be performed every hour in the ICU. Peripheral pulses and blood pressure should be compared on both the left side and the right side. Pressure differences exceeding 20 mm Hg in the upper extremities may indicate the possibility of dissection (McCoy & Livingston, 1999). To confirm faint or absent pulses, a Doppler may be used. Frequent assessment of a bruit over the dressing site should be included with the assessment of bowel sounds. Accurate urinary output data should be collected to rule out the possibility of acute renal failure caused by decreased renal cortical blood flow from the surgical procedure. A complete neurologic assessment is important to evaluate the patient's recovery from general anesthesia and to monitor for spinal cord ischemia or stroke (Phillips, 1998b).

Nitroprusside and dopamine are titrated to keep blood pressure values within prescribed limits (Urden, 1998). Nitroprusside is used to decrease the systemic vascular resistance by dilating the venous and arterial beds. By decreasing the afterload, the heart will have less resistance to work against in ejecting its stroke volume. Renal tonic dopamine is used for its positive inotropic effects, which ultimately dilate the renal vessels and decrease the potential for renal complications.

β-Blockers or calcium channel blockers may also be administered to maintain an acceptable mean arterial blood pressure value. Moreover, frequent hemodynamic monitoring of heart rate, blood pressure, pulmonary artery wedge pressure, and cardiac output is an essential element in the care of a patient after surgery.

Serial hemodynamic assessments are imperative to detect bleeding or massive fluid shifts. Assessing distal pulses in the lower extremities can be pivotal in detecting circulation disturbances. A decrease in heart rate, blood pressure, and hemoglobin level can be a red flag for a postoperative third-space fluid shift (Phillips, 1998b). Careful monitoring for fluid loss and hemorrhage is incorporated in the plan of care, and these are usually detected within the first 24 hours after the AAA repair.

ABDOMINAL AORTIC ANEURYSM

References

Ferri, F. F. (1999). *Clinical advisor.* St Louis: Mosby.

Lessig, M., & Lessig, P. M. (1998). The cardiovascular system. In Grif-Alspach, J. (Ed.), *American Association of Critical-Care Nurses: Core curriculum for critical care nursing* (5th ed., pp. 137-336). Philadelphia: Saunders.

McCance, K. L., & Huether, S. E. (1998). *Pathophysiology: The biologic basis for disease in adults and children* (3rd ed.). St Louis: Mosby.

McCoy, C. & Livingston, N. (1999). Cardiovascular laboratory and diagnostic tests. In L. Bucher & S. Melander (Eds.), *Critical care nursing*. Philadelphia: Saunders.

Nowak, T. J., & Handford, A. G. (1999). *Essentials of pathophysiology* (2nd ed.). Boston: McGraw-Hill.

Pearce, W. H., Zarins, C. & Hallett, J. W. (1999). Diagnosis and management of aneurysmal disease [WWW document]. URL: http://www.vascsurg.org/doc/1466.html (visited 1999, June 1).

Phillips, J. K. (1998a). Abdominal aortic aneurysm. *Nursing, 28*(5), 34-40.

Phillips, J. K. (1998b). Diagnosing abdominal aortic aneurysm: An update. *Hospital Medicine, 34*(2), 42-51.

Thelan, L., Urden, L., Lough, M., & Stacy, K. (1998). *Critical care nursing: Diagnosis and management* (3rd ed.). St Louis: Mosby.

Urden, L. D. (1998). *Critical care nursing: Diagnosing and management* (3rd ed.). St Louis: Mosby.

CHAPTER 28

BLUNT ABDOMINAL TRAUMA

Joan E. King, RN, PhD, ACNP

CASE PRESENTATION

Mr. Packard is a 35-year-old man who was involved in a motor vehicle accident. Mr. Packard was wearing a seat belt and was driving at a high rate of speed when he lost control of the car and hit an abutment. He was initially awake at the scene, but his level of consciousness declined while in transport to the hospital. Upon arrival at the hospital, he was already intubated and he had received 3 L of normal saline en route.

Mr. Packard's medical history was noncontributory. His family history was negative for heart disease, diabetes, or cancer. Mr. Packard has a 15-pack-year history of smoking, and he drinks socially.

Upon arrival at the hospital, Mr. Packard was on a backboard with a cervical collar. His vital signs were the following:

BP	110/80 mm Hg
HR	113 bpm
Sao_2	95% (with 100% oxygen)

His pupils were 3 cm and equal and reacted briskly to light. Mr. Packard did not have a Battle's sign nor raccoon eyes, and no abnormalities ("step-offs") were noted over his skull or down his spine. The tympanic membranes were clear, and the trachea was midline. Examination of the chest revealed no flailing and no subcutaneous emphysema. Breath sounds were diminished in the lower lobes bilaterally. The patient was tachycardic with normal S_1 and S_2 and no murmurs, rubs, or gallops. Peripheral pulses were 2+ bilaterally. His abdomen was soft and moderately distended with hypoactive bowel sounds. There were no palpable masses and no hepatosplenomegaly. The pelvis was stable. Genitourinary examination revealed no gross hematuria. Rectal tone was normal, and stool was guaiac negative. The patient was able to move all four extremities spontaneously, but orientation to time, person, and place was difficult to assess because he had been sedated.

Initially, Mr. Packard was taken for a computed tomographic (CT) scan, which revealed a grade III liver laceration. No splenic or renal injuries were noted. A CT scan of the head revealed no hematoma. Because of the patient's unstable condition, his spine could not be fully evaluated. Chest x-ray examination revealed bilateral pulmonary contusion with bilateral rib fractures.

His initial laboratory values after fluid resuscitation were the following:

WBCs	21.7×10^3 mm^3	CO_2	22 mmol/L
PCVs	34	Cl$^-$	119 mmol/L
Platelets	217,000/mm^3	BUN	9 mg/dl
PT	21.0 sec	Creatinine	1.0 mg/dl
INR	1.7	Glucose	170 mg/dl
PTT	41.9 sec	AST (SGOT)	635 U/L
Na$^+$	135 mmol/L	Bilirubin	0.9 mg/dl
K$^+$	4.2 mmol/L	Albumin	1.8 g/dl

Arterial blood gas (ABG) values were as follows:

pH	7.1	Pao$_2$	82 mm Hg (with
Paco$_2$	51 mm Hb		100% oxygen)
		Base deficit	14.4

A toxicology screen was negative for drugs, but Mr. Packard's blood alcohol level was 171 g/dl.

Mr. Packard's problem list upon admission to the trauma center was the following:

1. Blunt abdominal trauma
2. No closed head injury (CHI) as revealed by CT scan
3. Bilateral pulmonary contusions with bilateral rib fractures
4. Relative hypoxia with a Pao$_2$ value of 80 with inhalation of 100% oxygen
5. Metabolic acidosis
6. Hypovolemic shock

Mr. Packard was taken directly to the trauma intensive care unit, where he was given synchronized intermittent mechanical ventilation (SIMV) with positive end-expiratory pressure (PEEP) and pressure support (PS). A pulmonary artery (PA) catheter, nasogastric tube (NGT), and Foley catheter were inserted. Because of his hyperchloremia, his fluid infusions were changed from normal saline to lactated Ringer's solution. His acidosis was treated with three runs of sodium bicarbonate. Over the next 12 hours, Mr. Packard's abdomen became very firm and distended, with less than 300 ml of drainage from the NGT. In addition, his peak inspiratory pressures rose from 35 to 60 mm Hg, and his bladder pressure rose to 35 mm Hg.

At this time, his vital signs were as follows:

BP	100/80 mm Hg
HR	130 bpm
Respirations	14 breaths/min

The diagnosis of abdominal compartment syndrome (ACS) was made. Mr. Packard was immediately taken to the operating room, and a decompression celiotomy was performed. At that time, the laceration on the right dome of the liver was assessed and packed. No other injuries were noted, but the small bowel was edematous and distended. Because of the edema, the abdomen could not be closed, and the intestines were covered with a sterile towel and a large sterile transparent dressing was placed over the wound.

When Mr. Packard was returned to the trauma unit, vital signs were the following:

PIP	35 mm Hg	PAP	50/27
BP	120/64 mm Hg	CI	5.5 L/min/m²
HR	112 bpm		

His ventilator settings were the following:

SIMV rate	14	PEEP	10 cm H_2O
Respirations	14 breaths/min	PS	5
V_T	750 ml	Sao_2	97%
Fio_2	40%	Svo_2	83%

Antibiotics (gentamicin and trovafloxacin/alatrofloxacin [Trovan]) were started with fentanyl (Sublimaze) for pain control. Peptic ulcer prophylaxis with famotidine (Pepcid) was begun. Because of his pulmonary contusions and the need to control his respiratory status, Mr. Packard was also receiving cisatracurium (Nimbex). This was accompanied by conscious sedation using lorazepam (Ativan).

Two days after his initial surgery, Mr. Packard returned to the operating room for reexploration of his abdomen, and an assessment of his liver laceration. When the packing was removed, hemostasis had been maintained and there was no necrosis of the liver or any signs of active bleeding. On day 6, he was returned to the operating room, and his abdominal fascia was closed using stay sutures. The skin was not closed because the wound had been open for 6 days, and instead the wound was packed with sterile wet to dry dressings. Other significant events that occurred included the start of enteral feedings on day 3 with progression to 90 ml of Perative every hour by day 5. On day 6, Mr. Packard underwent a tracheotomy, and weaning from the ventilator began on day 8. Nineteen days after Mr. Packard was in the accident, he was transferred to a rehabilitation facility, where he required only supplementary oxygen through a tracheotomy collar with minimal suction every 2 hours.

BLUNT ABDOMINAL TRAUMA

Questions

1. What are the initial assessment priorities for a patient with blunt abdominal trauma?
2. What is meant by a *secondary survey*?
3. What is meant by a *tertiary survey*?
4. What diagnostic tests are done to evaluate and treat patients who have sustained a blunt abdominal trauma?
5. What are the management guidelines for a patient with blunt abdominal trauma?
6. What is meant by *ACS*?

7. What is a pulmonary contusion?
8. What other factors may be contributing to Mr. Packard's poor oxygenation status?
9. Why was Mr. Packard pharmacologically paralyzed and what are the nursing implications?
10. What other complications is Mr. Packard at risk for, and how should they be monitored?
11. What are the nutritional needs of a patient with a blunt abdominal trauma?

BLUNT ABDOMINAL TRAUMA

Questions and Answers

1. **What are the initial assessment priorities for patients with blunt abdominal trauma?**

Trauma is the fourth leading cause of death in the United States (Klein, 1995), with the mortality rate for blunt abdominal trauma ranging from 10% to 30% (Smith, 1994). Blunt abdominal trauma is particularly challenging because assessment of the injuries is often difficult and injuries can be missed (Sommers, 1995). Assessment of the patient with blunt abdominal trauma can be divided into primary survey, secondary survey, and tertiary survey.

The primary survey focuses on an initial assessment of airway, breathing, and circulation and a rapid neurologic assessment to identify spinal injuries or a CHI. Airway management and oxygenation are of prime importance. This includes assessing for a patent airway, life-threatening facial injuries, the patient's ability to breathe spontaneously, and the presence and quality of breath sounds. Absent or diminished breath sounds may indicate a hemothorax or pneumothorax. Absent breath sounds with a deviated trachea are signs of a tension pneumothorax, which requires immediate management with the insertion of a chest tube or decompression with a 14- to 16-gauge needle. Further assessment of the chest for rib fractures, flail chest, sucking, open wounds, or subcutaneous emphysema should be rapidly performed. If the patient is responsive to pain, palpation of the chest anteriorly and laterally may help identify possible rib fractures (Prentice & Ahrens, 1994). A flail chest can be assessed by noting the paradoxical movement of the chest wall caused by multiple rib fractures in two or more places. Portable chest x-ray units will provide added data about rib fractures and document the presence of a hemothorax or pneumothorax. Many patients with a pneumothorax or a flail chest may require intubation to provide ventilatory support and improve oxygenation.

Although ABG values give the most definitive assessment of the patient's respiratory status, pulse oximetry can provide a quick assessment of the patient's oxygen saturations. It should be noted that pulse oximetry will often overestimate the patient's true oxygen saturation (Prentice & Ahrens, 1994). For example, if a patient's oxygen saturation is 95%, the peripheral pulse oximeter may register 96% to 100%. However, important information can still be obtained with pulse oximetry, including oxygen saturation trends and critically low saturations below 90%.

While a rapid assessment of the respiratory system is performed, the circulatory status is also assessed, including heart rate, rhythm, and blood pressure (BP). In the prehospital field, if a BP reading cannot be obtained, the following guidelines are used: (1) if a radial pulse is palpable the BP is estimated to be 80 mm Hg; (2) if the radial pulse is not palpable but the femoral artery is, the BP is estimated to be 70 mm Hg; and (3) if only the carotid pulse is palpable, the BP is estimated to be 60 mm Hg (Cardonna, Hurn, Mason, Scanlon, & Veise-Berry, 1994). During the primary survey, any overt signs of bleeding are assessed and controlled, if possible, with direct pressure.

Interventions to achieve stabilization of the circulatory system will include the administration of fluids, either normal saline or lactated Ringer's, and blood products. There is a great deal of controversy concerning the use of colloids during initial stabilization. It is important to realize that capillaries of patients in shock begin to leak fluid into the interstitial spaces as a result of increased capillary permeability. This implies that regardless of the type of fluid administered, a certain proportion will leave the circulatory system and enter the interstitial spaces. This phenomenon is called *third spacing,* and it contributes to the edema that trauma patients experience in the postresuscitation phase. Because it is believed that colloids may enhance the third spacing as a result of an increase in colloidal osmotic pressure in the interstitial spaces, crystalloids are preferred (Melio, 1998). However, because of the generalized increase in capillary permeability, during the initial resuscitation phase, patients will need rapid fluid administration to maintain an adequate circulatory status. For patients in hemorrhagic shock, 3 L of fluids are administered for every 1 L of estimated blood loss (Jacobs, 1994). Monitoring the BP serves as the key assessment parameter in determining the amount of fluid required.

Another factor that needs to be evaluated when determining fluid resuscitation is whether the bleeding is considered to be controlled or uncontrolled. *Controlled bleeding* refers to the ability to identify and stop the source of bleeding. *Uncontrolled bleeding* or *hemorrhage* refers to the inability to either identify or stop the source of the bleeding. According to Melio (1998) and Jacobs (1994), if the bleeding can be controlled, maximal fluid resuscitation is appropriate. However, if the bleeding is uncontrolled, rapid fluid resuscitation may promote additional bleeding and increase mortality. In patients with uncontrolled bleeding or hemorrhage, sufficient amounts of fluid should be administered to treat the shock, but not enough to restore full cardiovascular status and hence promote additional bleeding (Melio, 1998).

Patients with blunt trauma must also be assessed for cardiac tamponade, especially those involved in a motor vehicle accident. Because of the frequent presence of hypotension or hemorrhagic shock, the classic Beck's triad (elevated central venous pressure [CVP], pulsus paradoxus, and decreased heart sounds) may not be evident because muffled heart sounds may be difficult to hear. Melio (1998) recommends ultrasonography or echocardiography if the patient's condition is stable, and a pericardiocentesis if the patient's condition is unstable and a cardiac tamponade is suspected.

Although many trauma patients will enter the emergency department already intubated and sedated and with the cervical spine immobilized, it is important to perform a primary neurologic survey. The patient's level of responsiveness to verbal and painful stimuli should be assessed as well as the pupillary response to light and pupil size. In addition, the patient's ability to move all four extremities should be assessed quickly. At all times until the patient can have appropriate radiologic studies done to assess the cervical spine, all trauma patients must be considered to have a cervical spine injury, and a cervical collar should be applied. Flexion and extension of the neck must be avoided even during intubation.

2. What is meant by a *secondary survey?*

As the primary survey is completed and life-threatening diagnoses are managed, the secondary survey begins. The secondary survey is a more complete and focused head-to-toe assessment of the patient. For patients with blunt abdominal trauma, the purpose of the secondary survey is to identify the extent of internal injuries. Obtaining information about the mechanism of injury is often helpful in guiding clinicians with their assessment. For patients who were involved in a motor vehicle accident, such as Mr. Packard, it is important to determine whether the patient was wearing a seat belt, if an air bag was activated, or if the patient was thrown from the vehicle. Persons who had been wearing a seat belt are often protected from CHIs but, depending on whether the patient was a passenger or the driver, are more prone to liver and splenic injuries (Smith, 1994). A more thorough examination of the patient's abdomen, pelvis, and extremities is important during the secondary survey. Assessment of the abdomen should include auscultating for bowel sounds, percussion, and palpation. Abdominal tenderness is often difficult to assess in patients with blunt trauma, particularly if there is a CHI or if alcohol was involved. Both of these conditions diminish or alter the patient's response to pain and hence may provide misleading information about the absence of any abdominal trauma. Tests that may be performed to confirm or deny the presence of any abdominal injuries include a diagnostic peritoneal lavage (DPL) and an abdominal CT scan. Although the abdominal CT scan provides more exact information about the type and degree of injury a patient has sustained, it is often reserved for patients with more hemodynamically stable conditions. If the patient's condition is not hemodynamically stable, the DPL can be performed at the bedside and provides a quick assessment about the presence of abdominal bleeding. Although a DPL can provide a false-positive reading (Melio, 1998), it is considered to be 98% reliable (Pachter & Feliciano, 1996). It is important to also decompress the stomach as soon as possible by passing a NGT or orogastric tube, depending on the extent of any facial injuries.

Kidney and bladder injuries are also assessed during the secondary survey. Blood at the meatus and/or hematuria are indicators for additional tests to be performed to determine the extent of the injury and the definitive treatment. Hematuria is considered the hallmark of genitourinary injury. If urine tests show either microscopic or gross hematuria, subsequent diagnostic tests including a CT scan, an intravenous pyelogram, or a cystogram may be required (Ahn, Morey, & McAninch, 1998).

Additional assessments that will be made during the secondary survey include a continual assessment of cardiovascular and pulmonary function via vital signs and cardiac rhythm, and possibly echocardiography and CT scan of the thorax to assess for valvular problems, missed pneumothoraces, or missed injuries to the aorta or peripheral vasculature.

A more in-depth neurologic examination is also performed during the secondary survey, with attention being given to any skull or spinal abnormalities, usually referred to as *step-offs.* In addition, assessment of rectal tone can provide information about the integrity of the spinal nerves. Assessment for raccoon eyes (periorbital ecchymosis), a Battle's sign (mastoid ecchymosis), or rhinorrhea should also be performed. The presence of any of these conditions may indicate a basilar skull fracture.

3. What is meant by a *tertiary survey?*

Tertiary survey refers to an additional comprehensive assessment that is done either after the patient can talk, when the patient is about to ambulate, or in some institutions within 24 hours of admission (Janjua, Sugrue, & Deane, 1998). The focus of the tertiary survey is to identify previously missed injuries and to prevent possible complications caused by missed injuries. Studies have indicated great variability in the frequency of missed injuries for trauma patients, ranging from 2% to 50% (Sommers, 1995). However, patients with blunt abdominal trauma are at a higher risk for missed injuries than patients with penetrating trauma (Janjua et al, 1998). For all trauma patients, the most frequently missed injuries are musculoskeletal, with the most critically missed injury being a cervical spine injury. Although alterations in level of consciousness caused by either head injuries or drug or alcohol intake contribute to injuries being missed, hemodynamic instability and radiologic and technical errors also add to the problem. The guideline for assessing trauma patients is always to have a high degree of suspicion for missed injuries and to do frequent reassessments, looking for musculoskeletal injuries, additional pulmonary injuries (including rib fractures, cardiac and spinal injuries), and hidden abdominal injuries (Ferrera, Verdile, Bartfield, Snyder, & Salluzzo, 1998; Sommers, 1995). When a tertiary survey is being performed, external signs of injury should be noted, including any indication of soft tissue injury that may accompany skeletal, muscular, or nerve injury.

4. What diagnostic tests are done to evaluate and treat patients who have sustained a blunt abdominal trauma?

Routine laboratory tests performed for trauma patients include serial hematocrit measurements to assess the degree of bleeding; chemistry profiles to determine any imbalances particularly with sodium, chloride, and potassium as the result of fluid resuscitation; and serum glucose to assess for the degree of hyperglycemia that is often the result of insulin resistance caused by the trauma. The blood urea nitrogen (BUN) and creatinine levels should also be monitored to evaluate kidney function both at the time of admission and throughout the patient's hospitalization. ABG values also need to be monitored closely.

Mr. Packard had developed hyperchloremia caused by his metabolic acidosis and the administration of normal saline during his prehospital resuscitation. Correction of both metabolic acidosis and hyperchloremia involved administration of sodium bicarbonate and changing Mr. Packard's fluid infusions from normal saline, which has 154 mEq/L of both sodium and chloride, to lactated Ringer's solution, which has 130 mEq/L of sodium and 107 mEq/L of chloride. In addition, 4 mEq/L of potassium, 2.7 mEq/L of calcium, and 27 mEq/L of lactate were administered. Changing Mr. Packard's fluid infusions was beneficial in a number of ways. First, the lactate in lactated Ringer's solution is converted to bicarbonate and hence helps buffer the acidosis. Second, as the bicarbonate levels increase, the kidneys are able to exchange chloride ions for bicarbonate ions. Third, the lactated Ringer's solution contains less chloride. Thus the change not only addressed his hyperchloremia, but also helped address his metabolic acidosis.

Additional tests that may be ordered are serial cardiac enzyme measurements if chest trauma is suspected. Also 12-lead electrocardiograms will help document any patterns of ischemia or injury. Toxicologic analysis of blood and blood alcohol levels are important to determine whether altered mental status is related to a CHI or to drug or alcohol use. Mr. Packard had a blood alcohol level of 171 g/dl. Any value greater than 100 is considered intoxication.

As previously stated, for assessment of blunt abdominal trauma, either a DPL or abdominal CT scan may be ordered. For patients whose conditions are hemodynamically unstable, the DPL provides a bedside assessment of potential bleeding; however, it does not indicate the source of the bleeding. For a DPL, 1000 ml of IV fluid is instilled into the peritoneal cavity, and then the fluid is drained back out and assessed for the presence of red blood cells. A recent study indicates that at least 600 ml should be retrieved to obtain reliable results (Sullivan, Nelson, & Tandberg, 1997). A disadvantage of the DPL is that minor bleeding episodes that would not normally require surgical intervention are also detected, thus creating an incidence of 15% to 27% of unnecessary laparotomies (Melio, 1998). However, there is only a 0.2% incidence of false-positive findings (Pachter & Hofstetter, 1995).

With the advent of new capabilities for CT scanning, abdominal CT scans have become more widely used. Numerous studies have been done that indicate the reliability of using CT scans to determine not only the area of the bleeding, but also the degree of involvement (Brasel, DeLisle, Olson, & Borgstrom, 1997; Pachter & Hofstetter, 1995). CT scans are particularly useful in assessing solid organ damage such as liver lacerations, splenic involvement, and kidney injuries. CT scans are less reliable in assessing hollow organ damage, and CT scans cannot detect whether bleeding has stopped (Melio, 1998).

5. **What are the management guidelines for a patient with a blunt abdominal trauma?**

The liver and spleen are the most commonly injured organs in blunt abdominal trauma. However, because of refinements in CT scanning, all patients with abdominal traumas are no longer taken to the operating room for surgical treatment. Between 24% and 55% of all patients with blunt abdominal traumas are managed nonoperatively (Brasel et al, 1997). Liver injuries are graded I through VI, with grade I representing a hematoma involving less than 10% of the surface area or a laceration less than 1 cm in depth, and grade VI representing total avulsion (Box 28-1). The current trend is nonoperative management for patients who have sustained a blunt trauma to the abdomen, whose conditions are hemodynamically stable, and who have less than 500 ml of blood in the peritoneum as evidenced by CT scan. For patients with a grade I or grade II liver injury and some patients with a grade III injury, nonoperative management necessitates frequent abdominal assessments, including noting any increase in abdominal girth and tension and the presence or absence of bowel sounds. These patients are also closely assessed for a decrease in hematocrit, hemodynamic instability, and any increase in abdominal pain (Pachter & Hofstetter, 1995; Richardson & Brewer, 1996). A change in any of these parameters would indicate a reevaluation of the patient and possible surgery. For patients whose conditions are not hemodynamically stable or who have greater than 500 ml of blood in peritoneum (grade IV and grade V liver injuries), an emergency celiotomy is performed (Pachter & Hofstetter, 1995).

Mr. Packard's case illustrates the newest trend in managing abdominal blunt traumas. He had sustained a grade III liver laceration. After initial fluid resuscitation, Mr. Packard's condition was hemodynamically stable, thus making him a candidate for nonoperative management. However, over the course of 12 hours, Mr. Packard's

---

Box 28-1   Blunt Abdominal Trauma: Liver Injury Scale

GRADE I
Subcapsular hematoma <10% of surface area, or
Laceration <1 cm deep

GRADE II
Subcapsular hematoma between 10% and 50% surfaces area, or
Intraparenchymal hematoma <10 cm wide
Laceration between 1-3 cm deep or <10 cm long

GRADE III
Subcapsular hematoma >50% or expanding, or
Ruptured subcapsular or parenchymal hematoma
Intraparenchymal hematoma >10 cm or expanding or
Laceration >3 cm in parenchymal depth

GRADE IV
Laceration or parenchymal disruption involving 25%-75% of hepatic lobe, or
Between 1 and 33 Couinaud segments within a single lobe

GRADE V
Laceration or parenchymal disruption involving >75% of a hepatic lobe, or
>3 Couinaud segments within a single lobe, or
Juxtahepatic venous injury

GRADE VI
Hepatic avulsion

From Pachter, H. L., & Feliciano, D. V. (1996). Complex hepatic injuries. *Surgical Clinics of North America, 76*(4), 763-783.

abdomen became more distended and firm, and his ventilation became increasingly difficult with peak inspiratory pressures as high as 60 mm Hg. ACS was diagnosed, and subsequently he was taken to the operating room for a decompression celiotomy.

Another former trend had been for the patient to undergo total corrective surgery for any abdominal injuries at the time of the initial procedure. However, total corrective surgery usually involved extended operating time, which could lead to problems related to hypothermia, coagulopathies, and acidosis. The current trend is to do only a staged laparotomy, during which the major sources of bleeding are identified and are either ligated or packed, any bowel leakage is controlled, and the patient is returned to the intensive care unit for stabilization (Zacharias, Offner, Moore & Burch, 1999). Often, because of the edema from the trauma itself and the fluid resuscitation, the abdomen cannot be closed and either towel clips or occlusive dressings are used to protect the abdomen. Although this places the patient at risk for infection, the risk offset by the positive effects of preserving vascular integrity and function of the abdomen. Usually 12 to 48 hours after the initial celiotomy, the patient is returned to the operating room for surgical reexploration. There, the liver, spleen, and other organs can be assessed, and the viability of the intestines can be determined. If the edema has subsided, the abdomen may be closed at that time, or additional procedures may be required depending upon the patient's status.

6. What is meant by ACS?

ACS (abdominal compartment syndrome) refers to an increase in intraabdominal pressures greater than 25 mm Hg as the result of expanding abdominal contents (Ivatury, Porter, Simon, Isalm, John, & Stahl, 1998; Zacharias et al, 1999). The increase in abdominal contents can be the result of bleeding within the abdominal cavity or bowel edema caused by the injury itself or fluid resuscitation (Ivatury, Diebel, Porter, & Simon, 1997). Patients who have also had an emergency celiotomy or laparotomy are also at risk for developing ACS. Although additional bleeding and edema may contribute to the development of ACS in these patients, abdominal surgical packs used to control bleeding also place these patients at risk for developing ACS. Regardless of the cause of ACS, the increase in abdominal pressure can produce cardiovascular instability as a result of a decrease in preload from compression of the inferior vena cava and decrease the cardiac output (CO), resulting in hypotension. The increase in intraabdominal pressures can also transmit high pressure to the ventricles, which further reduces stroke volume and subsequent CO. Rising intraabdominal pressures also transmit the pressure to the pulmonary system and restrict alveolar ventilation and can dramatically increase peak inspiratory pressures. Renal function is also compromised as a result of the reduced CO and direct compression on the kidneys. The rise in abdominal pressures also reduces urinary flow and blood flow to the intestines and abdominal organs themselves and places them at risk for ischemia. Clinical signs and symptoms of ACS include a sudden rise in peak inspiratory pressures, elevated pulmonary artery pressures, and pulmonary capillary wedge pressures (PCWP), a drop in arterial blood oxygen saturation (Sao_2), a falsely high CVP, a decrease in CO, an increase in systemic vascular resistance (SVR), and either oliguria or anuria. If a sudden rise in peak inspiratory pressures and hemodynamic instability with a decrease in CO and BP occur in a patient such as Mr. Packard, decompression of the abdomen may be done as am emergency procedure either at the bedside or in the operating room (Eddy, Nunn, & Morris, 1997). For patients in whom development of ACS is suspected but whose conditions are not profoundly hemodynamically unstable, bladder pressures may be measured to document rising intraabdominal pressures. Bladder pressures may be obtained by instilling 50 ml of sterile fluid into the bladder via the Foley catheter and then measuring the bladder pressures with a manometer. Bladder pressures of 25 mm Hg or greater usually require an emergency celiotomy (Zacharias et al, 1999).

Although relief of ACS is critical, a sudden release of abdominal pressures also poses problems. Research has indicated that as the intraabdominal pressure is released, there is a sudden drop in BP and a sudden release of toxic anaerobic by-products into the systemic circulation. This predisposes the patient to cardiovascular complications including asystole. Eddy et al (1997) recommend infusing 2 L of saline mixed with mannitol and bicarbonate in order to reduce the incidence of what they define as "reperfusion syndrome" (p. 809).

7. What is a pulmonary contusion?

Although Mr. Packard did not sustain any trauma to his heart muscle or his aorta, he did sustain rib fractures and bilateral pulmonary contusions. *Pulmonary contusion* is a hemorrhage into the alveolar and interstitial spaces, resulting in reduced alveolar ventilation and subsequent hypoxemia. Of patients who sustain blunt trauma to the chest, 75% will have pulmonary contusions, with a 40% mortality (Prentice &

Ahrens, 1994). Chest injuries that accompany pulmonary contusion are rib fractures, flail chest, hemothorax, pneumothorax, and scapula fractures, all of which place the patient at risk for bruised or injured lung parenchyma. Depending on the extent of the contusion, the patient not only will develop hypoxemia from loss of ventilated alveoli but will also experience reduced pulmonary compliance and an increase in pulmonary vascular resistance. Assessment parameters include both monitoring ABGs and monitoring Sao_2. In addition, derived oxygen variables can help to determine the degree of alveolar capillary shunting. Normally, less than 5% of the total pulmonary blood flow is not oxygenated (Prentice & Ahrens, 1994). However, with pulmonary injury, the alveoli cannot be ventilated, and hence the blood flowing past those alveoli is not oxygenated. One formula that can be used to calculate the degree of alveolar-capillary shunting is to divide the arterial oxygen pressure (Pao_2) by the fraction of inspired oxygen (Fio_2): Pao_2/Fio_2. The normal value is 286 or greater. Mr. Packard's Pao_2 was 82 and his Fio_2 was 1.0. This indicates an alveolar capillary shunt of 82, which represents a extremely large shunt. Thus, although Mr. Packard appears to have a normal Pao_2 value, it is important for clinicians to interpret the ABG values in reference to the amount of supplementary oxygen the patient is receiving. For a patient with a Fio_2 of 1.0 not to have an alveolar capillary shunt, the Pao_2 should be 286 or higher. Thus, by correlating Mr. Packard's chest x-ray films, which revealed bilateral pulmonary contusions, with his ABG values and his alveolar capillary shunting, the clinician is able to understand the degree of damage to Mr. Packard's lungs, and the need for continual mechanical ventilation. Patients with greater than 28% pulmonary contusions require mechanical ventilation (Prentice & Ahrens, 1994). Nursing considerations for these patients include suctioning and positioning the patient to allow the good lung to receive maximum gas exchange. In some cases, this may require a semi-Fowler's position or reverse Trendelenburg or even prone position. Daily assessment of chest x-ray films and the characteristics of secretions is also important because 50% of patients who have pulmonary contusions may develop pneumonia (Prentice & Ahrens, 1994).

8. **What other factors may be contributing to Mr. Packard's poor oxygenation status?**

Although Mr. Packard's pulmonary contusion is contributing to his poor oxygenation status and his need for mechanical ventilation, trauma patients are also at risk for developing acute respiratory distress syndrome (ARDS). *ARDS* can be defined as noncardiogenic pulmonary edema. It is the accumulation of fluid in the interstitial spaces in the lungs from noncardiac causes. Often, trauma is accompanied by overactivation of the systemic inflammatory immune system. This overactivation results in neutrophils and macrophages migrating to the lungs. Although neutrophils and macrophages are part of the normal inflammatory response, when they are overactivated, these cells become very destructive. Much of the destruction that accompanies the neutrophils and macrophages is from chemicals that they release and also from a cascade effect as the chemicals from the neutrophils and macrophages cause other chemicals to be released. The chemicals, or chemical mediators as they are called, include oxygen radicals, interleukin-1, tissue necrosis factor, proteases, platelet-activating factor, thromboxane, leukotrienes, and prostaglandins. These chemical mediators produce vasodilation and increase capillary permeability. The increase in capillary permeability in turn allows fluid from the vascular bed to leak into the interstitial spaces. When this process occurs in the lungs, it is called *ARDS* (discussed fully in Chapter 1). ARDS is characterized by the lungs becoming wet and boggy, and oxygen exchange is dramatically reduced. Clinically, the patient's oxygen therapy is no longer effective, and a very high Fio_2 is required to maintain a Pao_2 within normal range. Because the lungs have an excess amount of fluid in the interstitial spaces, the lungs become very difficult to ventilate and high peak inspiratory pressures develop. To help facilitate ventilation, PEEP and PS are commonly used. Also while Mr. Packard was maintained on SIMV, other modes of ventilation may be used such as inverse inspiratory/expiratory ratio, jet ventilation, and pressure-regulated, volume-controlled ventilation.

9.   Why was Mr. Packard pharmacologically paralyzed and what are the nursing implications?

Because ventilation is difficult in patients who have ARDS, they often require high levels of PEEP and PS as well as a high Fio_2. High levels of both PEEP and PS are uncomfortable for the patient and may make the patient feel dyspneic. To facilitate ventilation and reduce their metabolic needs, these patients are often pharmacologically paralyzed. Cisatracurium (Nimbex) was the pharmacologic agent used for Mr. Packard. It is a neuromuscular blocker that produces skeletal muscle relaxation. It has a minimal effect on the cardiovascular system and no analgesic effect. The cisatracurium dose for paralysis with mechanical ventilation is 9 µg/kg/min as a continuous infusion (Wilson, Shannon, & Stang, 1998).

It is important to remember that cisatracurium does *not* alter consciousness or cerebration. Hence, it is important to provide adequate pain relieve and sedation because these patients are actually "awake" but paralyzed and are still aware of pain. For Mr. Packard, lorazepam (Ativan) was used to produce conscious sedation and fentanyl (Sublimaze) was given for pain management. When caring for patients who are pharmacologically paralyzed, the nurse must continually monitor their Sao_2 values and set the respiratory rate on the ventilator high enough to provide adequate minute ventilation. Failure to set the respiratory rate at the proper setting can be devastating to the patient because they no longer have a respiratory drive.

10.   What other complications is Mr. Packard at risk for, and how should they be monitored?

After stabilization, Mr. Packard was at risk for hemorrhage or rebleeding from his liver injury. Continual cardiac hemodynamic monitoring is vital. Changes in his CO, his pulmonary wedge pressures, BP, and SVR all provide data concerning his hemodynamic stability. Hemorrhage would be manifested as a drop in CO with a drop in BP. As the body attempts to compensate and epinephrine is released, there is an accompanying increase in SVR. The SVR can be calculated from the following formula:

$$[(MAP - CVP)/CO] \times 80.$$

The normal SVR is between 800 and 1200 dynes/cm^{-5}.

Rebleeding or continual bleeding from internal injuries is monitored most effectively by serial hematocrit measurements. However, as previously discussed, Mr. Packard's grade III liver laceration continued to bleed and he developed ACS. His ACS was assessed by his sudden increase in peak inspiratory pressures and increase in bladder pressures above 35 cm H_2O. He was then taken to the OR for a emergency celiotomy to relieve the pressure and control the bleeding. Because of the extent of his intestinal edema, Mr. Packard's abdomen was left open until the edema resolved.

Because Mr. Packard's abdomen was not surgically closed at the time of his first operation, he was at risk for developing an infection. White blood cell (WBC) count and temperature are important parameters to monitor to determine whether an infection has developed. Daily chest x-ray films are also important to assess whether the patient has developed pneumonia in addition to ARDS. Once a patient's temperature begins to increase, blood, urine, and sputum cultures need to be obtained to determine the origin of the infection and the type of antibiotic therapy needed.

Often, patients with blunt abdominal trauma are at risk for developing sepsis. Sources of the sepsis include invasive monitoring lines, the Foley catheter, pulmonary infections, and abdominal abscesses. An additional problem, called *translocation of bacteria,* may also cause sepsis (Faries, Simon, Martella, Lee, & Machiedo, 1998). Bacterial translocation occurs when the villi in the intestinal wall become ischemic as a result of hypoperfusion. The ischemic villi allow bacteria from the gut to travel across the membrane into either the blood or the lymph system and seed these systems with their own native gastrointestinal (GI) flora. Steps to prevent translocation of bacteria include restoring perfusion as quickly as possible and use of the GI tract as soon as possible. Although initial tube feedings for patients with abdominal trauma will not support their nutritional needs, research as shown that 15 to 25 ml of tube feeding per hour is sufficient to keep the GI tract functional and reduce the chance of translocation of bacteria (Wachtel, 1994).

However, despite all efforts to prevent a systemic infection, many trauma patients develop septic shock. Septic shock can be differentiated clinically from hemorrhagic or hypovolemic shock by monitoring the SVR in addition to monitoring the BP, heart rate, CO, and PCWP. With septic shock, the SVR will drop. The drop in SVR is attributed to the vasodilation that accompanies the release of the bacterial toxins, especially endotoxins. Management of septic shock will include treatment of the infection as well as vasopressor therapy to maintain the BP and restore the SVR.

Early in the resuscitative phase, all trauma patients are at risk for "the trauma triad of death" (Zacharias et al, 1999). The trauma triad is hypothermia, coagulopathy, and acidosis. Because of the events surrounding the trauma and vasoconstriction caused by shock, patients often are hypothermic on arrival in the emergency department. Removal of clothing and the administration of large amounts of IV fluids can contribute to their hypothermia. In addition, if patients are taken to the operating room and their intestines are exposed to room air, they can lose as much as 4.6° C/hr (Zacharias et al, 1999). Administration of cool blood can also contribute to their hypothermia. Hypothermia can produce a number of negative sequelae: reduced platelet activity that can lead to the development of coagulopathies; altered respiratory status, making patients unable to compensate for rising levels of arterial carbon dioxide pressure ($Paco_2$); and affects on the cardiovascular system that predispose patients to develop arrhythmias that are refractory to drugs such as lidocaine and procainamide (Fritsch, 1995). Coagulopathy and acidosis are additional problems that can develop as the result of the ensuing shock after the trauma. Coagulopathy can also occur as the result of massive blood transfusions.

Prevention of hypothermia and early detection of bleeding problems and acidosis are key elements in reducing the mortality associated with these conditions. Specific nursing interventions that can be used to treat these problems are first to remove all wet clothing upon admission to the hospital and keep the patient as covered and protected as possible even during primary and secondary surveys. Second, IV fluids should be warmed before administration. If large amounts of fluid and blood are needed, a rapid infuser may be used that will not only allow for the administration of fluid at a rate of 1.5 L/min, but also warm the fluids and blood. Third, warming units, head wraps, or heat shields should be used to warm the patient. To assess for any coagulopathies, the nurse should closely monitor the patient's clotting studies, including prothrombin time (PT) and partial thromboplastin time (PTT), and platelet levels. If large amounts of blood are needed, it is important to be prepared to also administer fresh frozen plasma (FFP) and platelets. One rule of thumb is that 6 to 10 units of platelets are administered for every 8 to 10 units of pack red blood cells, and 1 to 2 units of FFP are administered for every 5 units of pack red blood cells (Cardonna et al, 1994). To correct the metabolic acidosis, administration of sodium bicarbonate may be required as well as reestablishment of respiratory function.

Once the patient has survived the initial resuscitative phase, bleeding problems can still occur. As previously stated, trauma patients often have overactive inflammatory immune systems, and they can develop systemic inflammatory immune response syndrome (SIRS). *SIRS* is overactivation of the inflammatory-immune system as manifested by tachycardia greater than 90, $Paco_2$ less than 32 mm Hg, temperature either above 38° C or less than 36° C, and a WBC count either greater than 12,000 or less than 4000. When these signs and symptoms cannot be attributable to any other cause, the patient has developed SIRS. One of the outcomes of SIRS is the development of disseminated intravascular coagulation (DIC). DIC results in clotting in the patient's microvascular circulation and consumption of clotting factors, including platelets. The result is organ failure secondary to the microvascular clotting and bleeding secondary to the consumption of clotting factors. In addition, because of the extensive clotting, patients also have increased fibrinolytic activity and hence fibrin split product levels are elevated. DIC is a coagulopathy that is manifested by prolonged PTs and PTTs, a drop in the platelet count, and an increase in fibrin split product levels. To assess whether a patient has developed a coagulopathy either from hypothermia, massive blood transfusions, or DIC, PT and PTT and platelet levels should be measured. If DIC is suspected, fibrin split product levels should also be monitored.

Because patients with multiple trauma, including abdominal traumas, are often immobile for an extended period, they are at risk for the development of deep vein thrombosis (DVT) and subsequent pulmonary embolus. To prevent the development of DVT, sequential compression stockings or similar devices should be used as soon as possible. These devices help maintain normal venous return and prevent venous status. Heparin therapy should also be started. For DVT prophylaxis, Mr. Packard was given enoxaparin (Lovenox) on day 3. Because the calf or thigh is often the site of a DVT, nursing assessment should include monitoring for an increase in calf or thigh size and the presence of a warm, tender area. Although the absence of a positive Homans' sign does not rule out the presence of a DVT, the presence of a positive Homans' sign is considered clinically significant. Because a DVT may develop into an embolus, signs and symptoms of a pulmonary embolus should also be monitored. These signs and symptoms include dyspnea, pleuritic chest pain, a decrease in Sao_2, hypoxia, tachycardia, arrhythmias, and hypotension.

11.   What are the nutritional needs of patients with blunt abdominal trauma?

Supporting the nutritional needs of every trauma patient is very important. As the result of the trauma, these patients are hypermetabolic and hyperglycemic and in a catabolic state. Failure to support the nutritional needs of these patients can predispose them to poor wound healing, sepsis, respiratory failure, an increased incidence of translocation of bacteria, and multisystem organ failure (Romito, 1995; Stamatos & Reed, 1994). Factors that need to be kept in mind are that the gut is the largest immune organ in the body, and failure to use the gut even on a short-term basis will result in atrophy of the intestinal villi. As previously stated, even small amounts of intestinal feeding have been shown to maintain gut integrity (Romito, 1995). Other factors that are important to consider when the body is in a catabolic state is that the body uses all muscle mass, including the diaphragm, as an energy source. Hence, while the patient is in a catabolic state, he or she has an additional risk of respiratory failure caused by a decrease in the strength of the diaphragm. Also if the patient is febrile, energy requirements increase by 7% for every 1° (Fahrenheit) increase in temperature (Stamatos & Reed, 1994).

With a stressful event, the metabolic demands of the body can be divided into two phases: the ebb phase and the flow phase. The *ebb phase* is the first 24 to 48 hours after an injury and is characterized by shunting of blood to the heart, lungs, and brain in an effort to maintain perfusion. During the ebb phase, the body's metabolism is reduced. After stabilization, the body's metabolic rate begins to climb. This is called the *flow phase* and is characterized by an increase in CO, oxygen consumption, body temperature, and catabolic activity (Stamatos & Reed, 1994).

Ideally, nutritional support should be started within 24 to 72 hours of admission or at the resolution of the ebb phase (Romito, 1995; Stamatos & Reed, 1994). For the patient with abdominal trauma, it is important to assess bowel and renal function to determine whether any pancreatic injury is present. However, even if bowel function is hypoactive, small amounts of enteral feedings are recommended to preserve bowel function.

Nutritional support may include both total parenteral nutrition and enteral feedings, but enteral feedings are preferred in a effort to maintain the function of the bowel and to prevent translocation of bacteria. A number of products for enteral feeding are on the market. Mr. Packard was given Perative on day 3. Perative contains 1.3 kcal/ml, and it has 66.6 g of protein per liter, plus supplemental arginine, medium chain triglycerides, and ω-fatty acids. Although there are a number of ways to institute enteral feedings, one approach is to begin with 25 to 30 ml/hr and increase the amount every 6 hours until the goal is reached. Mr. Packard's enteral feedings were gradually increased over a 48-hour period, until finally on day 5 he was receiving 90 ml of Perative per hour.

Once enteral feedings are started it is important to monitor electrolyte, glucose, BUN, and creatinine levels as well as daily weights. Weekly laboratory studies should include a liver function panel and triglyceride levels. For long-term management, anthropometric studies, including thigh and midarm circumferences, can help monitor the patient's progress, the patient's prealbumin levels, and the patient's weight.

BLUNT ABDOMINAL TRAUMA

References

Ahn, J. Morey, A., & McAninch, J. (1998). Workup and management of traumatic hematuria. *Emergency Medicine Clinics of North America, 16*(1), 145-165.

Brasel, K., DeLisle, C., Olson, C., & Borgstrom, D. (1997). Trends in the management of hepatic injury. *American Journal of Surgery, 174*(6), 674-677.

Cardonna, V., Hurn, P., Mason, P., Scanlon, A. & Veise-Berry, S. (1994). *Trauma nursing: From resuscitation through rehabilitation.* Philadelphia: Saunders.

Eddy, V., Nunn, C., & Morris, J. (1997). Abdominal compartment syndrome. *Surgical Clinics of North America, 77*(4), 801-813.

Faries, P., Simon, R., Martella, A., Lee, M., & Machiedo, G. (1998). Intestinal permeability correlates with severity of injury. *Journal of Trauma Injury Infection and Critical Care, 44*(6), 1031-1035.

Ferrera, P., Verdile, V., Bartfield, J, Snyder, H., & Salluzzo, R. (1998). Injuries distracting from intraabdominal injuries after blunt trauma. *American Journal of Emergency Medicine, 16*(2), 145-149.

Fritsch, D. (1995). Hypothermia in the trauma patient. *AACN Clinical Issues, 6*(2), 196-211.

Ivatury, R., Diebel, L., Porter, J., & Simon, R. (1997). Intra-abdominal hypertension and the abdominal compartment syndrome. *Surgical Clinics of North America, 77*(6), 783-799.

Ivatury, R., Porter, J., Simon, R., Isalm, S., John, R., & Stahl, W. (1998). Intra-abdominal hypertension after life-threatening penetrating abdominal trauma; prophylaxis, incidence, and clinical relevance to gastric mucosal pH and abdominal compartment syndrome. *Journal of Trauma Injury Infection and Critical Care, 44*(6), 1016-1023.

Jacobs, L. (1994). Timing of fluid resuscitation in trauma. *The New England Journal of Medicine, 331*(17), 1153-1154.

Janjua, K., Sugrue, M., & Deane, S. (1998). Prospective evaluation of early missed injuries and the role of tertiary trauma survey. *The Journal of Trauma, Injury, Infection and Critical Care, 44*(6), 1000-1007.

Klein, D. (1995). Trauma. *AACN Clinical Issues, 6*(2), 173-174.

Melio, F. (1998), Priorities in the multiple trauma patient. *Emergency Medicine Clinics of North America, 16*(1), 29-43.

Pachter, H. L., & Feliciano, D. V. (1996). Complex hepatic injuries. *Surgical Clinics of North America, 76*(4), 763-783.

Pachter, H. L., & Hofstetter, S. (1995). The current status of nonoperative management of adult blunt hepatic injuries. *American Journal of Surgery, 169*(4), 442-454.

Prentice, D., & Ahrens, T. (1994). Pulmonary complications of trauma. *Critical Care Nursing Quarterly, 17*(2), 24-33.

Richardson, D., & Brewer, M. (1996), Management of upper abdominal solid organ injuries. *AORN Journal, 63*(5), 907-916.

Romito, R. (1995). Early administration of enteral nutrients in critically ill patients. *AACN Clinical Issues, 6*(2), 242-257.

Smith, S. (1994). Treatment of abdominal trauma. *Emergency, 26*(10), 27-32.

Sommers, M. (1995), Missed injuries: A case study of trauma hide and seek. *AACN Clinical Issues, 6*(2), 187-195.

Stamatos, C., & Reed, E. (1994). Nutritional needs of the trauma patient. *Critical Care Nursing Clinics of North America, 6*(3), 501-514.

Sullivan, K., Nelson, M., & Tandberg, D. (1997). Incremental analysis of diagnostic peritoneal lavage fluid in adult abdominal trauma. *American Journal of Emergency Medicine, 15*(3), 277-279.

Wachtel, T. (1994). Critical care concepts in the management of abdominal trauma. *Critical Care Nursing Quarterly, 17*(2), 34-49.

Wilson, B., Shannon, M., & Stang, C. (1998). *Nurses drug guide*. Stamford, CT: Appleton & Lange.

Zacharias, S., Offner, P., Moore, E., & Burch, J. (1999). Damage control surgery. *AACN Clinical Issues, 10*(1), 95-103.

ABBREVIATIONS

AAA	Abdominal aortic aneurysm
ABG	Arterial blood gas
ACE	Angiotensin-converting enzyme
ACS	Abdominal compartment syndrome
ACTH	Adrenocorticotropic hormone
ADH	Antidiuretic hormone
ADP	Adenosine diphosphate
ADR	Adverse drug reaction
AHA	American Heart Association
ALT	Alanine aminotransferase
AMI	Acute myocardial infarction
ANH	Atrial natriuretic hormone
aPTT	Activated partial-thromboplastin time
ARDS	Acute respiratory distress syndrome
ARF	Acute renal failure
AST	Aspartate aminotransferase
ATN	Acute tubular necrosis
ATP	Adenosine triphosphate
AV	Atrioventricular; atriovenous
AZT	Azidothymidine
BGM	Blood glucose monitoring
BP	Blood pressure
BUN	Blood urea nitrogen
CABG	Coronary artery bypass graft
CAP	Community-acquired pneumonia
CAPD	Continuous ambulatory peritoneal dialysis
CAVHD	Continuous arteriovenous hemofiltration dialysis
CBC	Complete blood count
CCS	Corticosteroid
CCU	Cardiac care unit
CHF	Chronic heart failure
CI	Cardiac index
CICU	Cardiac intensive care unit
CK	Creatine kinase
CK-MB	Creatine kinase-myocardial band
CO	Cardiac output

COPD	Chronic obstructive pulmonary disease
CPP	Cerebral perfusion pressure
CRF	Chronic renal failure
CRH	Corticotropin-releasing hormone
CRRT	Continuous renal replacement therapy
CSF	Cerebrospinal fluid
CT	Computed tomography
CVA	Cerebrovascular accident
CVC	Central venous catheter
CVP	Central venous pressure
CVVHD	Continuous venovenous hemodialysis
D5W	5% dextrose in water
D5LR	5% dextrose in lactated Ringer's solution
DAI	Diffuse axonal injury
DI	Diabetes insipidus
DIC	Disseminated intravascular coagulation
DKA	Diabetic ketoacidosis
dl	Deciliter
DVT	Deep venous thrombosis
E	Epinephrine
ECG	Electrocardiogram
ED	Emergency department
EDH	Epidural hematoma
EF	Ejection fraction
EGD	Esophagogastroduodenoscopy
ELISA	Enzyme-linked immunoabsorbent assay
EPO	Erythropoietin
ES	Elastic stockings
ESRD	End-stage renal disease
ft	Feet
g	Gram
GCS	Glasgow Coma Scale
GFR	Glomerular filtration rate
GH	Growth hormone
GI	Gastrointestinal
GIs	Glycemic indices
GP	Glycoprotein
HAART	Highly active antiretroviral therapy
HAP	Hospital-acquired pneumonia
HAV	Hepatitis A virus
HBV	Hepatitis B virus
HCG	Human chorionic gonadotropin
Hct	Hematocrit
HCV	Hepatitis C virus
HCW	Health care worker
Hgb	Hemoglobin
HPV	Human papilloma virus
HR	Heart rate
HRP	Hormone replacement therapy
HSV	Herpes simplex virus
IABP	Intraaortic balloon pump

ICP	Intracranial pressure
ICU	Intensive care unit
IL	Interleukin
IM	Intramuscular
in	Inch
IMV	Intermittent mandatory ventilation
INR	International Normalized Ratio
IPC	Intermittent pneumatic compression
IV	Intravenous
IVC	Inferior vena cava
IVP	Intravenous push
JG	Juxtaglomerular
JGA	Juxtaglomerular apparatus
KS	Kaposi's sarcoma
KUB	Kidneys, ureters, and bladder (x-ray)
LAP	Left atrial pressure
LBBB	Left bundle-branch block
LDH	Lactate dehydrogenase
LDUH	Low-dose unfractionated heparin
LMWH	Low-molecular-weight heparin
LOC	Level of consciousness
LR	Lactated Ringer's solution
LVF	Left ventricular failure
μl	Microliter
MAP	Mean arterial pressure
MAST	Medical antishock trousers
MI	Myocardial infarction
MIDCABG	Minimally invasive direct coronary artery bypass graft
mm Hg	Millimeters of mercury
MODS	Multiple organ dysfunction syndrome
MOF	Multiple organ failure
MRI	Magnetic resonance imaging
MSH	Melanocyte-stimulating hormone
NE	Norepinephrine
NPO	Nothing by mouth
NRTI	Nucleoside analog reverse transcriptase inhibitor
NS	Normal saline
NSAIDs	Nonsteroidal antiinflammatory drugs
NSS	Normal saline solution
NTG	Nasogastric tube
PAC	Pulmonary artery catheter
PAD	Pulmonary artery diastolic (pressure)
PAF	Platelet-activating factor
PAOP	Pulmonary artery occlusive pressure
PAP	Pulmonary artery pressure
PAS	Pulmonary artery systolic (pressure)
PAWP	Pulmonary artery wedge pressure
PCA	Patient-controlled analgesia
PCV	Packed cell volume
PCWP	Pulmonary capillary wedge pressure
PEEP	Positive end-expiratory pressure

PI	Pulmonary infarction
PIP	Peak inspiratory pressure
PO	Orally
POMC	Proopiomelanocortin
PRBCs	Packed red blood cells
PS	Pressure support
PT	Prothrombin time
PTCA	Percutaneous transluminal coronary angioplasty
PTT	Partial thromboplastin time
PVC	Premature ventricular contraction
PVR	Peripheral vascular resistance
RAAS	Renin-angiotensin-aldosterone system
RAP	Right atrial pressure
RAS	Renin-angiotensin system
RBCs	Red blood cells
RN	Registered nurse
RVF	Right ventricular failure
SDH	Subdural hematoma
SIADH	Syndrome of inappropriate secretion of antidiuretic hormone
SICU	Surgical intensive care unit
SIMV	Synchronized intermittent mandatory ventilation
SIRS	Systemic inflammatory response system
SNS	Sympathetic nervous system
SOB	Shortness of breath
SV	Stroke volume
SVR	Systemic vascular resistance
T_3	Triiodothyronine
T_4	Tetraiodothyronine, thyroxine
TEE	Transesophageal echocardiography
THA	Total hip arthroplasty
THR	Total hip replacement
THK	Total knee replacement
TIA	Transient ischemic attack
TLC	Total lung capacity
TMP-SMX	Trimethoprim-sulfamethoxazole
TNF	Tumor necrosis factor
tPA	Tissue plasminogen activation
TPN	Total parenteral nutrition
TSH	Thyroid-stimulating hormone
VAD	Ventricular assist device
VTE	Venous thromboembolism
WBCs	White blood cells
WHO	World Health Organization

INDEX

Page numbers in italic indicate illustrations;
t indicates tables.